Frontiers in Anti-Infective Drug Discovery

Volume 3

Editor
Atta-ur-Rahman, *FRS*
Honorary Life Fellow
Kings College
University of Cambridge
UK

Co-Editor
M. Iqbal Choudhary
H.E.J. Research Institute of Chemistry
International Center for Chemical and Biological Sciences
University of Karachi
Pakistan

CONTENTS

PREFACE

Infectious diseases are slowly becoming a major threat to human survival. Many people predict the return of the pre-antibiotic period due to the emergence of resistance against all major classes of antibiotics. It is now more difficult to treat infectious diseases than it was in the last several decades. *Super-bugs*, XRDs and TRDs, now result in more deaths than ever before. Many nosocomial infections are now spread in communities, largely affecting the malnourished populations, living in poor hygienic conditions in densely populated regions of the world. Difficulty in treating infections is directly affecting the outcome of surgical intervention, pre-mature birth, and hospital care of elderly and immune compromised patients. The dwindling supply of effective medicines against prevailing infectious diseases is yet another challenge, as fewer and fewer pharmaceutical companies are interested to work in this field due to economic reasons. Yet fortunately academic and research communities continue to work towards understanding the infectious diseases and resistance in positive agents at the molecular level. The scientific literature is constantly being enriched with useful information and seminal discoveries. This is where we feel the eBook series such as the **"Frontier in Anti-Infective Drug Discovery"** can play an important role in updating the scientific community and providing them with an overview of key recent findings.

Volume 3 of the eBook series entitled, *"***Frontiers in Anti-Infective Drug Discovery***",* is a useful compilation of six scholarly reviews, contributed by some of the most eminent researchers in the field. We expect this volume to be a useful treatise for researchers interested in infections and their treatments.

In the first article, Marino *et al* skillfully review the success and failures in the discovery and development of anti-tuberculosis (TB) drugs. TB has been a major global threat, particularly in developing countries which has attracted major attention in the last two decades due to emergence of XRD TB, co-infection with HIV, and alarming increase in TB patients. The review focuses on major impediments in anti-TB drug discovery as well as some of the most promising leads currently in the process of development.

Bhardwaj *et al* have contributed a review on the growing understanding of the resistance mechanisms in infection causing microorganisms. The possibility of attacking the virulence of bacteria rather than the bug itself in order to circumvent the MDR has been discussed. The key factors responsible for fast emerging resistance are discussed, along with appropriate scientific and public response.

Vaccines have played an important role in controlling viral infections in the past five decades. However, the potential of virus expression vectors for generating vaccines against bacterial and fungal infections has not been fully explored. Hefferon reviews the potential of using the vectors based on viruses for the delivery of vaccines or other immunization agents against infectious diseases. The review also summarizes the current successes and future challenges in using virus vaccines against prevailing infections.

Zhang *et al* have contributed a comprehensive review on the use of Newcastle disease virus (NDV)-based vector vaccines against emerging and re-emerging pathogens. Newcastle disease is one of the most important diseases in the poultry industry. The oncolytic properties of certain strains of NDV have also been discussed as innovative therapy against cancers.

The vector-born protozoal tropical diseases cause major mortality and morbidity to a large segment of the world population in over 80 countries. Allahverdiyev *et al* review various aspects of leishmaniasis, a major disease caused by parasites of the genus *Leishmania*. Various approaches to combat this wide spread disease, including prospects of development of vaccines, chemotherapy, physical treatment, immunotherapy, phototherapy and nanotechnological products have been discussed.

Proantocynidins, polyphonolic natural products of plant origin, are known for diverse biological activities. Yamamoto *et al* have contributed an article, comprehensively reviewing the *in silico* and *in vitro* studies conducted on anti-viral activity of proanthcynidins, particularly dengue virus.

This volume of this eBook series is the result of hard work of so many eminent contributors, for which we express our profound gratitude. We would also like to acknowledge the commitment and hard work of the excellent team of Bentham Science Publishers, led by Mr. Mahmood Alam, Director Bentham Science Publishers. The efforts of Ms. Fariya Zulfiqar, Assistant Manager Publications, deserve special appreciation.

Prof. Atta-ur-Rahman, *FRS*
Honorary Life Fellow
Kings College
University of Cambridge
UK

Prof. M. Iqbal Choudhary
H.E.J. Research Institute of Chemistry
International Center for Chemical and Biological Sciences
University of Karachi
Pakistan

LIST OF CONTRIBUTORS

Adil M. Allahverdiyev
Yildiz Technical University, Department of Bioengineering, Istanbul, Turkey

Akiko Saito
Graduate School of Engineering, Osaka Electro-communication University (OECU), Osaka 572-8530, Japan

Ashima Kushwaha Bhardwaj
Department of Human Health and Diseases, Indian Institute of Advanced Research, Koba Institutional Area, Gandhinagar 382 007, Gujarat, India

Braj Mohan Ram Narayan Singh Kutar
Department of Human Health and Diseases, Indian Institute of Advanced Research, Koba Institutional Area, Gandhinagar 382 007, Gujarat, India

C.Q.F. Leite
School of Pharmaceutical Sciences – UNESP – University of Estadual Paulista, Department of Biological Sciences – Araraquara – SP, Brazil

Chao Gao
Key Laboratory of Zoonosis Research, Ministry of Education, Institute of Zoonosis, College of Veterinary Medicine, Jilin University, Changchun 130062, China

Donald L. Reynolds
Atlantic Veterinary College, University of Prince Edward Island, Prince Edward Island, Canada

Dylan Frabutt
Michigan State University, East Lansing, MI 48824, USA

Emrah Sefik Abamor
Yildiz Technical University, Department of Bioengineering, Istanbul, Turkey

F.R. Pavan
School of Pharmaceutical Sciences – UNESP – University of Estadual Paulista, Department of Biological Sciences – Araraquara – SP, Brazil

Kathleen L. Hefferon
Cornell University, Ithaca, NY 14886, USA

Kittappa Vinothkumar
Department of Human Health and Diseases, Indian Institute of Advanced Research, Koba Institutional Area, Gandhinagar 382 007, Gujarat, India

Koji Ichiyama
Translational ID Lab, Department of Microbiology, Yong Loo Lin School of Medicine, National University of Singapore, 14 Medical Drive, #15-02 Centre for Translational Medicine (MD6), 117599, Singapore

Lakshmi Chandrasekaran
Translational ID Lab, Department of Microbiology, Yong Loo Lin School of Medicine, National University of Singapore, 14 Medical Drive, #15-02 Centre for Translational Medicine (MD6), 117599, Singapore

Leonardo B. Marino
School of Pharmaceutical Sciences – UNESP – University of Estadual Paulista, Department of Biological Sciences – Araraquara – SP, Brazil

Liangxue Lai
Key Laboratory of Zoonosis Research, Ministry of Education, Institute of Zoonosis, College of Veterinary Medicine, Jilin University, Changchun 130062, China

M. Miyata
School of Pharmaceutical Sciences – UNESP – University of Estadual Paulista, Department of Biological Sciences – Araraquara – SP, Brazil

Melahat Bagirova
Yildiz Technical University, Department of Bioengineering, Istanbul, Turkey

Meral Miraloglu
Cukurova University, Vocational School of Health, Adana, Turkey

Mingming Han
Key Laboratory of Zoonosis Research, Ministry of Education, Institute of Zoonosis, College of Veterinary Medicine, Jilin University, Changchun 130062, China

Minhua Sun
Institute of Animal Health, Guangdong Academy of Agriculture Sciences, Guangzhou, China

Naoki Yamamoto
Translational ID Lab, Department of Microbiology, Yong Loo Lin School of Medicine, National University of Singapore, 14 Medical Drive, #15-02 Centre for Translational Medicine (MD6), 117599, Singapore

Neha Rajpara
Department of Human Health and Diseases, Indian Institute of Advanced Research, Koba Institutional Area, Gandhinagar 382 007, Gujarat, India

Nihan Aytekin
Acibadem University, School of Medicine, Department of Microbiology, Istanbul, Turkey

P.C. Souza
School of Pharmaceutical Sciences – UNESP – University of Estadual Paulista, Department of Biological Sciences – Araraquara – SP, Brazil

Priyabrata Mohanty
Department of Human Health and Diseases, Indian Institute of Advanced Research, Koba Institutional Area, Gandhinagar 382 007, Gujarat, India

Rabia Cakir Koc
Yildiz Technical University, Department of Bioengineering, Istanbul, Turkey

Renfu Yin
Key Laboratory of Zoonosis Research, Ministry of Education, Institute of Zoonosis, College of Veterinary Medicine, Jilin University, Changchun 130062, China

Serhat Elcicek
Firat University, Department of Bioengineering, Elazig, Turkey

Sezen Canim Ates
Yildiz Technical University, Department of Bioengineering, Istanbul, Turkey

Sinem Oktem
Acibadem University, School of Medicine, Department of Microbiology, Istanbul, Turkey

Tanıl Kocagoz
Acibadem University, School of Medicine, Department of Microbiology, Istanbul, Turkey

Vivian Feng Chen
Translational ID Lab, Department of Microbiology, Yong Loo Lin School of Medicine, National University of Singapore, 14 Medical Drive, #15-02 Centre for Translational Medicine (MD6), 117599, Singapore

Xiang Li
Key Laboratory of Zoonosis Research, Ministry of Education, Institute of Zoonosis, College of Veterinary Medicine, Jilin University, Changchun 130062, China

Xiaodong Zhang
Key Laboratory of Zoonosis Research, Ministry of Education, Institute of Zoonosis, College of Veterinary Medicine, Jilin University, Changchun 130062, China

Ying Chen
College of Animal Science and Technology, Guangxi University, Nanning, China

Yoshiyuki Yoshinaka
Department of Molecular Virology, Graduate 15 School, Tokyo Medical and Dental University, Tokyo 113-5819, Japan

Zhuang Ding
Key Laboratory of Zoonosis Research, Ministry of Education, Institute of Zoonosis, College of Veterinary Medicine, Jilin University, Changchun 130062, China

CHAPTER 1

Drug Discovery for TB: Frontiers and Perspectives

Leonardo B. Marino[*]**, M. Miyata, P.C. Souza, C.Q.F. Leite and F.R. Pavan**

School of Pharmaceutical Sciences - UNESP - University of Estadual Paulista, Department of Biological Sciences - Araraquara-SP, Brazil

Abstract: Despite advances in the treatment of tuberculosis (TB) and increased effort to discover new anti-TB drugs, 8.6 million people were affected by *Mycobacterium tuberculosis* infection, leading to 1.3 million deaths in 2013. Tuberculosis is a substantial threat to public health because of co-infection with HIV and the emergence of resistant strains (MDR and XDR). The main obstacles for the discovery of new drugs against TB include high cost, lack of investment by large pharmaceutical companies and lack of infrastructure in the countries affected by this disease. The global effort to eliminate tuberculosis includes contributions by the Global Alliance for TB Drug Development (TB Alliance), several research groups, regulatory agencies, and institutions such as the NIH (National Institutes of Health) and Bill and Melinda Gates Foundation. This chapter discusses factors that impede anti-TB drug discovery, which include the development of bacterial drug resistance, role of bacterial efflux pumps, cross-resistance, drug interactions with antiretrovirals and lack of investment by pharmaceutical industries; furthermore, new drugs that are being tested for the treatment of TB are discussed.

Keywords: Drug discovery, drug interactions, drug resistance, efflux pumps, HIV, isoniazid, investments, mycobacteria, rifampicin, tuberculosis.

1. INTRODUCTION

Tuberculosis (TB) is the leading global cause of death from a single infectious bacterial agent (*Mycobacterium tuberculosis*). In 2012 alone, 8.6 million cases and 1.3 million deaths occurred, mostly in developing countries (World Health Organization) [1]. There have been significant improvements in treatment statistics with 56 million cases successfully treated between 1995 and 2012 and a 45% decrease in mortality between 1990 and 2012 [1]; however, several factors

*Corresponding Author Leonardo B. Marino: School of Pharmaceutical Sciences - UNESP - University of Estadual Paulista, Department of Biological Sciences, Room 380 - Araraquara-SP, Brazil; Tel: +55 16 3301-4671; E-mail: leobmarino@hotmail.com

contributing to the prevalence of TB necessitate further studies. These factors include co-infection of TB and HIV (Human Immunodeficiency Virus) and the close relationship between these pathogens as well as the continuous appearance and persistence of MDR (multi-drug resistant) and XDR (extensively drug-resistant) strains. Among the new cases observed in 2012, 1.1 million involved individuals co-infected with HIV and 300,000 were HIV-positive, which can lead to mortality [1].

Infected individuals transmit the bacterium after aerosol inhalation of bacilli in droplet nuclei, and the bacterium exhibits lung tropism. Approximately 10 to 30% of exposed individuals become ill (primary TB), and 60 to 90% develop effective cellular immune responses that successfully contain the infection; in the latter individuals, *M. tuberculosis* can exist in a latent state (latent TB) [2, 3]. Individuals suffering from active pulmonary tuberculosis expel droplets containing the bacilli. Alveolar macrophages engulf these droplets but do not kill the pathogen. Specific T cells are stimulated in the draining lymph nodes and induce bacterial elimination by containment in small pulmonary granulomatous lesions; however, these cells fail to completely eradicate the bacteria, leading to primary tuberculosis [4]. The latent state is defined as the presence of pulmonary bacteria that are phagocytosed by alveolar macrophages, which induces a proinflammatory response and initiates the recruitment of mononuclear cells from neighboring blood vessels. The bacilli surrounded by T cells, monocytes, and macrophages cannot reproduce and exist in a latent state. The bacilli are not infectious in this state, and they can remain in this state for many years or undergo reactivation, which is the most common form of TB in adults. The reactivation is often associated with impaired immune function caused by conditions including co-infection with HIV, nutritional deficiency, advanced age, and stress [5].

The complexity of this disease poses seemingly insurmountable problems for treatment. According to the World Health Organization Guidelines [6], the standard treatment recommended for TB, which has been in effect since 1970 when it was proposed by the British Medical Research Council [7], consists of two phases: an intensive phase and a continuation phase. During the intensive phase, which lasts for two months, four main first-line drugs are used against the disease: Isoniazid (H or INH), rifampicin (R or RIF), pyrazinamide (P or PZA), and Ethambutol (E or EMB) (Fig. **1**). The continuous phase follows the intensive phase and is composed of the administration of Isoniazid and Rifampicin over a four-month period. The doses must be administered daily, but intermittent therapy (thrice a week) can be used for immunocompetent patients. For patients co-infected with HIV, the treatment involves daily doses in both the intensive and continuation phases. For these patients, ART (Antiretroviral therapy) is indispensable and must begin as soon as possible after the initiation of TB treatment, irrespective of the CD4 cell count of the individual. The stringency and elaborateness of this regimen often result in non-adherence. The lack of adherence is also associated with the high toxicity of these drugs and the considerable improvement of patients in the first few weeks of treatment, leading them to believe that they are cured and to discontinue treatment. An alternative regimen used in Bangladesh consists of a minimum of 9 months of initial treatment using gatifloxacin, clofazimine, ethambutol and pyrazinamide, followed by prothionamide, kanamycin and high-dose isoniazid; this method yields results comparable to treatment using the first-line drugs [8].

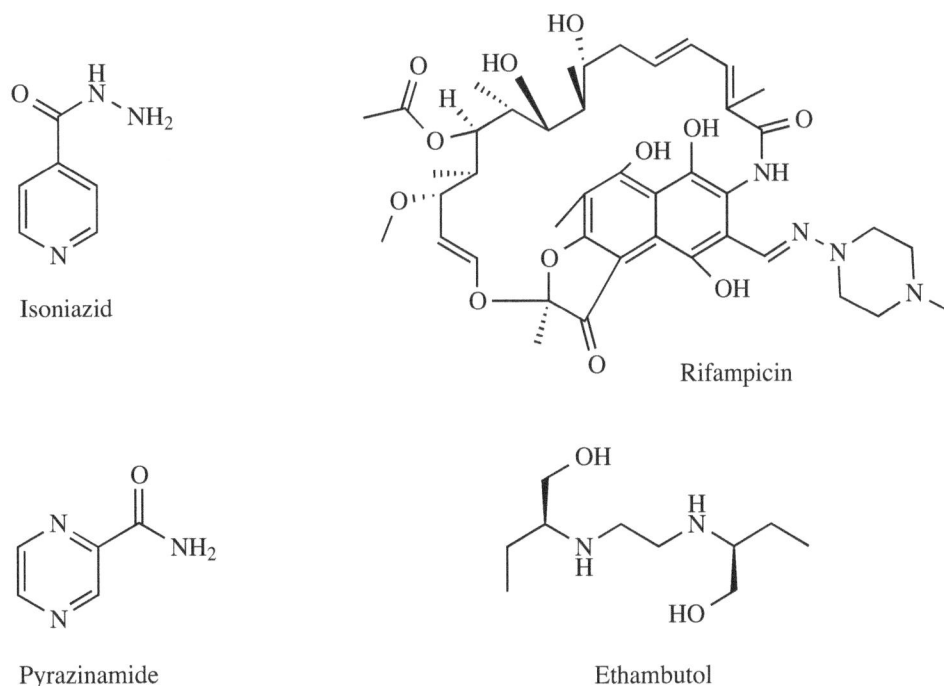

Fig. (1). Molecular structures of the four main drugs used against TB.

Treatment abandonment can lead to a process that is intrinsically favored in *M. tuberculosis*: the emergence of resistance. The micro-organism acquires resistance due to several factors, such as the high mycolic acid content of the cell envelope, the action of efflux pumps [9-11], and the occurrence of chromosomal mutations in genes encoding proteins that are the targets of the main treatment drugs, or proteins required for prodrug activation [12]. To inhibit the spread of disease, drug resistance must be rapidly and safely overcome; this requires new drugs that circumvent these resistance mechanisms by acting on novel targets or on known targets in different locations the formulation of therapies that target the maximum number of cellular pathways to comprehensively inhibit bacterial metabolism [12].

Studies on anti-TB drugs must consider another parameter: interaction between the drugs used to combat the bacillus and the drugs used to treat HIV in co-infected individuals. An important example of such an effect is the promiscuous induction of cytochrome P450 and phase II enzymes by rifampicin, a major drug used for TB treatment. The induction of these enzymes reduces the concentrations of co-administered drugs, such as antiretrovirals that are metabolized by this system [13, 14]. The alarming number of cases of co-infected patients, which reached 1.1 million in 2012 [1], reinforces the need for new anti-TB drugs that do not interact with antiretrovirals. The current treatment regimen for HIV-positive patients newly diagnosed with TB may vary depending on the individual, but certain factors must be considered: (1) the anti-TB treatment should be started immediately; (2) the antiretroviral therapy might need to be modified due to drug interactions or to reduce toxicity; and (3) the TB clinical presentation in the patient might be due to the failure of antiretroviral therapy [6]. Co-morbidities frequently occur in TB [7]. Therapy regimens for other diseases might clash with the anti-TB therapy, and perfect immune balance is required to control TB. Therefore, some individuals with these co-morbidities may develop worse clinical manifestations if they contract TB, for instance, patients with rheumatoid arthritis [15, 16], organ transplant recipients [17, 18], and type 2 diabetes [19, 20]. Another complication is the case of childhood TB, which is usually treated with sub-optimal drug concentrations, leading to the development of drug resistance. Therefore, pediatric studies must be performed using new pharmaceutical formulations for existing and novel drugs, and pediatric pharmacokinetic and safety studies must be performed after the safety and efficacy parameters have been established in adults [21].

Another factor that has impeded the discovery of new diagnostic methods and especially new drugs is the lack of investment. For several years, TB was "neglected" because it was considered a disease of the developing world, usually affecting individuals without the financial means to obtain proper treatment. However, with globalization, the migration of people between countries has increased, and the disease has affected developed countries at relatively high rates. In New York City, between 1978 and 1992, the number of TB cases tripled with the advent of HIV [22, 23]. Another notable example was the high TB incidence in cities such as Manchester (59.1/100,000) and London (44.4/100,000) in 2009, leading to London being called the "European Capital of TB" [23]. Such episodes highlighted the need for government action in developed countries; for instance, in New York, the situation could be reversed only by heavy investments in the program against TB (considered a priority policy) by investing primarily in professionals from the area and in DOT (Directly Observed Therapy) [23]. Although there are isolated exceptions, there is a major lack of investment in solving these problems. Many countries, even though they are considered "first world", do not have a strategy for controlling the spread of the disease with medical teams accompanying the patient in treatment. This fact is also reflected in the level of government investment in research to identify new drugs; these data are available in the current report of the WHO under the item "Financing TB control". For many countries (mostly developed), there are no data on how much is spent in this area, which may indicate a lack of investment control or lack of investment altogether. This is also evident in the main patent offices around the world; several patents with the keyword "tuberculosis" are related to the development of diagnostic kits but few describe molecules with anti-mycobacterial potential.

There have been several promising developments in the control of TB. Because of programs such as Stop TB, the death rate decreased by 45% from 1990 to 2012 [1]; furthermore there are currently 19 drugs in pre-clinical steps and clinical trials for disease treatment, and a new treatment regimen has been proposed, which is in phase II trials. Since the discovery of rifampicin in 1963, no new antituberculosis drugs have been developed [24], however, significant progress has been made. In 2013, compelled by the need to improve TB treatment (mainly MDR strains), the FDA (Food and Drug Administration) accelerated approval and granted a provisional license to a new drug, bedaquiline (TMC207, Sirturo™). This potentially marks the beginning of a new phase of discovery of compounds acting on novel mycobacterial targets, favoring a therapy that comprehensively limits bacterial metabolism. Bedaquiline (diarylquinoline) represents a class of drugs with novel molecular targets [25-27], another drug in this class, SQ109 (inhibits cell wall synthesis by targeting an unknown molecule) potentially has multiple targets because the rates of SQ109-resistance are extremely low [25]. In addition to the synthesis of novel drugs, some drugs initially created for other purposes were repurposed for TB and are currently under evaluation; these drugs include oxazolidinones, clofazimine, β-lactams, and fluoroquinolones [24]. Each of these candidate drugs is discussed below.

This chapter highlights the challenges to TB drug discovery including factors such as the features of TB (the skills of the organism and its virulence factors), drug resistance (against first-line drugs, either mutational origin or efflux pump action), interaction between drugs (TB therapy *versus* HIV therapy), cross-resistance between drugs, investments in the area, as well as an overview of the drugs that are in pre-clinical and clinical research for treatment.

2. TB/HIV CO-INFECTION AND THERAPY

TB is the most common cause of death in HIV-infected individuals among all HIV-related deaths globally. For patients with HIV and TB, mortality is decreased by treating both diseases concurrently rather than waiting until the TB treatment is completed to start antiretroviral drugs [28-30]. Therefore, co-treatment is now the standard care for most patients.

The Department of Health and Human Services and Infectious Diseases Society of America now recommend beginning antiretroviral treatment two weeks after the initiation of tuberculosis treatment for most patients with CD4 counts less than 50 cells/mm. Patients should be treated with daily or thrice-weekly therapy in both the initial and continuation phases. The duration of treatment for patients with TB/HIV is 6 months, even for patients with a negative TB culture in some cases, because late response to therapy may extend for up to 9 months [31].

The recommended treatment for TB in adults infected with HIV (susceptible to first-line drugs) is a six-month regimen consisting of

- An initial phase of INH, RIF, PZA, and EMB for the first 2 months;

- A continuation phase of INH and RIF for the last 4 months [32].

Unfortunately, the TB and HIV co-therapy generates adverse reactions that often lead to patient non-adherence to therapy; one such adverse reaction is hepatotoxicity [33], which affects the bioavailability of drugs due to enzymatic metabolism. Hepatotoxicity has significant economic impact and prolongs the duration of illness, morbidity, and mortality and might necessitate alteration of the drug dosage.

This hepatotoxic effect is mediated by the interaction of drugs with the cytochrome P450 enzyme complex. This complex has an important role in drug metabolism and drug interactions. Even if the medicines are not administered simultaneously, their bioavailability can have physiological effects on enzymes for hours to months.

RIF-based TB regimens have been used successfully to manage TB in HIV-positive patients and are most effective if administered throughout the course of TB treatment [34]. RIF is the main drug involved with possible interactions between the two therapies because it reduces the concentrations of companion drugs including antiretroviral treatments (ART), which are metabolized by the cytochrome (CYP) P450 enzyme [35]. The consequence is a decrease in plasma levels of ART [36, 37]. Interactions between nevirapine (NVP) and RIF can potentially lead to clinical decreases in NVP plasma concentrations and compromise HIV treatment. This effect depends on whether the patient can metabolize CYP2B6 [38, 39].

A study conducted at a hospital in Ethiopia with 296 patients assessed the incidence of hepatotoxicity in drug therapy for tuberculosis among patients co-infected with TB/HIV; this study observed that hepatotoxicity occurred in 11.5% of cases, the majority (93.9%) of which occurred during the initial phase. Therefore, the first 8 weeks are a critical period, during which toxicity indicators must be carefully monitored [40].

Another study examined the impact of antiretroviral therapy (ART) in a TB-infected population in sub-Saharan Africa and highlighted the importance of sustained adherence and immunological response to ART as well as the critical need for effective HIV-prevention measures, including early widespread implementation of ART [41]. This study highlighted the high rates of TB/HIV co-infection in developing countries and the problems involved in the control of these diseases.

Non-nucleoside reverse transcriptase inhibitors (NNRTIs) are widely prescribed as the backbone of first-line ART, particularly in developing countries. Efavirenz (EFV) and nevirapine (NVP) are metabolized by the cytochrome P450 enzyme system. The CYP2B6 isoform is primarily responsible for EFV metabolism, and the CY3A4 isoform is primarily responsible for NVP metabolism and, to a lesser extent, EFV metabolism. Both EFV and NVP also have the ability to induce the enzymes that function their own metabolism and may increase the clearance of co-administered drugs that share these metabolic pathways. The newest NNRTI, etravirine (ETV), is metabolized in a similar manner by CYP P450 and interacts with rifamycins [34].

2.1. HIV/MDR-TB

In some regions, the increasing incidence of MDR-TB is accelerated by the high rate of co-infection with HIV, which significantly increases progression to active disease after infection with *M. tuberculosis* [42, 43]. The lack of rapid detection of such cases in laboratories masks numerous outbreaks of MDR-TB associated with HIV, preventing these individuals from obtaining medical or health care [42].

Various factors contribute to this underestimation. First, surveys are generally performed only in public facilities, excluding patients in the private sector. Second, in some countries, data are gathered only in some states instead of the whole country, which leads to incomplete information [1].

The association between HIV and TB drug resistance is complex [44]. The occurrence of drug-resistant mutants increases the number of individuals with active tuberculosis [45]. In addition, co-infection with HIV can enhance the spontaneous selection of mutations in several ways. Without proper management, individuals with HIV-associated tuberculosis may not adhere to therapy due to the increased pill burden and toxic effects [46]. This can lead to sub-therapeutic concentrations of antituberculosis drugs because of low absorption [47] or drug interaction [48].

Therefore, these patients are more susceptible and more likely to develop active tuberculosis drug resistance, whereas TB in HIV-negative patients can remain in the latent state without undergoing reactivation or can be reactivated after several years.

HIV infection is not the only factor responsible for the increased rate of drug resistance, but it has the potential to increase the number of individuals infected by resistant strains, and these individuals serve as reservoirs of these strains.

2.2. Potential Interactions between New Drugs

There are several new TB drugs being tested that can potentially increase the effectiveness of treatment regimens. These studies also examine the potential benefit for HIV-positive cases.

Nitroimidazoles PA-824 (TB Alliance) and Delamanid (Formerly OPC-67683, Otsuka). PA-824 (TB Alliance) and Delamanid (Otsuka) are active against dormant and growing bacteria and against sensitive and resistant bacteria [49]. The metabolism of Delamanid is not dependent on human liver microsomal enzymes; therefore, it does not induce the P450 enzymes, which represents a relatively low risk of interactions with other drug therapies. PA-824 is a weak inhibitor of CYP 3A, 2C8, 2C9, and 2C19 and is not significantly metabolized by CYP3A4; therefore, interactions are unlikely.

A combination of PA-824, pyrazinamide, and moxifloxacin showed higher activity for the treatment of TB [50]. Although no drug interaction is expected, studies are evaluating the metabolic pathways involved in potential interactions among these three drugs.

SQ109 (Sequella). SQ109 or [1, 2] - ethylenediamine is a drug with structural similarities to EMB but is ten times more active than EMB in preclinical trials and has a different mechanism of action compared to EMB [51]. SQ109 is metabolized by CYP2D6 and CYP2C19 *in vitro*, and there is a moderate risk of interaction when it is co-administered with drugs that induce or inhibit these enzymes. Further studies are required to ensure the safety of this drug in combination with other drugs [52].

Oxazolidinones - Sutezolid (Pfizer) and AZD5847 (AstraZeneca). Sutezolid and AZD5847 (AstraZeneca) are new oxazolidinones in phase-2 development for TB. Sutezolid is extensively metabolized by flavin monooxygenases to sulfoxide and sulfone derivatives. CYP3A4 accounts for approximately 30% of sutezolid metabolism, but neither sutezolid nor its metabolites appear to be inhibitors or inducers of CYP3A4. Further studies are required to test whether the metabolites circulate at higher concentrations and are more active than the parent drug [53].

3. RESISTANCE IN *MYCOBACTERIUM TUBERCULOSIS*

The biggest global concern for TB is the development of resistance to the main drugs used. Drug resistance occurs mainly due to bacterial selection by factors such as the limited access to medicines in certain epidemic areas, physician errors in prescription dosages, lack of adherence or treatment abandonment by individuals [54], and lack of rapid and accurate diagnostic methods to identify the resistance profile of the bacteria affecting the individual. This fact is extremely important because the treatments for resistant strains are generally much less effective and more expensive.

Fitzpatrick *et al.* [55] analyzed studies from Estonia, Peru, Philippines, and Tomsk and observed that the costs of treating each patient with MDR-TB strain were US$ 10,880.00, US$ 2,423.00, US$ 3,613.00, and US$ 14,657.00, respectively. These costs can be even higher depending on the treatment model used, including some second-line drugs (often necessary) and/or the region and can increase to US$ 195,078.00.

Despite the existence of mono-resistant strains and the consequent amplification of resistance [56, 57], the main concern in TB is the emergence of three different types of strains: MDR-TB strains (multidrug-resistant; resistant to isoniazid and rifampicin), XDR-TB (extensively drug-resistant; resistant to INH, RIF, fluoroquinolones and all injectable second-line drugs), and TDR-TB (totally drug-resistant; resistant to all drugs that have been tested for TB; this is not a commonly accepted term and requires further studies) [1].

According to the WHO, in 2011, 0.5 million new cases of MDR-TB occurred globally, with 60% of the cases occurring in the "BRIC countries" (Brazil, Russia, India and China). Furthermore, 3.7% of new TB cases are caused by MDR-TB strains, and 20% of these occur in previously treated patients. Until December 2013, 92 countries reported at least one case of TB caused by XDR-TB strains. The severity of drug-resistant TB significantly increases the economic cost and the rate of patient mortality. The WHO estimated that in 2015, US$ 2 billion would be needed for the diagnosis and treatment of MDR-TB; between 2000 and 2011, this amount rose from US$ 0.5 billion to US$ 0.7 billion.

The emergence of drug-resistant strains necessitates the discovery of new drugs because molecules that act only on susceptible strains are not useful. Therefore, it is important to focus on the rational development of new compounds with novel molecular targets to avoid cross-resistance.

Because drug resistance is a critical issue, it is important to understand the mechanisms by which the bacilli evade treatment. Some mechanisms have been elucidated and are discussed below.

M. tuberculosis has inherent resistance largely due to a cell wall rich in mycolic acids, which lowers the permeability of compounds; furthermore, the cell wall has efflux pump activity. The atypical cell envelope constitution was considered an insurmountable obstacle in the first half of the 20th century because the first antibiotics developed, the penicillins and sulfonamides, had no activity against this bacillus [58]. However, cell envelope constitution is not the sole factor underlying its resistance; the bacillus responds effectively to selective pressure and often alters the expression of proteins involved in drug metabolism by chromosomal mutations (and not mobile genetic elements such as transposons, plasmids, and integrons) [54, 58]. Although not very common in *M. tuberculosis*, resistance caused by regulatory activity of the transposon IS*6110* in the inactivation of some genes has been observed [59, 60]. One possible explanation for the acquisition of mutations in *M. tuberculosis* is that this bacterium grows in stressful environments within cells and is therefore hyper-mutable [58, 61]. These mutations can cause loss of protein function (*e.g.*, a protein activating a pro-drug), physical alteration of the target, specifically the drug binding site, and enzymatic inactivation of the drug used for treatment [12].

Sandgren *et al.* [62] developed a database of major chromosomal mutations related to drug resistance in *M. tuberculosis*. The TB Drug Resistance Mutation Database (TBDReaMDB, http: //www.tbdreamdb.com/) enables rational analysis of new bacterial resistance mechanisms and provides a platform for targeted searches on the profiled of clinical isolates, allowing more rapid and accurate identification of their sensitivity or resistance to specific drug therapies.

To elucidate the occurrence of resistance in *M. tuberculosis*, we describe the mechanisms and mutations acquired by the bacteria to resist therapy. We discuss the mechanism of action of each drug currently used for treatment, which is important to understand how these mechanisms are evaded by the bacillus; furthermore, we discuss the major chromosomal changes that generate resistance and highlight the loci that are "hot spots" for such changes.

3.1. Isoniazid (INH)

INH activity against *M. tuberculosis* was discovered in 1952 [63] during an attempt to enhance the activity of nicotinamide and thiosemicarbazone compounds. A γ-pyridylaldehyde thiosemicarbazone intermediate, isonicotinic acid hydrazide, had a strong effect against the bacillus and continues to be one of the most important therapeutic drugs for TB [64, 65].

INH action involves inhibition of the biosynthesis of mycolic acid, which is an important component of the *M. tuberculosis* cell wall [66]. The activity of this prodrug requires its conversion to acyl radicals by the *KatG* enzyme [67]. These radicals bind to NAD^+, forming a covalent adduct, as described by Rozwarski *et al.*; this adduct potentially inhibits the FASII enoyl-ACP reductase InhA [65, 67-69]. This reductase reduces the *trans* double bond between positions C2 and C3 of a fatty acyl chain linked to the acyl carrier protein, hindering an important step in mycolic acid production [70]. The mechanism of INH action is also related to other pathways such as inhibition of nucleic acid synthesis [71], phospholipids [72], and NAD^+ metabolism [64, 73, 74].

Resistance to this drug has been observed since the early discovery of its action on TB, but in recent years, the number of cases has increased [75-77]. Among the drugs used for TB therapy, INH potentially has the greatest variability of mutations associated with resistance because a large number of genes are involved in its action.

INH is a prodrug that requires activation to function as an antibiotic; therefore, the first bacterial mechanism to evade INH action is to prevent its activation. Isoniazid is activated by its conversion to acyl radicals (isonicotinaldehyde, nicotinic acid and isonicotinamide) by the enzyme *KatG* (catalase-peroxidase-peroxynitritase T) [78]. In the mid-1950s, Middlebrook *et al.* [79, 80] observed INH-resistant isolates lacking catalase-peroxidase activity.

Subsequently, molecular studies showed that the loss of catalase-peroxidase activity was directly related to mutations in the gene *katG* encoding the protein [81, 82]. Subsequent studies examined the nature of these mutations and the most frequent sites at which they occurred. Most *katG* mutations were missense mutations in which a single nucleotide substitution caused a change in the corresponding amino acid of the protein. Changes such as small insertions or deletions in the gene sequence were observed less frequently [83, 84]. The database contains 272 different mutations spanning all 2223 bp of the gene and a single mutation in the promoter region; these mutations were identified in INH-resistant isolates, but it is not known whether several of these mutations cause the resistance phenotype.

One of the 272 mutations is prominent because it appears frequently in isolates with that profile. The serine at position 315 of the protein in wild-type strains was altered in many INH-resistant isolates worldwide, including South Africa [85], Finland [86], Sierra Leone [85], France [87], Russia [88], and Germany [89]. Together, these data reveal that the most common amino acid substitution is Ser->Thr, caused by mutation of the codon AGC to ACC; however, other nucleotide substitutions in this codon cause amino acid alterations, including ACA (Thr), ATC (Ile), AGA (Arg), CGC (Arg), AAC (Asp), and GGC (Gly) [84]. The Ser->Thr mutation is proposed to reduce INH susceptibility by affecting the CO re-connection kinetics to the *KatG* heme group by steric hindrance, reducing the access to the channel without altering the integrity of the mutated enzyme catalytic site (Fig. **2**) [90]. Wengenack *et al.* [91] expressed wild-type and Ser315Thr mutant *KatG* in *E. coli* and observed that the mutant protein had six-fold-lower catalase activity and two-fold-lower peroxidase activity compared to the wild-type protein [84]. These data suggest a model for drug resistance conferred by the bacillus adaptive mechanisms: loss of catalase/peroxidase activity, through mutations in this gene, that would increase exposure to free radicals; alternatively, bacteria may combat INH action by invoking other resistance mechanisms.

Other mutations in the *katG* gene confer drug resistance. One such mutation is Arg463Leu, which was originally considered to have little or no impact on the sensitivity/resistance profiles [92], but it was later observed to be important in this process [93]. Ramaswamy *et al.* [84] reviewed data obtained by Rouse *et al.* [94] in which complementation assays were used to identify nine mutations in catalase-peroxidase, which altered the response to the front-line drug INH: Arg104Leu, His108Gln, Asn138Ser, Leu148Arg, His270Gln, Thr275Pro, Ser315Thr (mentioned above), Asp381Gly, and Trp321Gly. These regions represent the catalytic site and the heme-binding site, which offers a possible explanation for the resistance phenotype [84].

The importance of each gene alteration in INH resistance was confirmed by Hazbón *et al.* [77]; in this highly representative study, a large number of isolates from several geographical regions were examined, including sensitive and resistant strains. The results revealed a high frequency of mutations at amino acid

315 of the *katG* gene in 221/403 (54.8%) INH-resistant isolates; among these, 184 contained the Ser315Thr (AGC->ACC) mutation.

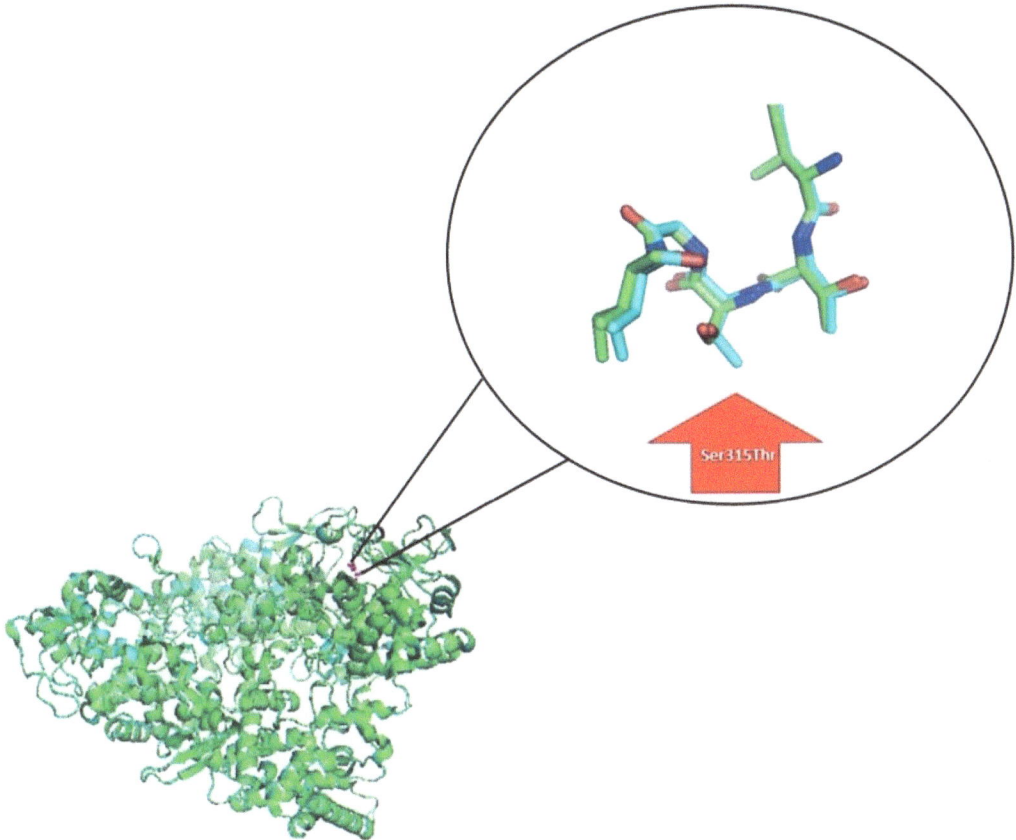

Fig. (2). Overlay of wild-type (green) and Ser315Thr mutant *KatG* (blue). The red arrow indicates the altered amino acid residue, which potentially causes steric hindrance in the enzyme. The structures were predicted by Zhao *et al*. [95].

Another mechanism for drug resistance in this bacillus is the occurrence of mutations in the gene encoding InhA, which binds the NAD$^+$-INH adduct. Such mutations might (1) cause overexpression of InhA, which binds the NAD$^+$-INH adduct and independently functions to promote mycolic acid synthesis and is essential for the cell envelope, and (2) reduce the affinity of protein binding to the adduct.

The *inhA* gene is located in an operon containing another gene, *mabA* [96], which encodes the 3- oxoacyl-[acyl-carrier protein] reductase [97]. Mutations that confer

INH resistance might cause overexpression of InhA, and these changes are located in the promoter region of the operon between the -15 and -8 positions, which is the region upstream of the *mabA* initiator codon and encodes the RBS (ribosome-binding site). The importance of these mutations in *M. tuberculosis* INH resistance was confirmed in studies by Musser *et al.* [98] in which 11/51 (21.57%) resistant isolates had a C- >T mutation in the RBS region (position -15) and no mutations in the *katG* gene. Miyata *et al.* [99] observed polymorphisms in the *inhA* promoter region in 10/56 (17.85%) INH-resistant isolates. Jnawali *et al.* [100] observed that 66/161 (41%) INH-resistant isolates in the Republic of Korea contained alterations in the promoter region, indicating that this region is a potential marker for the identification of TB resistance.

The most prominent mutation in the *inhA* ORF is Ser94Ala, which causes a five-fold increase in the MIC of a $H_{37}Rv$ reference strain to INH and ethambutol [101]. Other *inhA* mutations have been observed, including Ile16Thr, Ile21Thr, Ile21Val, Ile47Thr, Val78Ala, and Ile95Pro. These mutations cause resistance because they occur in regions of the protein related to NADH binding, lowering the NADH-binding affinity of InhA, which reduces the inhibition of InhA [102]. The following mutations were observed in a comprehensive study by Hazbón *et al.* [77]: Ile21Thr, Ile21Val, Ile47Thr, Ser94Ala, and Ile194Thr. However, the mutations Ile47Thr and Ile194Thr were also present in INH-susceptible isolates, which excludes their role in drug resistance.

Resistance to INH can be caused by other mechanisms involving specific mutations in other genes such as *ahpC*, *ndh*, and *kasA*. *ahpC* gene activity is closely related to the activity of *katG* and *oxyR* (induces an oxidative stress regulon in response to hydrogen peroxide stress), which is inherently mutated and inactive in *M. tuberculosis*. *oxyR* inactivity underlies the initial sensitivity of the bacillus strains to INH; this was observed by transforming sensitive $H_{37}Rv$ bacteria with a vector containing the wild-type native *oxyR* from *M. leprae*. This transformation conferred INH resistance (5 µg/mL) to the bacteria [103, 104]. The relationship between *katG* and *ahpC* involves complex regulatory activities in bacteria, but it has been elucidated. The *KatG* protein acts on protective mechanisms against oxidative stress within the macrophage, and this role might be inhibited by sequence-altering mutations. Why do these bacilli tolerate the existence of mutations that promote defense against antibiotics if these mutations might reduce fitness? The answer lies in the existence of compensatory mutations, which occur in the promoter of the *ahpC* gene, resulting in overexpression of AhpC, an alkyl hydroperoxide reductase, which can restore protective functions [105]. Although this hypothesis has not been verified [106, 107], drug-resistant isolates with mutations in the *ahpC* promoter and ORF were observed by Jnawali *et al.* [100] and Hoshide *et al.* [108]. In the latter study, mutations were observed only in the *ahpC* promoter region [position -46, G->A] in isolates from India. Hazbón *et al.* [77] observed a total of 73 different clinical isolates with resistance mutations in the *oxyR-ahpC* region, but the change at position -46 was not related to the acquisition of antibiotic resistance because this mutation was also observed in drug-sensitive isolates. Miyata *et al.* [99] observed mutations in the *oxyR-ahpC* region in 5/63 (7.9%) of Brazilian INH[r] isolates.

Mdluli *et al.* [109] sought to identify new targets for treatment with INH because mutations in genes such as *katG* and *inhA* were not present in all drug-resistant clinical isolates. Treatment with 1 μg/mL of INH generates accumulation of saturated hexacosanoic acid in the 12 kDa protein AcpM. The same study observed INH-dependent upregulation of an 80 kDa protein containing the same amino terminal as AcpM. This 80 kDa species was a complex formed by covalent interactions among AcpM, INH, and the β-ketoacyl ACP synthase KasA. By sequencing the *kasA* gene in 28 INH[r] isolates, 4 amino acid changes were identified that were not found in drug-susceptible strains: Asp66Asn, Gly269Ser, Gly312Ser, and Phe413Leu. Mutations in *katG* and *inhA* were not observed in two of these isolates, supporting the hypothesis that mutations in *kasA* might confer resistance to INH because the mutant KasA proteins with modified carboxyl-terminal regions would impair protein-protein interactions [84]. Lee *et al.* [110] identified *kasA* mutations in 10% of INH-resistant strains in Singapore; these included novel mutations such as Arg121Lys and Gly387Asp. The Gly312Ser mutation was also observed in drug-susceptible isolates, which excluded its role in drug resistance. Ramaswamy *et al.* [111] observed that the Met77Ile mutation was associated with mutations in other genes in the *kasA* operon, which is regulated by a gene homologous to *smrR*; however, the roles of these alterations in resistance profiles are not well understood.

Although there are other genes in which mutations can lead to INH resistance, the key gene in this context is *ndh*. This gene encodes a type II NADH dehydrogenase (NdhII), and it has been well characterized in organisms such as *E. coli* as a monomeric membrane-bound protein catalyzing NADH oxidation and electron transfer from reduced flavins to quinones [112-114]. Vilchèze *et al.* [114] proposed that *ndh* mutations cause drug-resistance because all NdhII mutants in their study showed an increase in the intracellular NADH/NAD+ conversion rate, leading to a higher level of free NADH, which in turn competitively inhibits the binding of the INH-NAD adduct to the InhA protein; this is consistent with the observations of Nguyen *et al.* [68]. Specific mutations related to this gene confer co-resistance to INH and ETH (ethionamide) (due to their similar mechanisms of action); these include the mutations Thr110Ala and Arg268His observed by Lee *et al.* [115] in 8 resistant isolates, and 7 of these had no mutations in other genes known to cause INH resistance. Cardoso *et al.* [116] observed two *ndh* mutations in resistant clinical strains from Brazil, which were not found in susceptible strains: Arg13Cys (CGT->TGT) and Val18Ala (GTG->GCG). Hazbón *et al.* [77] detected 30 *ndh* mutations in both sensitive and resistant strains. The most common mutation was Val18Ala [116]; however, this mutation was also present in susceptible strains. The study is consistent with the results of Lee *et al.* [115] who observed that the Arg268His mutation was present in only two INH^r isolates.

The mechanism of INH action is complex and involves inhibition of mycolic acid production, which is mediated by numerous enzymes; therefore, resistance to INH might be related to numerous alterations in the genes involved in this biosynthetic pathway. The multitude of resources used by bacilli to combat drug selection complicates the synthesis of new drugs and necessitates a search for new therapeutic targets. Furthermore, the identification of such mutations might facilitate the identification of novel markers for early diagnosis, which might significantly alter the course of treatment and improve patient prognosis.

3.2. Rifampicin (RIF)

Rifampicin was developed by the Dow-Lepetit Research Laboratories in Milan by modification of rifamycins, which are natural metabolites in *Nocardia mediterranei.* Notably, all metabolites with high antimicrobial activity were derived from the virtually inactive molecule rifamycin B [117].

The mechanism of rifampicin action was first described in *E. coli* by Hartmann *et al.* [118], and it involves inhibition of the bacterial RNA polymerase. Unlike other antibiotics, such as actinomycin and mitomycin, that inhibit the enzyme indirectly by interacting with the DNA template (causing high toxicity in humans), rifampicin selectively inhibits bacterial RNA polymerase at very low concentrations (~0.1 µg/mL), and targets mammalian RNA polymerase only at $>10^4$-fold higher concentrations [119]. Using ^{14}C-rifampicin, Wehrli *et al.* [120] were the first to observe a stable complex between RNA polymerase and rifampicin and demonstrated that *E. coli* strains phenotypically resistant to the antibiotic did not form this complex.

Other studies using *E. coli* elucidated the mechanism of rifampicin action on the RNA polymerase enzyme. This enzyme is composed of four subunits: α, β, β', and σ, and requires the core subunits (α, β, and β') to recruit the σ subunit to initiate gene transcription from promoter regions [121]. Transcription reconstitution experiments using α and β' RNA polymerase subunits from resistant strains and β from a susceptible strain generated a RIF-sensitive enzyme, whereas an enzyme with α and β' from a sensitive strain and β from a resistant strain was RIF-resistant [119], suggesting that the β subunit is a potential target for antibiotic binding [122]. RIF-induced abortive transcription initiation was observed in *M. smegmatis* [123].

In *M. tuberculosis*, the gene encoding the RNA polymerase β subunit is *rpoβ*. Recent data indicate that approximately 95% of all RIF-resistant isolates have mutations in an 81-bp region (RRDR - Rifampin Resistance Determining Region) between codons 507 and 533 of this gene [124]; these mutations most likely decrease the RIF binding affinity in the subunit (Fig. **3**). The TBDReaMD database contains 133 different mutations in the *rpoβ* ORF. The most common mutations and those responsible for the acquisition of resistance are in codons 531 and 526, which often involve the substitution of serine with leucine and histidine with tyrosine, respectively [84].

Position	507	508	509	510	511	512	513	514	515	516	517	518	519	520	521	522	523	524	525	526	527	528	529	530	531	532	533
Nucleotide sequence	GGC	ACC	AGC	CAG	CTG	AGC	CAA	TTC	ATG	GAC	CAG	AAC	AAC	CCG	CTG	TCG	GGG	TTG	ACC	CAC	AAG	CGC	CGA	CTG	TCG	GCG	CTG
Aminoacids sequence	Gly	Thr	Ser	Gln	Leu	Ser	Gln	Phe	Met	Asp	Gln	Asn	Asn	Pro	Leu	Ser	Gly	Leu	Thr	His	Lys	Arg	Arg	Leu	Ser	Ala	Leu

Fig. (3). The Rifampin Resistance Determining Region, the "hot spot" for mutations related to rifampicin resistance.

Recent studies, including those of Mohammed *et al.* [125] in Iraq and Makadia *et al.* [126] in India, observed high rates of *rpoβ* mutations conferring drug-resistance. Mohammed *et al.* [125] observed a total of 42/69 (60.87%) isolates with changes at codon 531 of the gene, but some susceptible strains also had these changes; the same was observed for codon 516. Only mutations at codon 526 were observed exclusively in resistant strains, reinforcing the idea that this position could be a marker of resistance. Makadia *et al.* [126] observed a high frequency of mutations at codon 531 (53.33%) in 30 cases of MDR-TB, and mutations in codons 516 and 526 were also observed in addition to a mutation at codon 529 and a deletion at position 509. Similar results were observed in other studies including Valim *et al.* [127] and Rahmo *et al.* [128].

Shi *et al.* [129] and Hazbón *et al.* [130] proposed that mutations at codon 306 of the *embB* gene, previously related to ethambutol resistance, are actually associated with very high resistance to RIF and the predisposition of isolates to acquire multi-drug resistance; however, this mechanism has not been elucidated.

3.3. Ethambutol (EMB)

Ethambutol is one of four first-line drugs for TB treatment, and its mechanism of action involves targeting various cellular activities; the most likely mechanism is that ethambutol acts as an inhibitor of arabinan cell wall biosynthesis [131]. Other studies, for instance, Plinke *et al.* [132], proposed that EMB functions in different ways, such as inhibition of nucleic acid metabolism [133], induction of accumulation of the trehalose dimycolate [134], spermidine biosynthesis [135], glucose metabolism [136], inhibition of the mycolic acid transfer in the cell wall [131], and phospholipid metabolism [137].

Consistent with the results of Takayama *et al.* [131], some studies observed an accumulation of B-D-L-arabinofuranosyl monophosphoryldecaprenol (DPA) in bacterial cells after EMB treatment [138], the inhibition of arabinan polymerization by DPA suggested that the target of EMB activity was arabinosyl transferase, which was subsequently confirmed [139].

Belanger *et al.* [139] and Telenti *et al.* [140] were the first to examine the molecular targets of EMB in *M. avium* and *M. smegmatis*, respectively, by screening genomic libraries. Telenti *et al.* [140] used a mutant library of *M. smegmatis* with high resistance to EMB and screened for genomic regions that conferred drug-resistance to the wild-type *M. smegmatis* mc²155 strain. The smallest region that conferred resistance to the wild-type strain was approximately 9 kb in length and contained three homologous regions and four potential coding regions. The Open Reading Frames (*embC*, *embA*, and *embB*) were each approximately 3200 bp in length; apart from the regions of homology, these results were inconsistent with the data of Belanger *et al.* [139], who observed that only two ORFs (*embA* and *embB*, and a putative transcriptional regulator *embR*) conferred drug resistance in *M. avium*.

Most studies examining the mechanism of EMB resistance have observed a mutation at codon 306 of the *embB* gene (mutations in Gly406 and Gln497 of *embB* are attributed to EMB resistance). Sreevatsan *et al.* [141] elucidated the role of this gene in the susceptibility profiles of the bacillus; the authors sequenced an 1892-bp gene region in 69 EMB[r] isolates and 30 EMB[s]. They observed the same wild-type profile for all susceptible strains, whereas in EMB[r] isolates, three individual mutations were observed: codon 285 (TTC->TTA, Phe3Leu), 330 (TTC->GTC, Phe->Val), and 630 (ACC->ATC, Thr->Ile). Mutations affecting the methionine at codon 306 accounted for 89% of all alterations in this gene, and five distinct changes were observed: GTG (Val), CTG (Leu), ATA (Ile), ATC (Ile), and ATT (Ile). By correlating phenotypic and genetic data, this study observed that all isolates with an amino acid substitution in this position exhibited an EMB MIC above 20 µg/mL.

Yoon *et al.* [142] examined the resistance profiles of 80 resistant strains in Korea and observed a total of 45 EMB[r] isolates; in 12 (26.7%) of these isolates, codon 306 was altered relative to a wild-type strain. They also observed a mutation at codon 319 in *embB* (Tyr319Ser) only in EMB[r] isolates, unlike the mutations at codon 306; this highlighted a potential new mechanism for drug resistance.

Consistent results were observed in a similar screen on Chinese isolates [143]; this study observed mutations in *embB* at codon 306 in ethambutol-sensitive strains, albeit at a much lower frequency than in resistant strains (54.7% in EMB^r and 19.2% in EMB^s isolates).

Although mutations at codon 306 are generally correlated with EMB resistance, some studies have presented evidence that contradicts this hypothesis because the same alterations are present in susceptible strains, which suggests the existence of additional mechanisms that mediate EMB resistance. Shi *et al.* [129] and Hazbón *et al.* [130] proposed that these mutations acted as facilitators by increasing the predisposition to development of multi-drug resistance. The data of Yoon *et al.* [142] confirms this hypothesis because mutations at codon 306 of *embB* also appeared in EMB^s isolates, but these isolates were INH^r and/or RIF^r.

Although most studies correlate ethambutol resistance with mutations in the *embB* gene, other genes have been associated with EMB resistance, including *embA* and *embC* (which is not surprising because these genes are in the same operon as *embB* and exhibit strong transcriptional corregulation) as well as the genes *iniA*, *iniB*, and *iniC*. These genes were first identified by Wilson *et al.* [144] using an assay for drug-induced changes in gene expression; this study identified the Rv0342 gene, also known as *iniA*, which encodes the Isoniazid-inducible protein IniA whose expression was induced by treatment with INH or EMB. However, the role of these genes, specifically *iniA*, in the acquisition of EMB resistance, was refuted by Jaber *et al.* [145] (in Kuwait) and Hazbón *et al.* [130] who observed that the *iniA*481 (His->Gln) and *iniA501* (Ser->Thr) mutations are highly uncommon and are not strong markers for EMB resistance.

3.4. Pyrazinamide (PZA)

PZA is a prodrug and requires activation; therefore, the mechanism of PZA action is very similar to that of the INH. The activity and efficacy of this drug were discovered by Chorine in 1945 [146] and McKenzie in 1948 [147]; these studies observed the activity of nicotinamide against the bacillus. Because PZA is analogous to nicotinamide, *in vivo* tests were performed using PZA, where it exhibited strong activity. These tests were performed even before the customary *in vitro* tests, where subsequently it was discovered that PZA was inactive [148]. The reason for this paradox was elucidated by McDermott *et al.* [149] who observed that PZA activation occurred only in acidic environments (pH ~5.5), which would occur during inflammation due to the production of lactic acid by inflammatory cells. The same group was also the first to show that pyrazinamide function required its conversion to pyrazinoic acid by a bacterial amidase, which was reported by Konno *et al.* [150].

PZA enters the bacillus by passive diffusion [151] or ATP-dependent transport [152] and is converted to pyrazinoic acid (POA) by nicotinamidase/pyrazinamidase (PZase). Subsequently, POA is excreted by an efflux pump. The protonated POA is reabsorbed by the bacillus during inflammatory conditions, and it accumulates in the intracellular environment and causes severe damage [148].

The identity of PZA targets is still somewhat controversial. Several hypotheses invoke mechanisms such as inhibition of fatty acid synthase type I (FASI) (involved in fatty acid synthesis [153, 154] and disruption of membrane potential and energy production) and trans-translation, suggesting an interaction with the ribosomal protein S1 (RpsA) [155], which was observed in a recent study. This study is promising for elucidation of the mechanism of PZA action because it was observed that a mutant with an alanine deletion in the RpsA C-terminal region was resistant to PZA and that overexpression of this protein in *M. tuberculosis* caused a five-fold increase in the PZA MIC.

Before the study of Shi *et al.* [155], the molecular basis for drug resistance was considered to involve mutations in the gene encoding the Pzase PncA (*pncA*); the mechanism was proposed to be similar to INH resistance mediated by the *katG* gene in which mutations in a particular enzyme prevent prodrug activation and consequently drug action. Several studies have examined mutations in the promoter and coding regions of *pncA*.

Among the mutations in the *pncA* promoter region, the following positions are important: -12 [156], -11 [156-158], and -7 [159]; the most common mutation is an A->G substitution at the -11 position. Various mutations have been observed in the *pncA* ORF, but the most commonly observed mutations are Trp68Leu [160],

Trp68Arg [161], Trp68Gly [161], Gly162Asp [160], Cys40Arg [157], Cys40His [162], Val139Met [163], Val139Leu [159], and Val139Ala [158]. Several other *pncA* mutations have been identified, suggesting that among the drug-resistance-related genes, *pncA* is the most susceptible to alterations in *Mycobacterium tuberculosis*. Two frameshift mutations have been observed in this gene: the insertion of two guanines at position 391 of the gene, observed by Lee *et al*. [161] and Lemaitre *et al*. [60] and a guanine deletion at codon 24, observed Sreevatsan *et al*. [158] and Hou *et al*. [164]. All *pncA* mutations impair PncA function and inhibit prodrug activation, which leads to resistance.

Tan *et al*. [165] confirmed the hypothesis of Shi *et al*. [155] that mutations in *rpsA* function in PZA-resistance; they observed three clinical isolates with alterations in *rpsA*: Arg474Leu, Arg474Trp, and Glu433Asp. Although some studies have suggested that the low frequency of *rpsA* mutations preclude its role in drug resistance, this study demonstrates that the 3' region of *rpsA* must be considered along with most mutations observed in *pncA*.

3.5. Other Drugs

As described above, *M. tuberculosis* is extremely skilled at surviving in hostile environments, which necessitates the use of poly-chemotherapy for treatment. This bacterium acquires resistance to the 4 first-line drugs used in treatment (INH, RIF, PZA, and EMB) as well as other drugs, which are discussed below.

Streptomycin is an aminoglycoside discovered in 1943 and was the first drug used to treat TB. It has a reduced bactericidal spectrum and interferes with translational proofreading, impairing protein synthesis by binding to the 16S rRNA [166]. Streptomycin resistance is related to mutations in two genes: *rpsL* (encoding the ribosomal protein S12) and *rrs* (encoding the 16S rRNA). Changes in RpsL destabilize the structure of the highly conserved 16S rRNA, and *rrs* mutations might affect binding of the 16S rRNA to streptomycin; both these mechanisms would confer streptomycin resistance [166, 167].

Fluoroquinolones are promising compounds for TB treatment and were introduced into clinical practice in the 1980s; these compounds have a broad antimicrobial spectrum [168]. Compounds belonging to this class such as levofloxacin, moxifloxacin, and gatifloxacin have MICs ranging from 0.12-1.0 mg/mL and can be valuable in therapy. Their mechanism of action involves inhibition of DNA gyrase, which is maintains the supercoiled DNA structure that is essential for chromosomal replication [169]. Therefore, fluoroquinolone resistance occurs is acquired by mutations in *gyrA* and *gyrB*, which respectively encode the A and B subunits of DNA gyrase, a type II DNA topoisomerase. A region known as the QRDR (quinolone resistance-determining region) was identified in both genes; missense mutations in the QRDR are associated with resistance, and the most common mutation is a substitution at codon 94 of the *gyrA* gene [167, 170].

Injectable drugs, such as amikacin (AMK), capreomycin (CAP), and kanamycin (KAN), are considered second-line drugs for TB treatment, but they are important allies in combating the disease. However, the use of these drugs has led to the emergence of XDR strains. The action of the aminoglycosides (AMK and KAN) involves binding to the 16S rRNA of the 30S ribosomal subunit, which interferes with protein synthesis [171]; CAP acts by methylation-dependent binding at the interface between the 16S and 23S rRNA subunits, which also interferes with protein synthesis [172]. Resistance to injectable drugs might be related to mutations in *rrs* (as described for streptomycin) and *tlyA* (which encodes the methyltransferase that enables CAP action) and the promoter region of the *eis* gene (which encodes an aminoglycoside acetyltransferase); the *eis* promoter mutations confer increased KAN resistance [173, 174]. Reeves *et al.* [175] observed that mutations in t'e 5'-UTR of the transcriptional activator *whiB7* might be related to cross-resistance to streptomycin and kanamycin.

Together, these data suggest that it is imperative to develop new drugs against TB because the bacillus has great versatility in acquiring mutations. Furthermore, poly-chemotherapy and the identification of new targets for drug action are important strategies to combat this disease.

3.6. Resistance Mediated by Efflux Pump Activity

The resistance in *Mycobacterium tuberculosis* can be divided into two groups: acquired resistance and intrinsic resistance. As discussed above, resistance can be acquired by selective pressure, which selects chromosomal mutations that affect proteins related to drug activation or drug targets. However, intrinsic resistance is conferred by two mycobacterial characteristics: the highly lipophilic, mycolic acid-rich cell wall that decreases drug permeability (natural barrier) and the increased activity of efflux pumps [9, 176, 177].

On average, 30% of INH^r isolates and 5% of RIF^r isolates do not have alterations in genes related to drug resistance [178], which suggests that the increased activity of efflux pumps mediates drug resistance [179]; this has been observed in several Gram-positive and Gram-negative bacteria [180]. Bacterial efflux pumps consist of five families, two of which are major because they are larger and developed earlier during evolution: the ATP-binding cassette superfamily (ABC) and Major Facilitator Superfamily (MFS). The other three families are smaller and have developed more recently: the Small Multidrug Resistance (SMR), Resistance-Nodulation-cell Division (RND), and Multidrug and Toxic Compounds Extrusion (MATE) families [181].

ABC transporters are present in both prokaryotes and eukaryotes and are responsible for the transport of various molecules (ions, amino acids, peptides, antibiotics, polysaccharides, and proteins) in an ATP hydrolysis-dependent manner [182-184]. These transporters consist of two hydrophobic membrane domains (MSDs - Membrane Spanning Domains) associated with two cytoplasmic domains that have nucleotide-binding activity (NBDs - Nucleotide Binding Domains) [183]. In prokaryotes, in addition to exporting molecules, this family of transporters imports molecules in the presence of the Substrate-Binding Protein (SBP); in *Mycobacterium tuberculosis*, the SBP is associated with the cytoplasmic membrane *via* a lipid tail similar to the Gram-positive bacteria [183]. Some pumps in this family are responsible for the decreased susceptibility of MDR strains to certain drugs, including DrrABC [185], Rv2686c-Rv2687c-Rv2688c [186], Rv0194 [187], and Rv1217c-Rv1218c [188], which confer resistance to ethambutol, fluoroquinolones, streptomycin, isoniazid, and rifampicin, respectively.

MFS transporters transport simple sugars, oligosaccharides, inositols, drugs, amino acids, nucleosides, organophosphate esters, Krebs cycle metabolites, and a variety of inorganic anions and cations between the mycobacterial cell and the environment using the proton motive force [189]; [181]. These transporters are divided into subfamilies based on the transported substrate and have conserved regions, suggesting that they have vital structural and functional roles apart from substrate interaction. Based on bioinformatic analyses, these proteins generally have 12 (up to 15) transmembrane segments and the C- and N-terminal domains are in the cytoplasm. Despite the small structural variations in different subfamilies, these transporters have a typical conformational feature known as the MFS fold [181, 190]. This efflux pump family is involved in the resistance of mycobacterial strains to drugs such as rifampicin, isoniazid, streptomycin, ofloxacin, fluoroquinolone, ethambutol, and ethionamide, and the pumps involved are Rv1258c [191]; [192], Rv1410c [188, 192], Rv1634 [181], Rv2459 [193], and Rv2846 [144], respectively.

The role of efflux pumps in mycobacterial resistance was first studied in *M. smegmatis*, and Liu *et al.* [194] discovered the first efflux system LfrA in this microorganism in 1996. In this study, the *lfrA* gene was cloned from the *Mycobacterium smegmatis* mc2-552 strain resistant to quinolones; overexpression of this gene on a plasmid conferred resistance to a sensitive strain. This observation led to studies on the role of efflux pumps in resistance to drugs other than quinolones. De Rossi *et al.* [195] identified the TetV system conferring tetracycline resistance, and Aínsa *et al.* [191] identified that the Tap transporter mediated resistance to tetracycline and aminoglycoside when overexpressed in *M. smegmatis*.

The importance of efflux pump activity in resistance is more evident when comparing the resistance/sensitivity patterns of *M. smegmatis* and *M. tuberculosis* to PZA. *M. smegmatis* is naturally resistant to PZA but has normal pyrazinamidase activity. This discrepancy was resolved by Zhang *et al.* [147] in 1999; they observed that POA is efficiently expelled from this organism, and this process can be inhibited by addition of the EPI (Efflux Pump Inhibitor) reserpine.

There are two aspects to the roles of efflux pumps: these efflux systems constitute real barriers in the discovery of new anti-TB drugs, and they are potential targets for TB therapy; therefore, it is important to identify molecules that inhibit efflux pump action and allow the retention of other drugs within the mycobacteria, which would increase the intracellular lifetime and therapeutic efficacy of these drugs.

Efflux pumps can be inhibited in several ways: (1) interfering with the regulation of efflux pump expression, (2) altering the chemical structures of the substrate antibiotics to prevent pump binding, (3) interfering with the folding of efflux pump components, (4) inhibiting substrate (antibiotic) binding by competitive or non-competitive mechanisms using other compounds, (5) blocking the pump pores through which efflux occurs, and (6) interfering with the availability of the energy required for pump function (Fig. **4**) [196].

Several efflux pump inhibitors have been identified; for instance, reserpine increases the sensitivity of *Bacillus subtilis* to toxic compounds [197], and in *Mycobacterium tuberculosis* (as mentioned above), this compound increases pyrazinoic acid accumulation [151], leading to increased pyrazinamide sensitivity [198]. Verapamil functions in a similar manner; this compound blocks ABC transporters and increases the susceptibility of quinolone-resistant bacilli to ofloxacin [11]. Efflux pump action can be inhibited in other ways by drugs such as chlorpromazine and thioridazine, which decrease the resistance of *Staphylococcus aureus* to methicillin [199] and increase the susceptibility of *Mycobacterium avium* ATCC 25291 and *Mycobacterium smegmatis* mc^{2}155 strains to erythromycin [200]. In this study, CCCP (Carbonyl cyanide m-chlorophenyl hydrazine), a drug that destabilizes the proton gradient and interferes with ATP production (essential for the efflux pump activity), increased the sensitivity of *Mycobacterium avium* ATCC 25291 to amikacin, ethambutol, and thioridazine. Plasmid-based expression of the P55 efflux pump genes (that naturally occur in *Mycobacterium bovis*) in *Mycobacterium smegmatis* mc^{2}155 revealed the role of CCCP, reserpine, and verapamil in reducing the minimum inhibitory concentrations (MIC) of tetracycline and streptomycin [189]. Despite the promising *in vitro* results using such compounds, they are problematic when used as therapeutics because they generate side effects; for instance, phenothiazine causes arrhythmia [200].

Gupta *et al.* [201] tested whether EPI can be used for TB treatment and observed that the use of verapamil with TMC (Bedaquiline) caused an 8- to 16-fold reduction in the MIC of TMC.

Therefore, although bacillus drug resistance is complicated and impedes the development of new drugs, knowledge of the resistance mechanisms can be used for the rational design of drugs to overcome these barriers.

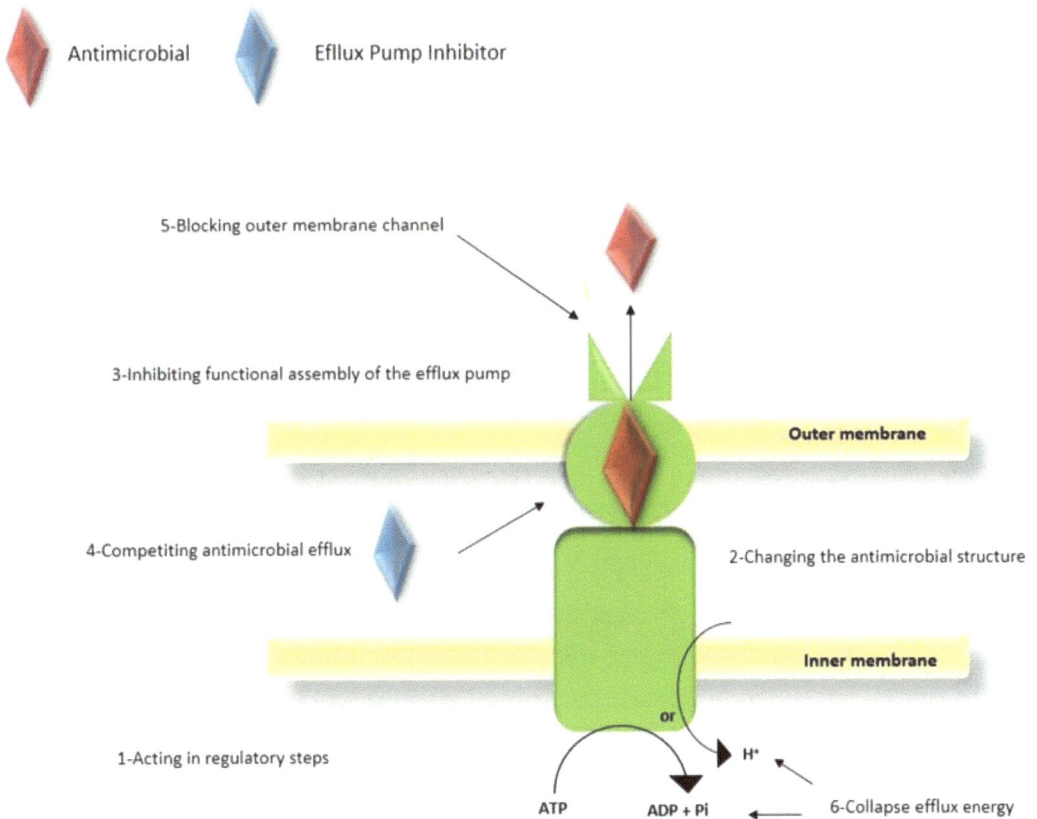

Antimicrobial   Efllux Pump Inhibitor

5-Blocking outer membrane channel

3-Inhibiting functional assembly of the efflux pump

Outer membrane

4-Competing antimicrobial efflux   2-Changing the antimicrobial structure

Inner membrane

or

1-Acting in regulatory steps

H+

ATP   ADP + Pi   6-Collapse efflux energy

Fig. (4). Possible mechanisms of action of an E.P.I. (Efflux Pump Inhibitor). Adapted from Askoura *et al.* [196].

4. INVESTMENTS IN TB

Infectious diseases cause high morbidity and mortality worldwide [202]. In less than 20 years, approximately 100 global health initiatives (GHIs) have been created to meet the Millennium Development Goals [MDGs]. These GHIs, often established as public-private partnerships, have leveraged and mobilized unprecedented levels of funding channeled through governments and civil society organizations for specific diseases and targeted interventions [203-205].

Since the early 2000s, there have been large increases in donor financing of human resources for health (HRH) [206]. This increase has been a major focus of global health investments, coinciding with the expansion of large scale Global Health Initiatives (GSI) [206-208]. For example, the G-Finder project originally commissioned by the Bill & Melinda Gates Foundation in 2007 has annually examined globally neglected disease research and development expenditures [202]. UK is the second largest investor in global health, but there was no detailed analysis of their investment in research. There are large gaps in the global data related to the expenditure on research of infectious diseases and the impact of development policies and health practices [202].

Among other efforts, the Global Plan to Stop TB estimates necessary financing in low and middle-income countries to achieve the TB control targets of the Stop TB Partnership [209].

The Global Plan to Stop TB from 2011 to 2015 (Global Plan), developed by the Stop TB Partnership with major inputs from the World Health Organization (WHO), specifies the level of TB interventions and funding that National TB Control Programs (NTPs) will need to reach the Millennium Development Goals (MDG). The Plan's cost projections are based on estimates of TB cases and deaths, intervention targets, and service implementation costs in low and middle-income countries (LMIC) [210].

The program results are encouraging. Between 2003 and 2011, the PNT Global Fund enabled the treatment of 8.6 million people with smear-positive TB sputum. In 2011, the Global Fund provided 76% of the external financing for control of TB and multi-drug resistant TB (MDR-TB) in LMIC and 11% of the total funding for TB in these countries. From its launch in 2002 and until 2011, the Global Fund invested US$2.3 billion in TB grants in 116 countries and disbursed US$512 million in TB grants in 2010 [211].

These actions were implemented to meet the following recommended goals:

By 2015: Reduce prevalence and death rates by 50% compared with their levels in 1990

By 2050: Eliminate TB as a public health problem, defined as a global incidence of active TB of less than one case per 1 million of population per year

The corresponding funding requirements are an overall US$ 47 billion from 2011 to 2015, including almost US$ 37 million for implementation and almost US$ 10 billion for research and development. Specific funding requirements include:

- DOTS (Directly Observed Therapy Short-course): US$ 22.6 billion;

- MDR-TB: US$ 7.1 billion;

- TB/HIV: US$ 2.8 billion.

In 2011, over 40 countries reported adherence to the WHO TB planning and budgeting tool in the planning of international strategies according to the recommendations and goals of the Comprehensive Plan. In 2011, all 27 countries with high MDR-TB rates developed new national MDR-TB strategies based on the comprehensive plan [210].

Projections of TB program expenditures funded by the Global Fund were based on 2010 donor pledges and the projected income of US$ 11.7 billion for the replenishment period between 2011 and 2013. Using the regional distribution of Global Fund disbursements from 2007 to 2009, we expect that 16% of the financing will be allocated to TB over the next five years, with the rest allocated to HIV/AIDS (49%), malaria (34%), and stronger health systems (captured within the three disease areas). These projections assume a one-year time lag between disbursements and program expenditures [210].

In China and India, DOTS treatments have decreased slowly, whereas TB/HIV cases have increased slowly (reflecting a stable, low prevalence of HIV), but there is a large increase in the number of patients treated for MDR-TB. The required funding will be increased from US$ 1.2 billion in 2010 to US$ 1.9 billion in 2015, mainly reflecting the cost of treating increasing cases of MDR-TB [210, 212].

Because MDR-TB is more costly to treat, overall funding needs will increase by 25% between 2010 and 2015. By 2015, 62% of the total funding will be allocated to drug-susceptible TB, 37% to MDR-TB, and less than 1% to TB/HIV [210].

In 2010, the Global Fund's total TB expenditure of US$ 387 million covered 7.7% of DOTS, MDR, and TB/HIV funding needs in LMIC. This contribution increased to 12.8% in 2012 and should decline to 8.4% by 2015 [210].

Fig. (5) illustrates the failure of donor communities to satisfy the funding targets established by the 2011-2015 Global Plan. With the exception of basic science, where investments increased by 6.5% from 2011 to 2012, the gap between actual and desired spending is widening in most research categories. Table 1 illustrates how the funding organizations invested in TB in the 2005-2012 period [213].

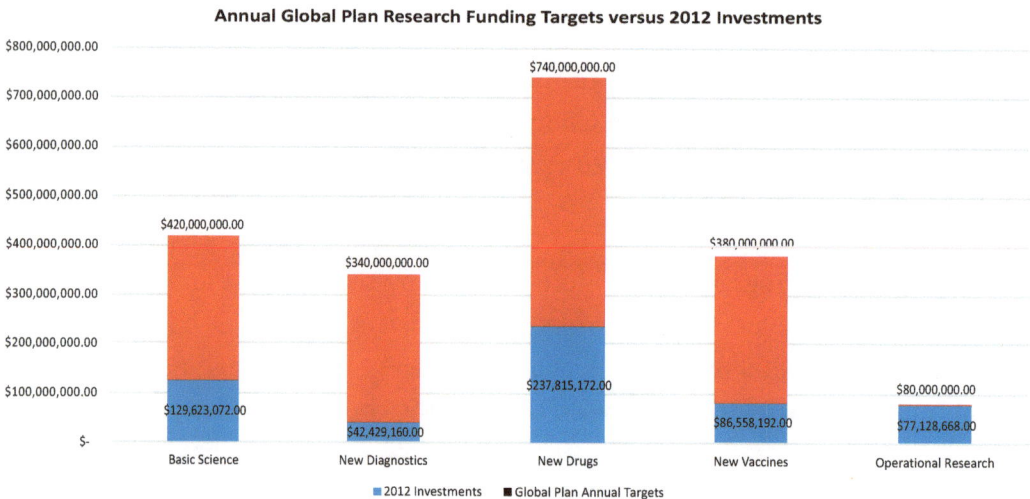

Annual Global Plan Research Funding Targets versus 2012 Investments

Fig. (5). Distance between the investments made in 2012 and the targets proposed by the 2011-2015 Global Plan. Adapted from TUBERCULOSIS RESEARCH AND DEVELOPMENT: 2013 Report on Tuberculosis Research Funding Trends, 2005-2012. Mike Frick and Eleonora Jiménez-Levi, 2013.

Despite the modest increase in basic-science investment, there is a deficit of US$ 290.4 million compared to the annual target. Diagnostics funding suffered the greatest percent decline, falling by 23.4% to US$ 42.4 million in 2012. Investments in diagnostics research will need to increase by US$ 297.6 million to meet the 2011-2015 Global Plan funding target. For the first time since 2005, funding for drug research has decreased, falling by 6.7% to US$ 237.8 million. This creates a gap of US$ 502.2 million in the US$ 740 million annual target. Investments in TB vaccines dropped by 9.3% to US$ 86.6 million, creating a shortfall of US$ 293.4 million. After exceeding the 2011-2015 Global Plan target in 2011, funding for operational research dropped back below this level in 2012, with total spending of US$ 77.1 million-US$ 2.9 million [213].

Table 1.   Investments in TB in the 2005-2012 Period

2012 Rank	Funding Organization	Funder Type	Total
1	U.S. National Institute of Allergy and Infectious Diseases [NIAID]	P	U$169,092,971
2	Bill & Melinda Gates Foundation (BMGF)	F	U$111,601,679
3	Otsuka	C	U$60,034,956
4	U.S. Other NIH Institutes and Centers (Other NIH ICs)	P	U$36,646,883
5	European Commission (EC)	P	U$27,260,036
6	Company X	C	U$22,844,099
7	U.S. Centers for Disease Control and Prevention (CDC)	P	U$18,481,592
8	U.K. Department for International Development	P-D	U$16,852,323
9	U.K. Medical Research Council (MRC)	P	U$14,790,087
10	Wellcome Trust	F	U$13,418,817
11	U.S. Agency for International Development (USAID)	P-D	U$12,174,064
12	U.S. National Heart, Lung, and Blood Institute (NHLBI)	P	U$11,831,219
13	AstraZeneca	C	U$10,303,559
14	India (reported)	P	U$8,684,341
15	U.S. President's Emergency Plan for AIDS Relief (PEPFAR)	P	U$6,606,609
16	Dutch Ministry of Foreign Affairs Directorate-General of Development Cooperation (DGIS)	P-D	U$6,195,582
17	Canadian Institutes of Health Research (CIHR)	P	U$6,017,561
18	Global Fund to Fight AIDS, Tuberculosis and Malaria (GFATM)	M	U$6,000,000
19	German Federal Ministry of Education and Research (BMBF)	P	U$5,232,441
20	Company Z	C	U$5,178,920
21	Company W	C	U$4,529,539

(Table 1) contd…..

2012 Rank	Funding Organization	Funder Type	Total
22	Company V	C	U$4,297,934
23	Institut National de la Santé et de la Recherche Médicale (INSERM)	P	U$4,173,870
24	Emergent Biosolutions	C	U$4,157,360
25	Australian National Health and Medical Research Council (NHMRC)	P	U$4,060,791
26	Sweden (reported)	P	U$3,719,138
27	Korea (reported)	P	U$3,279,378
28	Max Planck Institute for Infection Biology (MPIIB)	P	U$2,950,000
29	Institut Pasteur	P	U$2,553,445
30	Agence Nationale de la Recherches sur le Sida et les hepatites virales (ANRS)	P	U$2,527,027
31	Carlos III Health Institute	P	U$1,814,951
32	World Health Organization (WHO)	M	U$1,707,923
33	Canadian International Development Agency (CIDA)	P-D	U$1,684,379
34	Health Research Council of New Zealand (HRC)	P	U$1,683,781
35	U.S. Food and Drug Administration (FDA)	P	U$1,642,584
38	Bloomberg Philanthropies	F	U$1,500,000
40	Australian Research Council (ARC)	P	U$1,412,237
41	Agence Nationale de la Recherche (ANR)	P	U$1,385,878
42	Irish Aid	P-D	U$1,284,370
43	South African Department of Science and Technology (DST)	P	U$1,217,500
44	Swiss National Science Foundation (SNSF)	P	U$824,473
45	Sequella	C	U$642,350
46	UBS Optimus Foundation	F	U$632,262
47	German Research Foundation (DFG)	P	U$555,326
48	KNCV Tuberculosis Foundation (KNCV)	F	U$499,817
49	Danish International Development Agency (DANIDA)	P-D	U$323,250
50	OPEC Fund for International Development (OFID)	M	U$279,810
51	Danish National Advanced Technology Foundation	P	U$233,863
52	Departamento Administrativo de Ciencia, Tecnologia e Innovación (Colciencias)	P	U$220,000
53	Danish Council for Independent Research/ Medical Sciences	P	U$210,469
54	Company Y	C	U$196,239
55	BioDuro	C	U$180,000

(Table 1) contd…..

2012 Rank	Funding Organization	Funder Type	Total
57	Statens Serum Institut (SSI)	P	U$153,252
59	Netherlands Organization for Health Research and Development (ZonMw)	P	U$140,013
61	Gulbenkian	F	U$122,055
62	WHO Stop TB Partnership	M	U$112,500
68	GSK Biologicals	C	U$63,298
69	Fondation Mérieux	F	U$63,298
70	FIT Biotech	C	U$63,298
71	Pfizer Laboratories Ltd	C	U$56,566
77	Sandoz	C	U$30,476
78	GlaxoSmithKline (GSK)	C	U$29,123
79	Korea LG Life Sciences	C	U$26,100
80	Thrasher Research Fund	F	U$21,710
82	AP Moller Foundation	F	U$7,663
83	Faber Daeufer Itrato & Cabot	C	U$7,500
84	European Centre for disease Prevention and control (ECDC)	P	U$4,113
85	Corporate Donors to TB Alliance	C	U$1,680
	New Funders under $500K		U$42,665
	Grand Total		**$627,389,725**

P= Public-sector; R&D agency; C= Corporation/private sector; M= Multilateral; F= Foundation/philanthropy; P-D= Public-sector development agency.
Adapted from TUBERCULOSIS RESEARCH AND DEVELOPMENT: 2013 Report on Tuberculosis Research Funding Trends, 2005-2012. Mike Frick and Eleonora Jiménez-Levi, 2013.

To overcome the barriers in TB treatment, the WHO endorsed a new rapid molecular test called Xpert MTB/RIF (Cepheid, Sunnyvale, CA, USA) in December 2010. The test can identify and diagnose resistance of pulmonary TB to rifampicin. In five locations, the sensitivity of the test (in comparison with culture) for TB was 91%, with a specificity of 99%, and the sensitivity of the test for rifampicin resistance was 95%, with a specificity of 98%. In May 2011, the WHO published a guideline for the Xpert MTB/RIF that was used as an initial diagnostic test in two groups of people: those suspected of multidrug resistance (MDR-TB) and those living with HIV who are suspected of having TB. This would introduce a cost of US$ 70-90 million per year in the U.S.; in countries with a higher burden of TB, this test has a lower cost than conventional diagnoses.

In European countries, Brazil, and South Africa, the cost would represent 10% of TB funding [214].

Despite the clear goals and actions of the WHO, the need for an intense policy to eradicate tuberculosis is evident. The 2050 goal will not be achieved without efforts in low-income countries that still have high rates of the disease. Although it is important to discover new therapies and diagnostic methods, these must be easily accessible to reach the 2050 goal.

5. OVERVIEW OF POTENTIAL NEW DRUGS

Discovery and development of new TB drugs. As discussed, the discovery and development of new high-quality TB drug candidates is widely recognized as one of the major global health emergencies and a major pharmaceutical challenge [24, 25, 215-217]. The pipeline for the discovery of new anti-TB drugs includes projects based on phenotypic screening and target-specific assays of millions of compounds [218] with the following objectives: shortening and simplifying treatment regimens [21, 24, 25, 211, 219], identifying drugs with acceptable toxicity profiles that are active against MDR/XDR TB as well as drugs that are useful in HIV-TB coinfection and active against latent TB [25]. To shorten the duration of TB treatment, a drug must have sterilizing rather than bactericidal properties [220]. The new drugs must help the immune system combat *M. tuberculosis* or prevent the reactivation of latent TB [218]. In addition, synergistic drug combinations might eradicate different bacterial subpopulations and prevent the development of resistance [215, 221, 222].

5.1. New "old drugs" on the Block

Many TB drug candidates in clinical trials were designed for other diseases. Drugs used for the treatment of parasitic and cardiovascular diseases have been repurposed [216]. Some of these drugs are listed below.

5.1.1. Fluoroquinolones

These are a promising class of antimicrobials that are second-line drugs targeting the mycobacterial topoisomerase II DNA gyrase [215], which is required for chromosomal replication [223-227]. Fluoroquinolones have lower MICs and greater bactericidal activity [25, 226, 228-230], which is relevant for reduction of the TB treatment duration [216, 231]. Resistance to fluoroquinolones is characterized by mutations in the quinolone-resistance-determining region (QRDR), a conserved region of the *gyr*A and *gyr*B genes [168, 226, 229] and has been observed in MDR strains and strains in HIV-TB co-infection [25, 231]. In a mouse model, the combined activity of rifampin, pyrazinamide, and moxifloxacin was better than standard regimen [231]. Moxifloxacin and gatifloxacin are fluoroquinolones with excellent bactericidal activity and low MIC values. Currently, these drugs are in Phase III clinical trials to treat drug-susceptible TB [215, 216, 231]. **Moxifloxacin:** This is a promising drug that inhibits bacterial DNA gyrase (Fig. **6**) [232]. It is used to treat latent TB and shorten TB treatment [232]. Pharmacodynamic complications occur when moxifloxacin is used in combined therapy because it has a long half-life and is rapidly absorbed [232, 233]. The bactericidal activity of moxifloxacin is superior to rifampin and comparable to isoniazid [231]. Moxifloxacin has structural differences compared to ofloxacin, which decreases the efflux of moxifloxacin from bacteria and consequently lowers the MIC and increases the intracellular activity compared to ofloxacin [230, 233]. **Gatifloxacin:** This drug acts by blocking the bacterial DNA gyrase, which is required for chromosomal replication [25]. Gatifloxacin has strong bactericidal activity (Fig. **7**) [227, 234], which is slightly lower than isoniazid [229] and slightly better than moxifloxacin [215]. The combination of gatifloxacin and ethambutol was the most promising [234], and the replacement of ethambutol with gatifloxacin accelerated killing of *M. tuberculosis* in TB patients [229]. In a general way, drug interactions have been observed among fluoroquinolones but not among fluoroquinolones and first-line TB drugs [25].

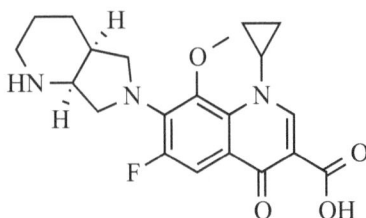

Fig. (6). Molecular structure of moxifloxacin.

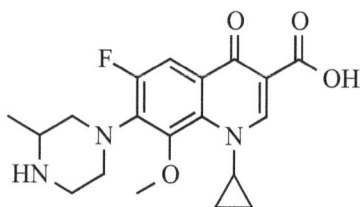

Fig. (7). Molecular structure of gatifloxacin.

5.1.2. Rifamycins

These antimicrobials are potent inhibitors of RNA polymerase [25, 216, 224, 235]. Microbial infections can be treated using semisynthetic rifamycins (rifampicin, rifapentine, rifabutin) [235]. **Rifampicin:** This is a first-line TB drug [235] that is cheap and widely available [25] and targets the beta subunit of RNA polymerase to inhibit transcription [216, 224]. Currently, high daily doses of rifampicin are used to shorten TB treatment [25]. **Rifapentine:** This drug has the same mechanism of action as rifampicin but has a longer half-life and is considered the analog with best activity (Fig. **8**) [236]; it is an important drug candidate to treat TB [25, 235] because it can be combined with oxifloxacin for the treatment of latent TB [25]. However, rifapentine induces the expression of P450 enzymes, which might cause interactions with protease inhibitors and other

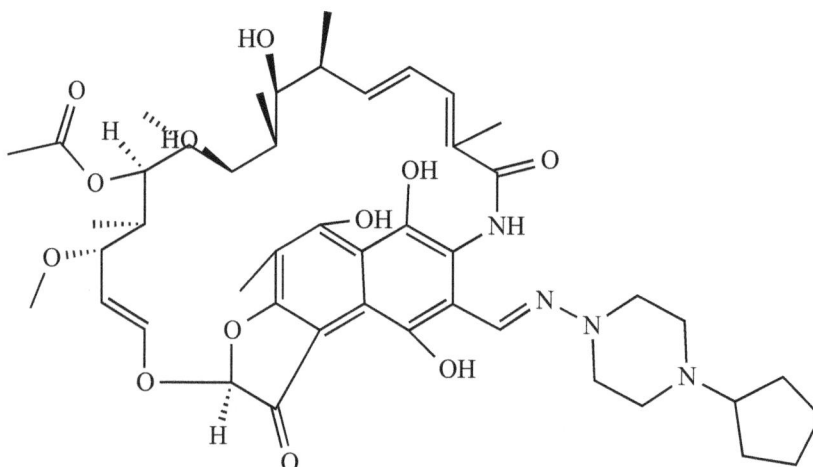

Fig. (8). Molecular structure of rifapentine.

TB drugs such as bedaquiline [26, 216, 235]. Therefore, there is significant interest in developing rifamycin-free regimens [216]. **Rifabutin:** The activity of this compound is comparable to that of rifampicin, but the use of higher rifabutin doses in TB treatment requires further study (Fig. **9**) [25].

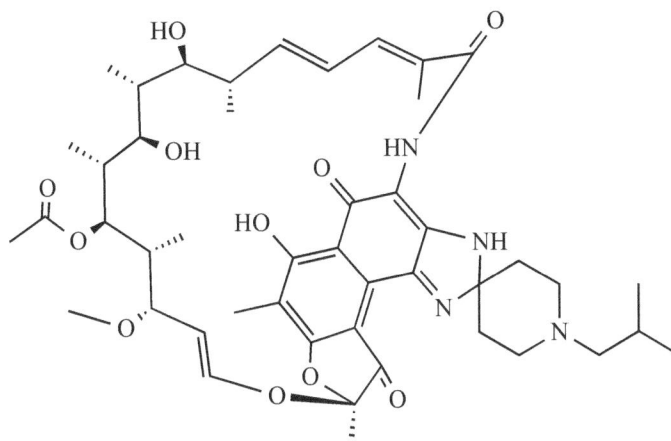

Fig. (9). Molecular structure of rifabutin.

5.1.3. Clofazimine

This is a riminophenazine antimicrobial derivative (Fig. **10**), which was initially developed for TB but is more widely used for leprosy treatment [24, 216]. Mycobacterial activity-deficient catalase is sensitive to clofazimine [237] because

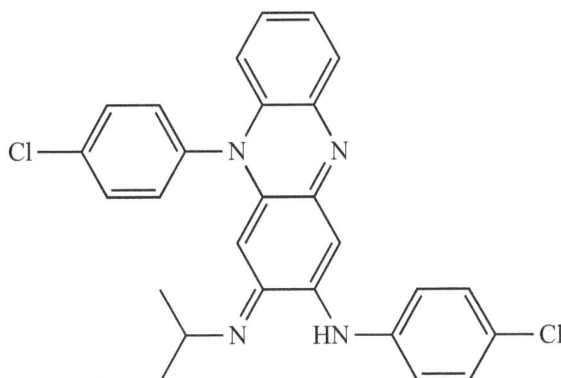

Fig. (10). Molecular structure of clofazimine.

reduced forms of this drug may target enzymes involved in the respiratory chain, resulting in the production of bacterial reactive oxygen species [237]. The use of clofazimine may shorten TB treatment [24], as observed in the Bangladesh regimen [8]; however, because it is a fat-soluble compound with a long half-life, it may accumulate in tissues including the lungs [238]. Further studies are required to optimize the dose as well as the duration and route of administration of therapy [24, 216].

5.1.4. Oxazolidinones

These are a new class of antimicrobial drugs with great potential for the treatment of drug-resistant TB; these drugs inhibit protein synthesis by binding to the bacterial 50S ribosomal subunit [24, 216]. **Linezolid:** This is a commercially available first-generation oxazolidinone that binds to ribosomal components such as the bacterial 23S rRNA in the 50S ribosomal subunit, resulting in inhibition of the initiation complex [24, 215, 216] during protein synthesis. Linezolid has tuberculostatic activity *in vitro* with a low MIC value (0.5 µg/mL), which enabled its use in combined regimens against MDR-TB with some success [216, 239-242]. The disadvantages of linezolid are the side effects caused by its potential toxicity [240] and the development resistance by mutations in the genes encoding ribosomal components [24, 216]. **Sutezolid:** This is a linezolid analog currently in Phase II studies and has promising antitubercular activity, which is stronger than linezolid in mice [24, 216] and similar to isoniazid [239]. **Posizolid:** This is a next-generation oxazolidinone that is not antagonistic with other TB drugs; it is safer than linezolid [235], and Phase II trials have revealed that its bactericidal activity is similar to linezolid [24, 216] (Fig. **11**).

5.1.5. β-Lactams

These are a highly important class of antimicrobial compounds [243]; they bind to transpeptidases and inhibit cell-wall synthesis [24]. Resistance to β-lactams is a natural characteristic of *M. tuberculosis*, which produces a highly active β-lactamase, resulting in the hydrolysis of β-lactams [24, 216]. Nevertheless, the antitubercular activity of various β-lactams, such as carbapenems (imipenem,

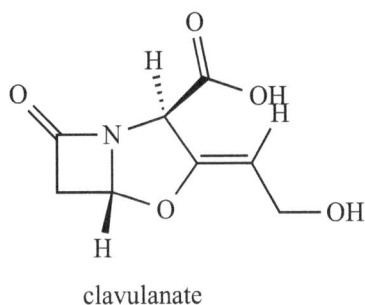

clavulanate

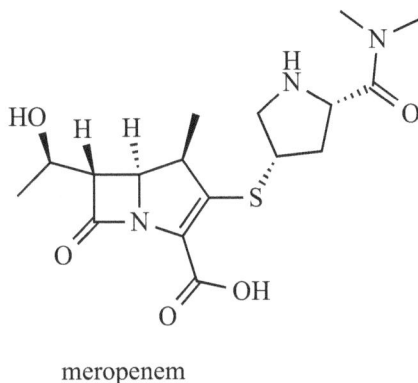

meropenem

Fig. (11). Molecular structures of linezolid, sutezolid and posizolid.

ertapenem, and meropenem), has been tested [24] because these compounds are relatively resistant to hydrolysis, and the MIC might be decreased by the addition of the FDA-approved β-lactamase inhibitor clavulanate [244] (Fig. **12**). **Clavulanate:** This compound irreversibly inhibits the β-lactamase BlaC [243] and enhances β-lactam activity [24]. **Meropenem:** This is a β-lactam that inhibits synthesis of peptidoglycan, which is a structural component of the cell wall [245]. Clavulanate and meropenem are FDA-approved drugs, and their combination has a synergistic effect [216, 244], which might be effective against drug-susceptible and XDR clinical strains of *M. tuberculosis* [24, 216, 244].

5.2. Promising Antituberculosis Agents

Some TB drug candidates with promising activity against *M. tuberculosis* are listed below. **Ruthenium complexes:** Two of the synthesized ruthenium (II)

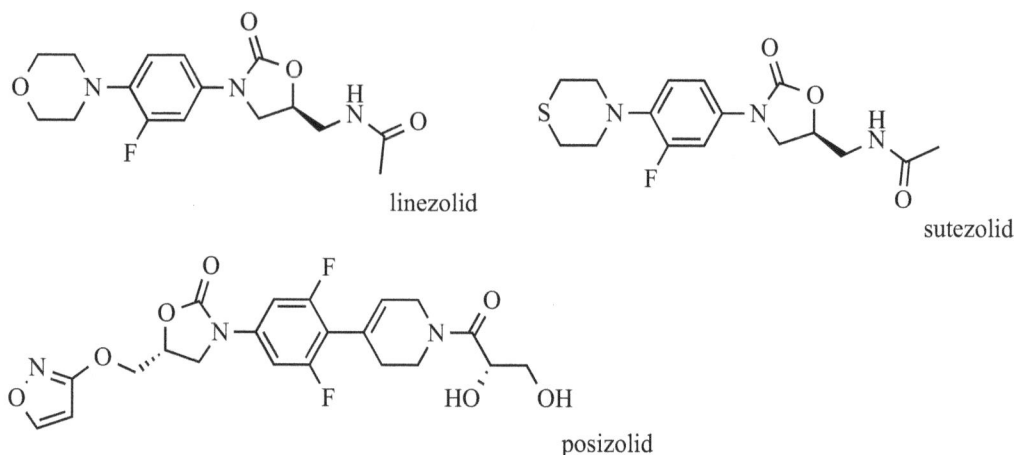

linezolid

sutezolid

posizolid

Fig. (12). Molecular structures of clavulanate and meropenem.

phosphine/picolinate complexes have potential antitubercular activity [246] with extremely promising biological results; these complexes meet all the criteria for a new drug and potentially constitute a new family of anti-TB drugs [247]. Preliminary studies have suggested that these compounds function by targeting cell wall biosynthesis [247]. **Thiosemicarbazones:** These are manganese compounds with thiosemicarbazone ligands and exhibit high anti-MTB activity and low cytotoxicity; the compound with highest oxidation potential may represent a new antitubercular agent that uses manganese as the metal center [247]. **Hydrazide/hydrazones and thiosemicarbazones:** These compounds are considered promising anti-TB agents, with MIC values ranging from 0.78 to 3.13 mg/mL and SI values equal to or greater than 200; they are more active and less toxic than other drugs used for the treatment of TB [248]. **Chloroquinolines and derivatives:** Seven such compounds have shown promising antitubercular activity, with MIC values lower than some drugs commonly used to treat TB; addition of ligands to the intermediate amino compounds increases their antitubercular activity [249]. **Indole-2-carboxamides:** Two leading candidates have shown improved *in vitro* and *in vivo* activity as well as pharmacokinetic properties and efficacy [250]. **Q203:** This compound targets ATP synthesis; its potency at low doses in a chronic mouse model and its effect on energy metabolism suggest that Q203 might shorten the tuberculosis treatment duration [251, 252]. **Triazoles derivatives:** Two leading compounds exhibited potency with MIC values of 2.5 mg/mL and low cytotoxicity against susceptible/MDR strains, making these compounds promising anti-TB agents; further studies are required to identify the targets of these molecules [253]. **Pyrroles derivatives:** Three molecules exhibited interesting activities against MDR strains and strongly inhibited the InhA protein and/or *M. tuberculosis* growth; therefore, these molecules represent new promising candidates for TB therapy [254].

5.3. New drugs in development.

The design of new treatment regimens poses the main obstacle to the discovery of new TB drugs. Furthermore, the discovery of new antimycobacterial drugs is complicated because (1) new TB agents must be developed and approved for use in combination with first-line anti-TB drugs [255, 256], (2) it is difficult to distinguish the effect of a candidate drug in a multidrug combination [257] and (3) new regimens must be compared to the current regimen (which uses four efficient drugs) [257]. Currently, there are promising candidates and new treatment regimens in clinical trials (Fig. **13**) [216]. An alternative strategy is the addition of a new drug to a regimen using second-line agents [258]. The TB Alliance is currently coordinating the development of regimens that combine old and repurposed drugs with new agents such as bedaquiline [255], which was approved by the FDA as a new drug after a 40-year interval [24]; this potentially represents the beginning of a new era of TB therapy [255]. TB drug candidates are briefly described below.

5.3.1. Diarylquinolines

By screening nitroimidazopyrans in *Mycobacterium smegmatis* [215, 256], bedaquiline was selected for its antimicrobial action due to a quinolinic central heterocyclic nucleus and side chains of tertiary alcohol and tertiary amine groups [259]. **Bedaquiline** (Sirturo™, Janssen Therapeutics) (TMC-207, formerly known as R207910) is the first TB drug of the novel diarylquinolines class (Fig. **14**) [24, 26, 215, 220, 223, 231, 260-265]. This drug was approved by the FDA in an accelerated approval program after a 40-year interval [216, 264]; its approval was based on two Phase II trials [255]. ***In vitro* activity:** Bedaquiline has MIC values

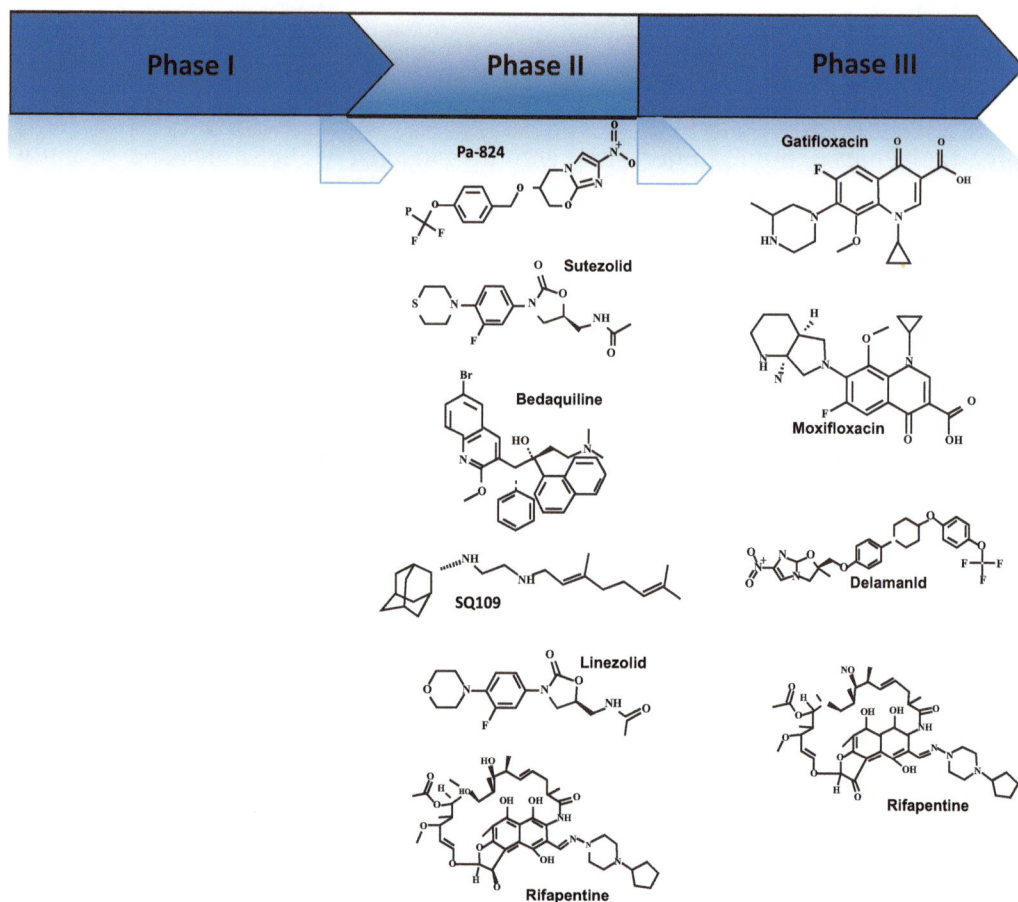

Fig. (13). Anti-TB drugs in development. Figure adapted from the Working Group on New TB Drugs (http: //www.newtbdrugs.org/).

ranging from 0.002 to 0.13 µg/mL [220, 263] and a MIC_{50} of 0.03 µg/mL [256], with no cross-resistance to the first-line TB drugs [263]; it is highly specific to *M. tuberculosis* because of its unique mechanism of action [231, 256, 263, 266]. Combinations of bedaquiline and pyrazinamide displayed synergistic effects, reducing the bacterial load by 7 log_{10}, with higher activity compared to the current first-line regimen of rifampicin, isoniazid and pyrazinamide [255, 256, 267, 268]. *In vivo activity:* In a murine model, bedaquiline exhibited greater bactericidal activity than the first-line drugs [24, 26, 216, 220, 223, 261, 264, 266] and enhanced the antibacterial activity of second-line drug combinations [256].

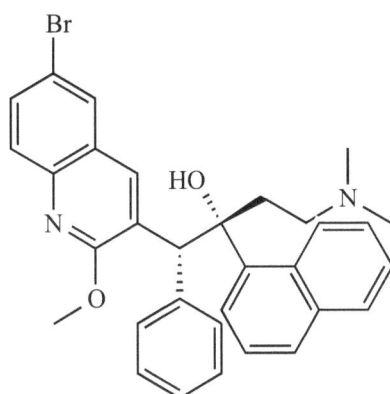

Fig. (14). Molecular structure of bedaquiline.

Bedaquiline is synergistic with pyrazinamide [219, 269]; however, the mechanism of its action complicates co-administration with rifampicin [256]. A combination of bedaquiline, rifampicin, and pyrazinamide was more effective than a combination of moxifloxacin, rifampin, and pyrazinamide [220] but not as effective as rifampin and isoniazid in humans [25]. ***Mechanism of action:*** Bedaquiline acts against susceptible/MDR and replicating/dormant strains by inhibiting the F0-subunit proton transfer chain (a transmembrane component comprising subunits a, b and c); bedaquiline interferes with the rotary movement of the central region of subunit c of the mycobacterial ATP synthase [27, 215, 219, 220, 231, 261-263, 265-267, 270-273] and leads to bacterial death [256]. Although there are human analogs of the bacterial target protein [256, 274], bedaquiline specifically targets the bacterial protein because of a three-amino acid difference in the binding site compared to the human protein [24]. ***Bedaquiline resistance:*** The *atpE* gene encodes the c subunit of ATP synthase [257], which synthesizes ATP [231, 263]. Mutations have been identified near the glutamic acid residue E61 [263] at position 63 (proline instead of alanine) or at position 66 (methionine instead of leucine), which disrupt the binding of bedaquiline to the c subunit of ATP synthase [26, 256], leading to bedaquiline resistance [223, 264]. ***Clinical trials:*** Based on its efficacy in two Phase II trials, the FDA approved bedaquiline for treatment of MDR-TB in adults when other alternatives are not available [216, 266, 272]; however, there are safety concerns because of unexplained deaths and drug interactions with rifampicin and antiretrovirals [24, 256, 264]. A large Phase III trial is planned to examine its potential long-term effect in a subset of patients with MDR-TB who are HIV-positive and on antiretroviral therapy [255, 265].

5.3.2. Nitroimidazopyrans

PA-824 and delamanid (OPC-67683) are two bicyclic nitroimidazole pro-drugs (Fig. **15**) with great potential in TB therapy [231]; these drugs require enzymatic activation by the deazaflavin cofactor F420 and mycobacterial glucose-6-phosphate dehydrogenase [25, 275]. **PA-824:** This compound is a metronidazole derivative of the nitroimidazopyran class [24, 25, 276]; it was selected by screening 328 compounds in a nitroimidazopyran chemical library [215, 263]. *In vitro activity:* PA-824 is specific to the *M. tuberculosis* complex [277] and is active (MIC of 0.015 to 0.25 µg/ml) against both susceptible/resistant [25, 231, 263, 277, 278] and replicating/non-replicating *M. tuberculosis* strains [279-284]. This drug does not interact with cytochrome P450 [24] and has no additive/synergistic effect or cross-resistance with the first-line drugs [25, 277, 278]. A PA-824-moxifloxacin-pyrazinamide combination was more effective than the current TB drugs for treating drug-sensitive and multidrug-resistant TB [24, 276, 280, 285] and might decrease the duration of treatment [282, 283]. *In vivo activity:* Murine studies have shown that PA-824 has bactericidal activity that is comparable to [231, 277, 279] or greater than INH [263]. It was active against persistent bacilli, and the combination of PA-824 and moxifloxacin was active against latent TB [25, 283]. *Mechanism of action:* The pro-drug PA-824 has a very complex mechanism of action that includes inhibition of a step in the synthesis of cell wall mycolates (analogous to isoniazid and ethionamide); this inhibition occurs by its significant effects on the transcription of genes responsive to known inhibitors of cell wall synthesis and causes hypoxia by the generation of radicals, which have toxic effects similar to cyanide [277, 278, 231, 275, 280-282, 286]. *PA-824-resistance:* Resistance to PA-824 is usually mediated by the loss of a specific glucose-6-phosphate dehydrogenase enzyme (fgd1) or its deazaflavin cofactor F420 through mutations in the PA-824 targets genes, such as Rv1173 (involved in F420 biosynthesis) and Rv3547 (encodes a protein with high structural specificity for binding to PA-824) [275, 284]. *Clinical trials:* PA-824 is one of two novel bicyclic nitroimidazoles in phase II clinical trials for TB

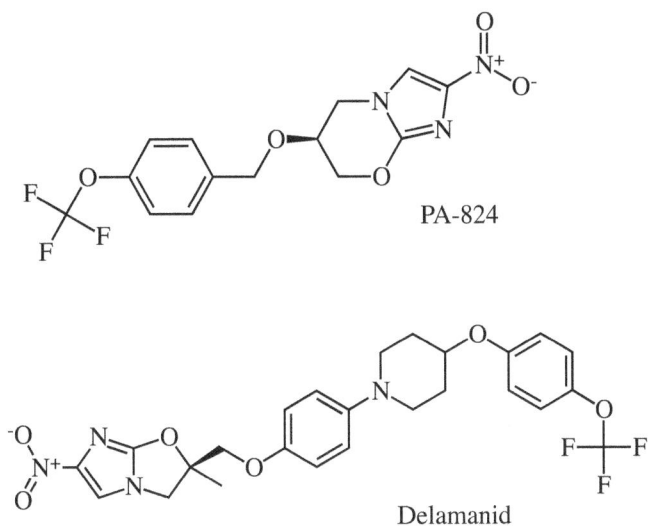

Fig. (15). Molecular structures of PA-824 and delamanid.

treatment [263, 280, 282]. **Delamanid:** This compound is another prodrug derivative of metronidazole and is structurally analogous to PA-824; Delamanid also requires metabolic activation by *M. tuberculosis*, and it was identified by screening a series of 6-nitro-2,3-dihydroimidazo[2,1-b]oxazoles [215, 231, 255, 263, 283, 286-288]. *In vitro activity:* Delamanid has excellent bactericidal and sterilizing activity and exhibits no cross resistance to any of the current first line drugs [215, 231, 287, 288]; its MIC values range between 0.006-0.024 µg/ml, which are approximately 10-fold lower than PA-824 [283, 289]. It is active against replicating/nonreplicating bacterial cells [215, 263, 281, 288, 289] and also has intracellular activity that may kill latent TB [287]. The activity of delamanid combined with rifampin and pyrazinamide was better than the standard four-drug regimen [24, 215, 263, 287]. *In vivo activity:* In a mouse model, delamanid exhibited the most potent anti-tubercular activity compared to the first-line drugs [215, 231, 287-289]. When combined with RIF, PZA [263, 283] and the first-line drugs [290], delamanid decreased the rapid culture conversion of lung tissue, displaying powerful sterilizing ability and the potential to reduce the treatment duration [263, 290]. *Mechanism of action:* Delamanid and PA-824 have similar mechanisms of action [231, 275]; Delamanid inhibits the incorporation of ^{14}C-acetate and fatty acid during mycolic acid biosynthesis [215, 283, 286, 290]. *Delamanid-resistance:* Mutations in the Rv3547 gene were observed in resistant strains [25], indicating that Rv3547 is required for delamanid activation [263, 286, 287]. *Clinical trials:* Delamanid has entered Phase III trials to test its safety and efficacy against MDR-TB and to test its role in HIV treatment combined with antiretroviral drugs [24, 215, 255, 288, 289, 291]. Delamanid is a promising drug for shortening the duration of treatment, improving patient attendance and accelerating sputum-culture conversion [291].

5.3.3. Diamines

By high-throughput screening of 63,238 ethylenediamine analogs [215, 231, 292-295], the second-generation agent SQ109 [296] was selected. **SQ109:** This compound is a member of a new class of ethylenediamine compounds (Fig. **16**) [295]; it is a synthetic analog of ethambutol [25, 215, 231, 289, 297, 298] with lipophilicity and low aqueous solubility [52]. It has bactericidal activity and a different intracellular target compared to the original pharmacophore; therefore, it is a novel potent antimicrobial compound [231, 297]. *In vitro activity:* It has strong bactericidal activity [222, 295] with low MICs (0.63 to 1.56 mM) against MDR and XDR-TB clinical strains [25]; it [49] effectively kills *M. tuberculosis* inside murine host macrophages with a potency and efficacy equivalent to INH and superior to EMB [222, 299, 300]. The synergistic effect of SQ109 with isoniazid and especially rifampin has been observed in both *in vitro* [including RIF-resistant strains] and *in vivo* trials [25, 215, 222, 289, 292, 294, 301], and it does not exhibit cross-resistance with ethambutol [289, 297]. *In vivo activity:* SQ109 has high efficacy in mice inoculated with *M. tuberculosis* [299] and was more effective than ethambutol [215] but less potent than INH [299, 300]. It has synergistic effects with isoniazid and rifampicin, which suggests new combination therapies for future clinical trials [297, 298]. The oral bioavailability of SQ109 was higher than ETH, and the tissue concentrations were 120-fold higher than in plasma [299]; it is poorly absorbed in rats and dogs (12% and 3.8-5%, respectively) [296]. *Mechanism of action:* SQ109 targets the mycolic acid transporter MmpL3 that transports the trehalose monomycolate, which is a component of the mycobacterial cell wall [51, 222, 289, 295] and cytoplasmic contents [222]. *SQ-109-resistance:* Specific mechanisms of resistance to SQ109 have not been observed [295, 297]. It is active against RIF-resistant *M. tuberculosis* clinical isolates [297] with a low resistance rate of 2.55 x 10^{-11} [25]. *Clinical trials:* SQ109 is currently in phase 2 clinical trials for TB treatment in adults [25, 215, 222, 298, 301]; phase 1 studies verified the safety, tolerability and pharmacokinetics of multiple doses of SQ109 in healthy volunteers [215, 289].

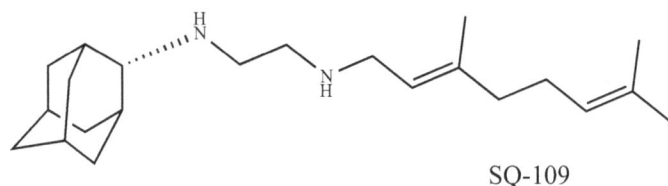

SQ-109

Fig. (16). Molecular structure of SQ-109.

5.3.4. Pyrroles

The pyrrole class was described in 1998; compounds of this class have bactericidal activity against susceptible/MDR strains and are effective *in vivo* [302]. A screen for potential anti-TB drug candidates identified a series of pyrroles [302], one of which showed promising activity [231, 289]. **Sudoterb (LL3858)** is a pyrrole derivative (Fig. **17**) that was first reported and evaluated in India [289]. *In vitro activity:* Sudoterb has low MIC values of 0.06-0.5 mg/mL; it has a synergistic effect with rifampin and is not affected by resistance to isoniazid and rifampicin [218, 231]. *In vivo activity:* In a mouse model of TB, this compound had sterilizing activity in the lungs and spleen similar to current TB drugs [218, 231]. *Mechanism of action:* The mechanism of sudoterb action remains unknown [218]. *Sudoterb-resistance:* There is no information on resistance to sudoterb. *Clinical trials:* Phase I clinical testing of sudoterb has been completed, and phase II tests are being performed to examine its early and extended bactericidal activity and pharmacokinetic properties.

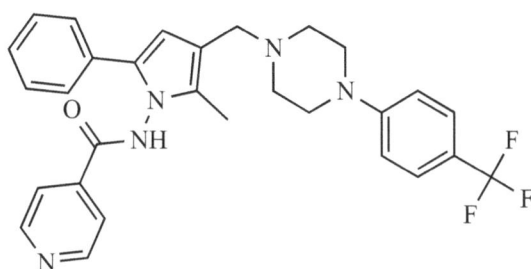

Fig. (17). Molecular structure of sudoterb.

CONCLUSION

This chapter highlights the major concerns regarding TB, many of which represent true barriers for drug discovery. Several pharmaceutical companies and universities have performed massive drug discovery studies to develop new compounds. Promising agents are in clinical trials, and strategies for the development of new molecules are being enhanced. New targets have been identified and validated, as in the case of bedaquiline, to shorten TB regimens.

However, a major shift in perception is required to combat this disease. The disease is not limited to regions where the lack of resources to be treated is evident. The bacillus constantly evolves resistance mechanisms to new drugs, which poses a challenge to current knowledge and necessitates intense scientific effort. Furthermore, this requires increased investment in the search for new anti-TB drugs. Unfortunately, the closure of the anti-infectives research division of Pfizer shows the evasion of potential investors.

A change in the global mindset towards TB will enable the development of novel and powerful drugs that act on different bacterial targets and successfully combat this disease.

The best prospects for curing this disease include increased investment in the rational development of new drugs, optimization of disease diagnosis and improving the accessibility of any new advances in all affected regions, but negligence regarding the real threat posed by this disease may allow the spread of resistant strains, which might have significant negative consequences.

ACKNOWLEDGEMENTS

This work was supported by the National Council for Scientific and Technological Development (CNPq), the Brazilian Federal Agency for Support and Evaluation of Graduate Education (CAPES) and the São Paulo Research Foundation (FAPESP ref. Process: 2011/21232-1).

CONFLICT OF INTEREST

The authors confirm that this chapter contents have no conflict of interest.

REFERENCES

[1]   Baddeley A, Dean A, Dias HM, Falzon D, Floyd K, Garcia I, *et al*. Global Tuberculosis Report 2013. Geneva: World Health Organization, 2013.

[2]   Ward SK, Hoye EA, Talaat AM. The global responses of *Mycobacterium tuberculosis* to physiological levels of copper. J Bacteriol. 2008; 190(8): 2939-46.

[3]   Manabe YC, Bishai WR. Latent *Mycobacterium tuberculosis* - persistence, patience, and winning by waiting. Nat Med. 2000; 6(12): 1327-9.

[4]   Kaufmann SH. How can immunology contribute to the control of tuberculosis? Nat Rev Immunol. 2001; 1(1): 20-30.

[5]   Russell DG. Who puts the tubercle in tuberculosis? Nat Rev Microbiol. 2007; 5(1): 39-47.

[6]   World Health Organization WHO. Guidelines for treatment of tuberculosis. 4th ed. Geneva: WHO Press; 2010.

[7]   Balganesh TS, Alzari PM, Cole ST. Rising standards for tuberculosis drug development. Trends Pharmacol Sci. 2008; 29(11): 576-81.

[8]   Van Deun A, Maug AK, Salim MA, Das PK, Sarker MR, Daru P, *et al*. Short, highly effective, and inexpensive standardized treatment of multidrug-resistant tuberculosis. Am J Respir Crit Care Med. 2010; 182(5): 684-92.

[9]   da Silva PEA, Von Groll A, Martin A, Palomino JC. Efflux as a mechanism for drug resistance in *Mycobacterium tuberculosis*. FEMS Immunol Med Microbiol. 2011; 63(1): 1-9.

[10]   Banerjee SK, Bhatt K, Rana S, Misra P, Chakraborti PK. Involvement of an efflux system in mediating high level of fluoroquinolone resistance in *Mycobacterium smegmatis*. Biochem Biophys Res Commun. 1996; 226(2): 362-8.

[11]   Singh M, Jadaun GPS, Ramdas, Srivastava K, Chauhan V, Mishra R, *et al*. Effect of efflux pump inhibitors on drug susceptibility of ofloxacin resistant *Mycobacterium tuberculosis* isolates. Indian J Med Res. 2011; 133(5): 535-40.

[12]   Green KD, Garneau-Tsodikova S. Resistance in tuberculosis: what do we know and where can we go? Front Microbiol. 2013; 4: 208.

[13]   Dooley KE, Kim PS, Williams SD, Hafner R. TB and HIV Therapeutics: Pharmacology Research Priorities. AIDS Res Treat. 2012; 2012: 874083.

[14]   Niemi M, Backman JT, Fromm MF, Neuvonen PJ, Kivisto KT. Pharmacokinetic interactions with rifampicin - Clinical relevance. ClinPharmacokinet. 2003; 42(9): 819-50.

[15]   Gomez-Reino JJ, Carmona L, Valverde VR, Mola EM, Montero MD, Grp B. Treatment of rheumatoid arthritis with tumor necrosis factor inhibitors may predispose to significant increase in tuberculosis risk - A multicenter active-surveillance report. Arthritis Rheum. 2003; 48(8): 2122-7.

[16]   Furst DE, Breedveld FC, Kalden JR, Smolen JS, Antoni CE, Bijlsma JWJ, *et al*. Updated consensus statement on biological agents for the treatment of rheumatoid arthritis and other rheumatic diseases (May 2002). Ann Rheum Dis. 2002; 61: 2-7.

[17] Haas C, Le Jeunne C. *Mycobacterium tuberculosis* infection following organ transplantation. Bulletin De L Academie Nationale De Medecine. 2006; 190(8): 1711-21.

[18] Rizvi SA, Naqvi SA, Hussain Z, Hashmi A, Akhtar F, Hussain M, *et al.* Renal transplantation in developing countries. Kidney Int Suppl. 2003(83): S96-100.

[19] Stevenson CR, Forouhi NG, Roglic G, Williams BG, Lauer JA, Dye C, *et al.* Diabetes and tuberculosis: the impact of the diabetes epidemic on tuberculosis incidence. BMC Public Health. 2007; 7.

[20] Leung CC, Lam TH, Chan WM, Yew WW, Ho KS, Leung GM, *et al.* Diabetic control and risk of tuberculosis: A cohort study. Am J Epidemiol. 2008; 167(12): 1486-94.

[21] Lienhardt C, Raviglione M, Spigelman M, Hafner R, Jaramillo E, Hoelscher M, *et al.* New drugs for the treatment of tuberculosis: needs, challenges, promise, and prospects for the future. J Infect Dis. 2012; 205 Suppl 2: S241-9.

[22] Frieden TR, Fujiwara PI, Washko RM, Hamburg MA. Tuberculosis in New York City - turning the tide. N Engl J Med. 1995; 333(4): 229-33.

[23] Cayla JA, Orcau A. Control of tuberculosis in large cities in developed countries: an organizational problem. BMC Med. 2011; 9.

[24] Wong EB, Cohen KA, Bishai WR. Rising to the challenge: new therapies for tuberculosis. Trends Microbiol. 2013; 21(9): 493-501.

[25] van den Boogaard J, Kibiki GS, Kisanga ER, Boeree MJ, Aarnoutse RE. New drugs against tuberculosis: problems, progress, and evaluation of agents in clinical development. Antimicrob Agents Chemother. 2009; 53(3): 849-62.

[26] Andries K, Verhasselt P, Guillemont J, Gohlmann HWH, Neefs JM, Winkler H, *et al.* A diarylquinoline drug active on the ATP synthase of *Mycobacterium tuberculosis*. Science. 2005; 307(5707): 223-7.

[27] de Jonge MR, Koymans LH, Guillemont JE, Koul A, Andries K. A computational model of the inhibition of *Mycobacterium tuberculosis* ATPase by a new drug candidate R207910. Proteins. 2007; 67(4): 971-80.

[28] Karim SSA, Naidoo K, Grobler A, Padayatchi N, Baxter C, Gray AL, *et al.* Integration of Antiretroviral Therapy with Tuberculosis Treatment. N Engl J Med. 2011; 365(16): 1492-501.

[29] Blanc F-X, Sok T, Laureillard D, Borand L, Rekacewicz C, Nerrienet E, *et al.* Earlier *versus* Later Start of Antiretroviral Therapy in HIV-Infected Adults with Tuberculosis. N Engl J Med. 2011; 365(16): 1471-81.

[30] Havlir DV, Kendall MA, Ive P, Kumwenda J, Swindells S, Qasba SS, *et al.* Timing of Antiretroviral Therapy for HIV-1 Infection and Tuberculosis. N Engl J Med. 2011; 365(16): 1482-91.

[31] CDC. Managing Drug Interactions in the Treatment of HIV-Related Tuberculosis [online]. 2013.

[32] Kaplan JE, Benson C, Holmes KK, Brooks JT, Pau A, Masur H. Guidelines for prevention and treatment of opportunistic infections in HIV-infected adults and adolescents: recommendations from CDC, the National Institutes of Health, and the HIV Medicine Association of the Infectious Diseases Society of America. MMWR Recomm Rep. 2009; 58(Rr-4): 1-207; quiz CE1-4.

[33] Burman WJ. Issues in the management of HIV-related tuberculosis. Clin Chest Med. 2005; 26(2): 283-94.

[34]   Gengiah TN, Gray AL, Naidoo K, Karim QA. Initiating antiretrovirals during tuberculosis treatment: a drug safety review. Expert Opin Drug Saf. 2011; 10(4): 559-74.

[35]   Cohen K, van Cutsem G, Boulle A, McIlleron H, Goemaere E, Smith PJ, *et al*. Effect of rifampicin-based antitubercular therapy on nevirapine plasma concentrations in South African adults with HIV-associated tuberculosis. J Antimicrob Chemother. 2008; 61(2): 389-93.

[36]   Jindani A, Nunn AJ, Enarson DA. Two 8-month regimens of chemotherapy for treatment of newly diagnosed pulmonary tuberculosis: international multicentre randomised trial. Lancet. 2004; 364(9441): 1244-51.

[37]   Khan FA, Minion J, Pai M, Royce S, Burman W, Harries AD, *et al*. Treatment of active tuberculosis in HIV-coinfected patients: a systematic review and meta-analysis. Clin Infect Dis. 2010; 50(9): 1288-99.

[38]   Cohen K, Grant A, Dandara C, McIlleron H, Pemba L, Fielding K, *et al*. Effect of rifampicin-based antitubercular therapy and the cytochrome P450 2B6 516G>T polymorphism on efavirenz concentrations in adults in South Africa. Antivir Ther. 2009; 14(5): 687-95.

[39]   Ngaimisi E, Mugusi S, Minzi O, Sasi P, Riedel KD, Suda A, *et al*. Effect of rifampicin and CYP2B6 genotype on long-term efavirenz autoinduction and plasma exposure in HIV patients with or without tuberculosis. Clin Pharmacol Ther. 2011; 90(3): 406-13.

[40]   Ali AH, Belachew T, Yami A, Ayen WY. Anti-Tuberculosis Drug Induced Hepatotoxicity among TB/HIV Co-Infected Patients at Jimma University Hospital, Ethiopia: Nested Case-Control Study. Plos One. 2013; 8(5): 8.

[41]   Dodd PJ, Knight GM, Lawn SD, Corbett EL, White RG. Predicting the Long-Term Impact of Antiretroviral Therapy Scale-Up on Population Incidence of Tuberculosis. Plos One. 2013; 8(9).

[42]   Gandhi NR, Shah NS, Andrews JR, Vella V, Moll AP, Scott M, *et al*. HIV Coinfection in Multidrug- and Extensively Drug-Resistant Tuberculosis Results in High Early Mortality. Am J Respir Crit Care Med. 2010; 181(1): 80-6.

[43]   Wells CD, Cegielski JP, Nelson LJ, Laserson KF, Holtz TH, Finlay A, *et al*. HIV infection and multidrug-resistant tuberculosis - The perfect storm. J Infect Dis. 2007; 196: S86-S107.

[44]   Soeters M, de Vries AM, Kimpen JLL, Donald PR, Schaaf HS. Clinical features and outcome in children admitted to a TB hospital in the Western Cape - the influence of HIV infection and drug resistance. S Afr Med J. 2005; 95(8): 602-6.

[45]   Dye C, Watt CJ, Bleed D. Low access to a highly effective therapy: a challenge for international tuberculosis control. Bull World Health Organ. 2002; 80(6): 437-44.

[46]   Havlir DV, Getahun H, Sanne I, Nunn P. Opportunities and challenges for HIV care in overlapping HIV and TB epidemics. JAMA. 2008; 300(4): 423-30.

[47]   Chideya S, Winston CA, Peloquin CA, Bradford WZ, Hopewell PC, Wells CD, *et al*. Isoniazid, rifampin, ethambutol, and pyrazinamide pharmacokinetics and treatment outcomes among a predominantly HIV-infected cohort of adults with tuberculosis from Botswana. Clin Infect Dis. 2009; 48(12): 1685-94.

[48]   Weiner M, Benator D, Peloquin CA, Burman W, Vernon A, Engle M, *et al*. Evaluation of the drug interaction between rifabutin and efavirenz in patients with HIV infection and tuberculosis. Clin Infect Dis. 2005; 41(9): 1343-9.

[49] Ginsberg AM, Laurenzi MW, Rouse DJ, Whitney KD, Spigelman MK. Safety, Tolerability, and Pharmacokinetics of PA-824 in Healthy Subjects. Antimicrob Agents Chemother. 2009; 53(9): 3720-5.

[50] Dutta NK, Alsultan A, Gniadek TJ, Belchis DA, Pinn ML, Mdluli KE, *et al.* Potent Rifamycin-Sparing Regimen Cures Guinea Pig Tuberculosis as Rapidly as the Standard Regimen. Antimicrob Agents Chemother. 2013; 57(8): 3910-6.

[51] Sacksteder KA, Protopopova M, Barry CE, Andries K, Nacy CA. Discovery and development of SQ109: a new antitubercular drug with a novel mechanism of action. Future Microbiol. 2012; 7(7): 823-37.

[52] Jia L, Noker PE, Coward L, Gorman GS, Protopopova M, Tomaszewski JE. Interspecies pharmacokinetics and *in vitro* metabolism of SQ109. Br J Pharmacol. 2006; 147(5): 476-85.

[53] Williams K, Minkowski A, Amoabeng O, Peloquin CA, Taylor D, Andries K, *et al.* Sterilizing Activities of Novel Combinations Lacking First- and Second-Line Drugs in a Murine Model of Tuberculosis. Antimicrob Agents Chemother. 2012; 56(6): 3114-20.

[54] Zhang Y, Yew WW. Mechanisms of drug resistance in *Mycobacterium tuberculosis*. Int J Tuberc Lung Dis. 2009; 13(11): 1320-30.

[55] Fitzpatrick C, Floyd K. A Systematic Review of the Cost and Cost Effectiveness of Treatment for Multidrug-Resistant Tuberculosis. Pharmacoeconomics. 2012; 30(1): 63-80.

[56] Meyssonnier V, Bui TV, Veziris N, Jarlier V, Robert J. Rifampicin mono-resistant tuberculosis in France: a 2005-2010 retrospective cohort analysis. BMC Infect Dis. 2014; 14: 18.

[57] Coovadia YM, Mahomed S, Pillay M, Werner L, Mlisana K. Rifampicin mono-resistance in *Mycobacterium tuberculosis* in KwaZulu-Natal, South Africa: a significant phenomenon in a high prevalence TB-HIV region. PLoS One. 2013; 8(11): e77712.

[58] Gillespie SH. Evolution of drug resistance in *Mycobacterium tuberculosis*: Clinical and molecular perspective. Antimicrob Agents Chemother. 2002; 46(2): 267-74.

[59] Dale JW. Mobile genetic elements in mycobacteria. Eur Respir J. 1995; 8: S633-S48.

[60] Lemaitre N, Sougakoff W, Truffot-Pernot C, Jarlier V. Characterization of new mutations in pyrazinamide-resistant strains of *Mycobacterium tuberculosis* and identification of conserved regions important for the catalytic activity of the pyrazinamidase PncA. Antimicrob Agents Chemother. 1999; 43(7): 1761-3.

[61] Karunakaran P, Davies J. Genetic antagonism and hypermutability in *Mycobacterium smegmatis*. J Bacteriol. 2000; 182(12): 3331-5.

[62] Sandgren A, Strong M, Muthukrishnan P, Weiner BK, Church GM, Murray MB. Tuberculosis drug resistance mutation database. PLoS Med. 2009; 6(2): e2.

[63] Robitzek EH, Selikoff IJ. Hydrazine derivatives of isonicotinic acid (rimifon marsilid) in the treatment of active progressive caseous-pneumonic tuberculosis; a preliminary report. Am Rev Tuberc. 1952; 65(4): 402-28.

[64] Kolyva AS, Karakousis PC. Old and New TB Drugs: Mechanisms of Action and Resistance. Understanding Tuberculosis - New Approaches to Fighting Against Drug Resistance. Dr. Pere-Joan Cardona ed2012.

[65] Vilcheze C, Jacobs WR, Jr. The mechanism of isoniazid killing: clarity through the scope of genetics. Annu Rev Microbiol. 2007; 61: 35-50.

[66] Winder FG, Collins PB. Inhibition by isoniazid of synthesis of mycolic acids in *Mycobacterium tuberculosis*. J Gen Microbiol. 1970; 63(1): 41-8.

[67]   Lei B, Wei CJ, Tu SC. Action mechanism of antitubercular isoniazid. Activation by *Mycobacterium tuberculosis KatG*, isolation, and characterization of inha inhibitor. J Biol Chem. 2000; 275(4): 2520-6.

[68]   Nguyen M, Quemard A, Broussy S, Bernadou J, Meunier B. Mn(III) pyrophosphate as an efficient tool for studying the mode of action of isoniazid on the InhA protein of *Mycobacterium tuberculosis*. Antimicrob Agents Chemother. 2002; 46(7): 2137-44.

[69]   Rawat R, Whitty A, Tonge PJ. The isoniazid-NAD adduct is a slow, tight-binding inhibitor of InhA, the *Mycobacterium tuberculosis* enoyl reductase: adduct affinity and drug resistance. Proc Natl Acad Sci USA. 2003; 100(24): 13881-6.

[70]   Rozwarski DA, Vilcheze C, Sugantino M, Bittman R, Sacchettini JC. Crystal structure of the *Mycobacterium tuberculosis* enoyl-ACP reductase, InhA, in complex with NAD+ and a C16 fatty acyl substrate. J Biol Chem. 1999; 274(22): 15582-9.

[71]   Gangadharam PR, Harold FM, Schaefer WB. Selective inhibition of nucleic acid synthesis in *Mycobacterium tuberculosis* by isoniazid. Nature. 1963; 198: 712-4.

[72]   Brennan PJ, Rooney SA, Winder FG. The lipids of *Mycobacterium tuberculosis* BCG: fractionation, composition, turnover and the effects of isoniazid. Ir J Med Sci. 1970; 3(8): 371-90.

[73]   Zatman LJ, Kaplan NO, Colowick SP, Ciotti MM. Effect of isonicotinic acid hydrazide on diphosphopyridine nucleotidases. J Biol Chem. 1954; 209(2): 453-66.

[74]   Bekierkunst A. Nicotinamide-adenine dinucleotide in tubercle bacilli exposed to isoniazid. Science. 1966; 152(3721): 525-6.

[75]   Middlebrook G. Sterilization of tubercle bacilli by isonicotinic acid hydrazide and the incidence of variants resistant to the drug *in vitro*. Am Rev Tuberc. 1952; 65(6): 765-7.

[76]   Pansy F, Stander H, Donovick R. *In vitro* studies on isonicotinic acid hydrazide. Am Rev Tuberc. 1952; 65(6): 761-4.

[77]   Hazbon MH, Brimacombe M, Bobadilla del Valle M, Cavatore M, Guerrero MI, Varma-Basil M, *et al*. Population genetics study of isoniazid resistance mutations and evolution of multidrug-resistant *Mycobacterium tuberculosis*. Antimicrob Agents Chemother. 2006; 50(8): 2640-9.

[78]   Cade CE, Dlouhy AC, Medzihradszky KF, Salas-Castillo SP, Ghiladi RA. Isoniazid-resistance conferring mutations in *Mycobacterium tuberculosis KatG*: catalase, peroxidase, and INH-NADH adduct formation activities. Protein Sci. 2010; 19(3): 458-74.

[79]   Middlebrook G. Isoniazid-resistance and catalase activity of tubercle bacilli; a preliminary report. Am Rev Tuberc. 1954; 69(3): 471-2.

[80]   Middlebrook G, Cohn ML, Schaefer WB. Studies on isoniazid and tubercle bacilli. III. The isolation, drug-susceptibility, and catalase-testing of tubercle bacilli from isoniazid-treated patients. Am Rev Tuberc. 1954; 70(5): 852-72.

[81]   Altamirano M, Marostenmaki J, Wong A, FitzGerald M, Black WA, Smith JA. Mutations in the catalase-peroxidase gene from isoniazid-resistant *Mycobacterium tuberculosis* isolates. J Infect Dis. 1994; 169(5): 1162-5.

[82]   Heym B, Alzari PM, Honore N, Cole ST. Missense mutations in the catalase-peroxidase gene, *katG*, are associated with isoniazid resistance in *Mycobacterium tuberculosis*. Mol Microbiol. 1995; 15(2): 235-45.

[83]   Musser JM. Antimicrobial agent resistance in mycobacteria: molecular genetic insights. Clin Microbiol Rev. 1995; 8(4): 496-514.

[84] Ramaswamy S, Musser JM. Molecular genetic basis of antimicrobial agent resistance in *Mycobacterium tuberculosis*: 1998 update. Tuber Lung Dis. 1998; 79(1): 3-29.

[85] Haas WH, Schilke K, Brand J, Amthor B, Weyer K, Fourie PB, *et al.* Molecular analysis of *katG* gene mutations in strains of *Mycobacterium tuberculosis* complex from Africa. Antimicrob Agents Chemother. 1997; 41(7): 1601-3.

[86] Marttila HJ, Soini H, Huovinen P, Viljanen MK. *katG* mutations in isoniazid-resistant *Mycobacterium tuberculosis* isolates recovered from Finnish patients. Antimicrob Agents Chemother. 1996; 40(9): 2187-9.

[87] Heym B, Alzari PM, Honore N, Cole ST. Missense mutations in the catalase-peroxidase gene, *katG*, are associated with isoniazid resistance in *Mycobacterium tuberculosis*. Mol Microbiol. 1995; 15(2): 235-45.

[88] Lipin MY, Stepanshina VN, Shemyakin IG, Shinnick TM. Association of specific mutations in *katG*, rpoB, rpsL and rrs genes with spoligotypes of multidrug-resistant *Mycobacterium tuberculosis* isolates in Russia. Clin Microbiol Infect. 2007; 13(6): 620-6.

[89] Dobner P, Rusch-Gerdes S, Bretzel G, Feldmann K, Rifai M, Loscher T, *et al.* Usefulness of *Mycobacterium tuberculosis* genomic mutations in the genes *katG* and inhA for the prediction of isoniazid resistance. Int J Tuberc Lung Dis. 1997; 1(4): 365-9.

[90] Kapetanaki SM, Chouchane S, Yu S, Zhao X, Magliozzo RS, Schelvis JP. *Mycobacterium tuberculosis KatG*(S315T) catalase-peroxidase retains all active site properties for proper catalytic function. Biochemistry. 2005; 44(1): 243-52.

[91] Wengenack NL, Uhl JR, St Amand AL, Tomlinson AJ, Benson LM, Naylor S, *et al.* Recombinant *Mycobacterium tuberculosis KatG*(S315T) is a competent catalase-peroxidase with reduced activity toward isoniazid. J Infect Dis. 1997; 176(3): 722-7.

[92] Cockerill FR, 3rd, Uhl JR, Temesgen Z, Zhang Y, Stockman L, Roberts GD, *et al.* Rapid identification of a point mutation of the *Mycobacterium tuberculosis* catalase-peroxidase (*katG*) gene associated with isoniazid resistance. J Infect Dis. 1995; 171(1): 240-5.

[93] Sreevatsan S, Pan X, Stockbauer KE, Connell ND, Kreiswirth BN, Whittam TS, *et al.* Restricted structural gene polymorphism in the *Mycobacterium tuberculosis* complex indicates evolutionarily recent global dissemination. Proc Natl Acad Sci USA. 1997; 94(18): 9869-74.

[94] Rouse DA, DeVito JA, Li Z, Byer H, Morris SL. Site-directed mutagenesis of the *katG* gene of *Mycobacterium tuberculosis*: effects on catalase-peroxidase activities and isoniazid resistance. Mol Microbiol. 1996; 22(3): 583-92.

[95] Zhao X, Yu H, Yu S, Wang F, Sacchettini JC, Magliozzo RS. Hydrogen peroxide-mediated isoniazid activation catalyzed by *Mycobacterium tuberculosis* catalase-peroxidase (*KatG*) and its S315T mutant. Biochemistry. 2006; 45(13): 4131-40.

[96] Lefford MJ. The ethionamide sensitivity of British pre-treatment strains of *Mycobacterium tuberculosis*. Tubercle. 1966; 47(2): 198-206.

[97] Banerjee A, Dubnau E, Quemard A, Balasubramanian V, Um KS, Wilson T, *et al.* inhA, a gene encoding a target for isoniazid and ethionamide in *Mycobacterium tuberculosis*. Science. 1994; 263(5144): 227-30.

[98] Sreevatsan S, Pan X, Stockbauer KE, Williams DL, Kreiswirth BN, Musser JM. Characterization of rpsL and rrs mutations in streptomycin-resistant *Mycobacterium tuberculosis* isolates from diverse geographic localities. Antimicrob Agents Chemother. 1996; 40(4): 1024-6.

[99]   Miyata M, Pavan FR, Sato DN, Marino LB, Hirata MH, Cardoso RF, *et al.* Drug resistance in *Mycobacterium tuberculosis* clinical isolates from Brazil: Phenotypic and genotypic methods. Biomed Pharmacother. 2011; 65(6): 456-9.

[100]   Jnawali HN, Hwang SC, Park YK, Kim H, Lee YS, Chung GT, *et al.* Characterization of mutations in multi- and extensive drug resistance among strains of *Mycobacterium tuberculosis* clinical isolates in Republic of Korea. Diagn Microbiol Infect Dis. 2013; 76(2): 187-96.

[101]   Vilcheze C, Wang F, Arai M, Hazbon MH, Colangeli R, Kremer L, *et al.* Transfer of a point mutation in *Mycobacterium tuberculosis* inhA resolves the target of isoniazid. Nat Med. 2006; 12(9): 1027-9.

[102]   Basso LA, Zheng R, Musser JM, Jacobs WR, Jr., Blanchard JS. Mechanisms of isoniazid resistance in *Mycobacterium tuberculosis*: enzymatic characterization of enoyl reductase mutants identified in isoniazid-resistant clinical isolates. J Infect Dis. 1998; 178(3): 769-75.

[103]   Deretic V, Philipp W, Dhandayuthapani S, Mudd MH, Curcic R, Garbe T, *et al.* *Mycobacterium tuberculosis* is a natural mutant with an inactivated oxidative-stress regulatory gene: implications for sensitivity to isoniazid. Mol Microbiol. 1995; 17(5): 889-900.

[104]   Dhandayuthapani S, Mudd M, Deretic V. Interactions of OxyR with the promoter region of the oxyR and ahpC genes from *Mycobacterium leprae* and *Mycobacterium tuberculosis*. J Bacteriol. 1997; 179(7): 2401-9.

[105]   Pym AS, Saint-Joanis B, Cole ST. Effect of *katG* mutations on the virulence of *Mycobacterium tuberculosis* and the implication for transmission in humans. Infect Immun. 2002; 70(9): 4955-60.

[106]   Heym B, Stavropoulos E, Honore N, Domenech P, Saint-Joanis B, Wilson TM, *et al.* Effects of overexpression of the alkyl hydroperoxide reductase AhpC on the virulence and isoniazid resistance of *Mycobacterium tuberculosis*. Infect Immun. 1997; 65(4): 1395-401.

[107]   Wilson T, de Lisle GW, Marcinkeviciene JA, Blanchard JS, Collins DM. Antisense RNA to ahpC, an oxidative stress defence gene involved in isoniazid resistance, indicates that AhpC of *Mycobacterium bovis* has virulence properties. Microbiology. 1998; 144 (Pt 10): 2687-95.

[108]   Hoshide M, Qian L, Rodrigues C, Warren R, Victor T, Evasco HB, 2nd, *et al.* Geographical Differences Associated with SNPs in Nine Gene Targets among Resistant Clinical Isolates of *Mycobacterium tuberculosis*. J Clin Microbiol. 2013.

[109]   Mdluli K, Slayden RA, Zhu Y, Ramaswamy S, Pan X, Mead D, *et al.* Inhibition of a *Mycobacterium tuberculosis* beta-ketoacyl ACP synthase by isoniazid. Science. 1998; 280(5369): 1607-10.

[110]   Lee AS, Lim IH, Tang LL, Telenti A, Wong SY. Contribution of kasA analysis to detection of isoniazid-resistant *Mycobacterium tuberculosis* in Singapore. Antimicrob Agents Chemother. 1999; 43(8): 2087-9.

[111]   Ramaswamy SV, Reich R, Dou SJ, Jasperse L, Pan X, Wanger A, *et al.* Single nucleotide polymorphisms in genes associated with isoniazid resistance in *Mycobacterium tuberculosis*. Antimicrob Agents Chemother. 2003; 47(4): 1241-50.

[112]   Yagi T. The bacterial energy-transducing NADH-quinone oxidoreductases. Biochim Biophys Acta. 1993; 1141(1): 1-17.

[113]   Kerscher SJ. Diversity and origin of alternative NADH: ubiquinone oxidoreductases. Biochim Biophys Acta. 2000; 1459(2-3): 274-83.

[114] Vilcheze C, Weisbrod TR, Chen B, Kremer L, Hazbon MH, Wang F, *et al*. Altered NADH/NAD+ ratio mediates coresistance to isoniazid and ethionamide in mycobacteria. Antimicrob Agents Chemother. 2005; 49(2): 708-20.

[115] Lee AS, Teo AS, Wong SY. Novel mutations in ndh in isoniazid-resistant *Mycobacterium tuberculosis* isolates. Antimicrob Agents Chemother. 2001; 45(7): 2157-9.

[116] Cardoso RF, Cardoso MA, Leite CQ, Sato DN, Mamizuka EM, Hirata RD, *et al*. Characterization of ndh gene of isoniazid resistant and susceptible *Mycobacterium tuberculosis* isolates from Brazil. Mem Inst Oswaldo Cruz. 2007; 102(1): 59-61.

[117] Sensi P. History of the development of rifampin. Rev Infect Dis. 1983; 5 Suppl 3: S402-6.

[118] Hartmann G, Honikel KO, Knusel F, Nuesch J. The specific inhibition of the DNA-directed RNA synthesis by rifamycin. Biochim Biophys Acta. 1967; 145(3): 843-4.

[119] Wehrli W. Rifampin: mechanisms of action and resistance. Rev Infect Dis. 1983; 5 Suppl 3: S407-11.

[120] Wehrli W, Knusel F, Staehelin M. Action of rifamycin on RNA-polymerase from sensitive and resistant bacteria. Biochem Biophys Res Commun. 1968; 32(2): 284-8.

[121] Ishihama A. Promoter selectivity of prokaryotic RNA polymerases. Trends Genet. 1988; 4(10): 282-6.

[122] Miller LP, Crawford JT, Shinnick TM. The rpoB gene of *Mycobacterium tuberculosis*. Antimicrob Agents Chemother. 1994; 38(4): 805-11.

[123] Levin ME, Hatfull GF. *Mycobacterium smegmatis* RNA polymerase: DNA supercoiling, action of rifampicin and mechanism of rifampicin resistance. Mol Microbiol. 1993; 8(2): 277-85.

[124] Zaczek A, Brzostek A, Augustynowicz-Kopec E, Zwolska Z, Dziadek J. Genetic evaluation of relationship between mutations in rpoB and resistance of *Mycobacterium tuberculosis* to rifampin. BMC Microbiol. 2009; 9: 10.

[125] Mohammed SH, Ahmed MM, Ahmed AR. First experience with using simple polymerase chain reaction-based methods as an alternative to phenotypic drug susceptibility testing for in Iraq. Int J Appl Basic Med Res. 2013; 3(2): 98-105.

[126] Makadia JS, Jain A, Patra SK, Sherwal BL, Khanna A. Emerging Trend of Mutation Profile of Gene in MDR Tuberculosis, North India. Indian J Clin Biochem. 2012; 27(4): 370-4.

[127] Valim AR, Rossetti ML, Ribeiro MO, Zaha A. Mutations in the rpoB gene of multidrug-resistant *Mycobacterium tuberculosis* isolates from Brazil. J Clin Microbiol. 2000; 38(8): 3119-22.

[128] Rahmo A, Hamdar Z, Kasaa I, Dabboussi F, Hamze M. Genotypic detection of rifampicin-resistant *M. tuberculosis* strains in Syrian and Lebanese patients. J Infect Public Health. 2012; 5(6): 381-7.

[129] Shi R, Zhang J, Otomo K, Zhang G, Sugawara I. Lack of correlation between embB mutation and ethambutol MIC in *Mycobacterium tuberculosis* clinical isolates from China. Antimicrob Agents Chemother. 2007; 51(12): 4515-7.

[130] Hazbon MH, Bobadilla del Valle M, Guerrero MI, Varma-Basil M, Filliol I, Cavatore M, *et al*. Role of embB codon 306 mutations in *Mycobacterium tuberculosis* revisited: a novel association with broad drug resistance and IS6110 clustering rather than ethambutol resistance. Antimicrob Agents Chemother. 2005; 49(9): 3794-802.

[131] Takayama K, Armstrong EL, Kunugi KA, Kilburn JO. Inhibition by ethambutol of mycolic acid transfer into the cell wall of *Mycobacterium smegmatis*. Antimicrob Agents Chemother. 1979; 16(2): 240-2.

[132] Plinke C, Walter K, Aly S, Ehlers S, Niemann S. *Mycobacterium tuberculosis* embB codon 306 mutations confer moderately increased resistance to ethambutol *in vitro* and *in vivo*. Antimicrob Agents Chemother. 2011; 55(6): 2891-6.

[133] Forbes M, Kuck NA, Peets EA. Effect of ethambutol on nucleic acid metabolism in *Mycobacterium smegmatis* and its reversal by poliamines and divalent cations. J Bacteriol. 1965; 89: 1299-305.

[134] Kilburn JO, Takayama K. Effects of ethambutol on accumulation and secretion of trehalose mycolates and free mycolic acid in *Mycobacterium smegmatis*. Antimicrob Agents Chemother. 1981; 20(3): 401-4.

[135] Paulin LG, Brander EE, Poso HJ. Specific inhibition of spermidine synthesis in Mycobacteria spp. by the dextro isomer of ethambutol. Antimicrob Agents Chemother. 1985; 28(1): 157-9.

[136] Silve G, Valero-Guillen P, Quemard A, Dupont MA, Daffe M, Laneelle G. Ethambutol inhibition of glucose metabolism in mycobacteria: a possible target of the drug. Antimicrob Agents Chemother. 1993; 37(7): 1536-8.

[137] Kilburn JO, Takayama K, Armstrong EL, Greenberg J. Effects of ethambutol on phospholipid metabolism in *Mycobacterium smegmatis*. Antimicrob Agents Chemother. 1981; 19(2): 346-8.

[138] Wolucka BA, McNeil MR, de Hoffmann E, Chojnacki T, Brennan PJ. Recognition of the lipid intermediate for arabinogalactan/arabinomannan biosynthesis and its relation to the mode of action of ethambutol on mycobacteria. J Biol Chem. 1994; 269(37): 23328-35.

[139] Belanger AE, Besra GS, Ford ME, Mikusova K, Belisle JT, Brennan PJ, *et al*. The embAB genes of *Mycobacterium avium* encode an arabinosyl transferase involved in cell wall arabinan biosynthesis that is the target for the antimycobacterial drug ethambutol. Proc Natl Acad Sci USA. 1996; 93(21): 11919-24.

[140] Telenti A, Philipp WJ, Sreevatsan S, Bernasconi C, Stockbauer KE, Wieles B, *et al*. The emb operon, a gene cluster of *Mycobacterium tuberculosis* involved in resistance to ethambutol. Nat Med. 1997; 3(5): 567-70.

[141] Sreevatsan S, Stockbauer KE, Pan X, Kreiswirth BN, Moghazeh SL, Jacobs WR, Jr., *et al*. Ethambutol resistance in *Mycobacterium tuberculosis*: critical role of embB mutations. Antimicrob Agents Chemother. 1997; 41(8): 1677-81.

[142] Yoon JH, Nam JS, Kim KJ, Choi Y, Lee H, Cho SN, *et al*. Molecular characterization of drug-resistant and -susceptible *Mycobacterium tuberculosis* isolated from patients with tuberculosis in Korea. Diagn Microbiol Infect Dis. 2012; 72(1): 52-61.

[143] Shi D, Li L, Zhao Y, Jia Q, Li H, Coulter C, *et al*. Characteristics of embB mutations in multidrug-resistant *Mycobacterium tuberculosis* isolates in Henan, China. J Antimicrob Chemother. 2011; 66(10): 2240-7.

[144] Wilson M, DeRisi J, Kristensen HH, Imboden P, Rane S, Brown PO, *et al*. Exploring drug-induced alterations in gene expression in *Mycobacterium tuberculosis* by microarray hybridization. Proc Natl Acad Sci USA. 1999; 96(22): 12833-8.

[145] Jaber AA, Ahmad S, Mokaddas E. Minor contribution of mutations at iniA codon 501 and embC-embA intergenic region in ethambutol-resistant clinical *Mycobacterium tuberculosis* isolates in Kuwait. Ann Clin Microbiol Antimicrob. 2009; 8: 2.

[146] Chorine V. Action de l'amide nicotinique sur les bacilles du genre *Mycobacterium*. C.R. Acad. Sci USA. 1945; p. 150-1.

[147] Mc KD, Malone L, *et al*. The effect of nicotinic acid amide on experimental tuberculosis of white mice. J Lab Clin Med. 1948; 33(10): 1249-53.

[148] Zhang Y, Wade MM, Scorpio A, Zhang H, Sun Z. Mode of action of pyrazinamide: disruption of *Mycobacterium tuberculosis* membrane transport and energetics by pyrazinoic acid. J Antimicrob Chemother. 2003; 52(5): 790-5.

[149] Mc DW, Tompsett R. Activation of pyrazinamide and nicotinamide in acidic environments *in vitro*. Am Rev Tuberc. 1954; 70(4): 748-54.

[150] Konno K, Feldmann FM, McDermott W. Pyrazinamide susceptibility and amidase activity of tubercle bacilli. Am Rev Respir Dis. 1967; 95(3): 461-9.

[151] Zhang Y, Scorpio A, Nikaido H, Sun Z. Role of acid pH and deficient efflux of pyrazinoic acid in unique susceptibility of *Mycobacterium tuberculosis* to pyrazinamide. J Bacteriol. 1999; 181(7): 2044-9.

[152] Raynaud C, Laneelle MA, Senaratne RH, Draper P, Laneelle G, Daffe M. Mechanisms of pyrazinamide resistance in mycobacteria: importance of lack of uptake in addition to lack of pyrazinamidase activity. Microbiology. 1999; 145 (Pt 6): 1359-67.

[153] Zimhony O, Cox JS, Welch JT, Vilcheze C, Jacobs WR, Jr. Pyrazinamide inhibits the eukaryotic-like fatty acid synthetase I (FASI) of *Mycobacterium tuberculosis*. Nat Med. 2000; 6(9): 1043-7.

[154] Boshoff HI, Mizrahi V, Barry CE, 3rd. Effects of pyrazinamide on fatty acid synthesis by whole mycobacterial cells and purified fatty acid synthase I. J Bacteriol. 2002; 184(8): 2167-72.

[155] Shi W, Zhang X, Jiang X, Yuan H, Lee JS, Barry CE, 3rd, *et al*. Pyrazinamide inhibits trans-translation in *Mycobacterium tuberculosis*. Science. 2011; 333(6049): 1630-2.

[156] Marttila HJ, Marjamaki M, Vyshnevskaya E, Vyshnevskiy BI, Otten TF, Vasilyef AV, *et al*. pncA mutations in pyrazinamide-resistant *Mycobacterium tuberculosis* isolates from northwestern Russia. Antimicrob Agents Chemother. 1999; 43(7): 1764-6.

[157] Scorpio A, Lindholm-Levy P, Heifets L, Gilman R, Siddiqi S, Cynamon M, *et al*. Characterization of pncA mutations in pyrazinamide-resistant *Mycobacterium tuberculosis*. Antimicrob Agents Chemother. 1997; 41(3): 540-3.

[158] Sreevatsan S, Pan X, Zhang Y, Kreiswirth BN, Musser JM. Mutations associated with pyrazinamide resistance in pncA of *Mycobacterium tuberculosis* complex organisms. Antimicrob Agents Chemother. 1997; 41(3): 636-40.

[159] Morlock GP, Plikaytis BB, Crawford JT. Characterization of spontaneous, *In vitro*-selected, rifampin-resistant mutants of *Mycobacterium tuberculosis* strain H37Rv. Antimicrob Agents Chemother. 2000; 44(12): 3298-301.

[160] Chan RC, Hui M, Chan EW, Au TK, Chin ML, Yip CK, *et al*. Genetic and phenotypic characterization of drug-resistant *Mycobacterium tuberculosis* isolates in Hong Kong. J Antimicrob Chemother. 2007; 59(5): 866-73.

[161] Lee KW, Lee JM, Jung KS. Characterization of pncA mutations of pyrazinamide-resistant *Mycobacterium tuberculosis* in Korea. J Korean Med Sci. 2001; 16(5): 537-43.

[162] Louw GE, Warren RM, Donald PR, Murray MB, Bosman M, Van Helden PD, *et al*. Frequency and implications of pyrazinamide resistance in managing previously treated tuberculosis patients. Int J Tuberc Lung Dis. 2006; 10(7): 802-7.

[163] McKinney JD, Honer zu Bentrup K, Munoz-Elias EJ, Miczak A, Chen B, Chan WT, *et al*. Persistence of *Mycobacterium tuberculosis* in macrophages and mice requires the glyoxylate shunt enzyme isocitrate lyase. Nature. 2000; 406(6797): 735-8.

[164] Hou L, Osei-Hyiaman D, Zhang Z, Wang B, Yang A, Kano K. Molecular characterization of pncA gene mutations in *Mycobacterium tuberculosis* clinical isolates from China. Epidemiol Infect. 2000; 124(2): 227-32.

[165] Tan Y, Hu Z, Zhang T, Cai X, Kuang H, Liu Y, *et al*. Role of pncA and rpsA Gene Sequencing in Diagnosis of Pyrazinamide Resistance in *Mycobacterium tuberculosis* Isolates from Southern China. J Clin Microbiol. 2013.

[166] Allen PN, Noller HF. Mutations in ribosomal proteins S4 and S12 influence the higher order structure of 16 S ribosomal RNA. J Mol Biol. 1989; 208(3): 457-68.

[167] De Stasio EA, Moazed D, Noller HF, Dahlberg AE. Mutations in 16S ribosomal RNA disrupt antibiotic--RNA interactions. EMBO J. 1989; 8(4): 1213-6.

[168] Ginsburg AS, Grosset JH, Bishai WR. Fluoroquinolones, tuberculosis, and resistance. Lancet Infect Dis. 2003; 3(7): 432-42.

[169] Sriram D, Aubry A, Yogeeswari P, Fisher LM. Gatifloxacin derivatives: synthesis, antimycobacterial activities, and inhibition of *Mycobacterium tuberculosis* DNA gyrase. Bioorg Med Chem Lett. 2006; 16(11): 2982-5.

[170] Takiff HE, Salazar L, Guerrero C, Philipp W, Huang WM, Kreiswirth B, *et al*. Cloning and nucleotide sequence of *Mycobacterium tuberculosis* gyrA and gyrB genes and detection of quinolone resistance mutations. Antimicrob Agents Chemother. 1994; 38(4): 773-80.

[171] Magnet S, Blanchard JS. Molecular insights into aminoglycoside action and resistance. Chem Rev. 2005; 105(2): 477-98.

[172] Johansen SK, Maus CE, Plikaytis BB, Douthwaite S. Capreomycin binds across the ribosomal subunit interface using tlyA-encoded 2'-O-methylations in 16S and 23S rRNAs. Mol Cell. 2006; 23(2): 173-82.

[173] Zaunbrecher MA, Sikes RD, Jr., Metchock B, Shinnick TM, Posey JE. Overexpression of the chromosomally encoded aminoglycoside acetyltransferase eis confers kanamycin resistance in *Mycobacterium tuberculosis*. Proc Natl Acad Sci USA. 2009; 106(47): 20004-9.

[174] Georghiou SB, Magana M, Garfein RS, Catanzaro DG, Catanzaro A, Rodwell TC. Evaluation of genetic mutations associated with *Mycobacterium tuberculosis* resistance to amikacin, kanamycin and capreomycin: a systematic review. PLoS One. 2012; 7(3): e33275.

[175] Reeves AZ, Campbell PJ, Sultana R, Malik S, Murray M, Plikaytis BB, *et al*. Aminoglycoside cross-resistance in *Mycobacterium tuberculosis* due to mutations in the 5' untranslated region of whiB7. Antimicrob Agents Chemother. 2013; 57(4): 1857-65.

[176] Jarlier V, Nikaido H. Mycobacterial cell wall: structure and role in natural resistance to antibiotics. FEMS Microbiol Lett. 1994; 123(1-2): 11-8.

[177] De Rossi E, Ainsa JA, Riccardi G. Role of mycobacterial efflux transporters in drug resistance: an unresolved question. FEMS Microbiol Rev. 2006; 30(1): 36-52.

[178] Louw GE, Warren RM, Gey van Pittius NC, McEvoy CR, Van Helden PD, Victor TC. A balancing act: efflux/influx in mycobacterial drug resistance. Antimicrob Agents Chemother. 2009; 53(8): 3181-9.

[179] Spies FS, da Silva PE, Ribeiro MO, Rossetti ML, Zaha A. Identification of mutations related to streptomycin resistance in clinical isolates of *Mycobacterium tuberculosis* and possible involvement of efflux mechanism. Antimicrob Agents Chemother. 2008; 52(8): 2947-9.

[180] Kohler T, Pechere JC, Plesiat P. Bacterial antibiotic efflux systems of medical importance. Cell Mol Life Sci. 1999; 56(9-10): 771-8.

[181] De Rossi E, Arrigo P, Bellinzoni M, Silva PEA, Martin C, Ainsa JA, *et al.* The multidrug transporters belonging to major facilitator superfamily (MFS) in *Mycobacterium tuberculosis.* Mol Med. 2002; 8(11): 714-24.

[182] Ames GFL. Bacterial periplasmic permeases as model systems for multidrug-resistance (MDR) and the cystic-fibrosis transmembrane conductance regulator (CFTR). Molecular Biology and Function of Carrier Proteins. 1993; 48: 77-94.

[183] Braibant M, Gilot P, Content J. The ATP binding cassette (ABC) transport systems of *Mycobacterium tuberculosis.* FEMS Microbiol Rev. 2000; 24(4): 449-67.

[184] Silva MLA, Martins CHG, Lucarini R, Sato DN, Pavan FR, Freitas NHA, *et al.* Antimycobacterial Activity of Natural and Semi-Synthetic Lignans. Zeitschrift Fur Naturforschung Section C-a Journal of Biosciences. 2009; 64(11-12): 779-84.

[185] Choudhuri BS, Bhakta S, Barik R, Basu J, Kundu M, Chakrabarti P. Overexpression and functional characterization of an ABC (ATP-binding cassette) transporter encoded by the genes drrA and drrB of *Mycobacterium tuberculosis.* Biochem J. 2002; 367: 279-85.

[186] Pasca MR, Guglierame P, Arcesi F, Bellinzoni M, De Rossi E, Riccardi G. Rv2686c-rv2687c-rv2688c, an ABC fluoroquinolone efflux pump in *Mycobacterium tuberculosis.* Antimicrob Agents Chemother. 2004; 48(8): 3175-8.

[187] Danilchanka O, Mailaender C, Niederweis M. Identification of a novel multidrug efflux pump of *Mycobacterium tuberculosis.* Antimicrob Agents Chemother. 2008; 52(7): 2503-11.

[188] Wang K, Pei H, Huang B, Zhu X, Zhang J, Zhou B, *et al.* The Expression of ABC Efflux Pump, Rv1217c-Rv1218c, and Its Association with Multidrug Resistance of *Mycobacterium tuberculosis* in China. Curr Microbiol. 2013; 66(3): 222-6.

[189] Silva PEA, Bigi F, Santangelo MD, Romano MI, Martin C, Cataldi A, *et al.* Characterization of P55, a multidrug efflux pump in *Mycobacterium bovis* and *Mycobacterium tuberculosis.* Antimicrobial Agents and Chemotherapy. 2001; 45(3): 800-4.

[190] Yan N. Structural advances for the major facilitator superfamily (MFS) transporters. Trends Biochem Sci. 2013; 38(3): 151-9.

[191] Ainsa JA, Blokpoel MCJ, Otal I, Young DB, De Smet KAL, Martin C. Molecular cloning and characterization of tap, a putative multidrug efflux pump present in *Mycobacterium fortuitum* and *Mycobacterium tuberculosis.* J Bacteriol. 1998; 180(22): 5836-43.

[192] Jiang X, Zhang W, Zhang Y, Gao F, Lu C, Zhang X, *et al.* Assessment of efflux pump gene expression in a clinical isolate *Mycobacterium tuberculosis* by real-time reverse transcription PCR. Microb Drug Resist. 2008; 14(1): 7-11.

[193] Gupta AK, Reddy VP, Lavania M, Chauhan DS, Venkatesan K, Sharma VD, *et al.* jefA (Rv2459), a drug efflux gene in *Mycobacterium tuberculosis* confers resistance to isoniazid & ethambutol. Indian J Med Res. 2010; 132(2): 176-88.

[194] Liu J, Takiff HE, Nikaido H. Active efflux of fluoroquinolones in *Mycobacterium smegmatis* mediated by LfrA, a multidrug efflux pump. J Bacteriol. 1996; 178(13): 3791-5.

[195] De Rossi E, Blokpoel MC, Cantoni R, Branzoni M, Riccardi G, Young DB, *et al.* Molecular cloning and functional analysis of a novel tetracycline resistance determinant, tet(V), from *Mycobacterium smegmatis.* Antimicrob Agents Chemother. 1998; 42(8): 1931-7.

[196]   Askoura M, Mottawea W, Abujamel T, Taher I. Efflux pump inhibitors (EPIs) as new antimicrobial agents against Pseudomonas aeruginosa. Libyan J Med. 2011; 6.

[197]   Neyfakh AA, Bidnenko VE, Chen LB. Efflux-mediated multidrug resistance in *Bacillus subtilis* - Similarities and dissimilarities with the mammalian system. Proc Natl Acad Sci USA. 1991; 88(11): 4781-5.

[198]   Zhang Y, Permar S, Sun ZH. Conditions that may affect the results of susceptibility testing of *Mycobacterium tuberculosis* to pyrazinamide. J Med Microbiol. 2002; 51(1): 42-9.

[199]   Kristiansen MM, Leandro C, Ordway D, Martins M, Viveiros M, Pacheco T, *et al*. Thioridazine reduces resistance of methicillin-resistant Staphylococcus aureus by inhibiting a reserpine-sensitive efflux pump. *In Vivo*. 2006; 20(3): 361-6.

[200]   Rodrigues L, Wagner D, Viveiros M, Sampaio D, Couto I, Vavra M, *et al*. Thioridazine and chlorpromazine inhibition of ethidium bromide efflux in *Mycobacterium avium* and *Mycobacterium smegmatis*. J Antimicrob Chemother. 2008; 61(5): 1076-82.

[201]   Gupta S, Tyagi S, Almeida DV, Maiga MC, Ammerman NC, Bishai WR. Acceleration of tuberculosis treatment by adjunctive therapy with verapamil as an efflux inhibitor. Am J Respir Crit Care Med. 2013; 188(5): 600-7.

[202]   Head MG, Fitchett JR, Cooke MK, Wurie FB, Hayward AC, Atun R. UK investments in global infectious disease research 1997-2010: a case study. Lancet Infect Dis. 2013; 13(1): 55-64.

[203]   Caines K. Key Evidence from Major Studies of Selected Global Health Partnerships London, U.K.: DFID Health Resource Centre 2005.

[204]   Samb B, Evans T, Dybul M, Atun R, Moatti J-P, Nishtar S, *et al*. An assessment of interactions between global health initiatives and country health systems. Lancet. 2009; 373(9681): 2137-69.

[205]   Warren AE, Wyss K, Shakarishvili G, Atun R, de Savigny D. Global health initiative investments and health systems strengthening: a content analysis of global fund investments. Global Health. 2013; 9.

[206]   Bowser D, Sparkes SP, Mitchell A, Bossert TJ, Barnighausen T, Gedik G, *et al*. Global Fund investments in human resources for health: innovation and missed opportunities for health systems strengthening. Health Policy Plan. 2013.

[207]   Ravishankar N, Gubbins P, Cooley RJ, Leach-Kemon K, Michaud CM, Jamison DT, *et al*. Financing of global health: tracking development assistance for health from 1990 to 2007. Lancet. 2009; 373(9681): 2113-24.

[208]   Atun R, Lazarus JV, Van Damme W, Coker R. Interactions between critical health system functions and HIV/AIDS, tuberculosis and malaria programmes. Health Policy Plan. 2010; 25 Suppl 1: i1-3.

[209]   Floyd K, Pantoja A. Financial resources required for tuberculosis control to achieve global targets set for 2015. Bull World Health Organ. 2008; 86(7): 568-76.

[210]   Korenromp EL, Glaziou P, Fitzpatrick C, Floyd K, Hosseini M, Raviglione M, *et al*. Implementing the Global Plan to Stop TB, 2011-2015-Optimizing Allocations and the Global Fund's Contribution: A Scenario Projections Study. Plos One. 2012; 7(6).

[211]   Malaria TGFtfATa. Approved grant amounts and disbursements: Disbursement in detail, commitments and disbursements - summary. 2012.

[212]   Vermund SH, Hayes RJ. Combination prevention: new hope for stopping the epidemic. Curr HIV/AIDS Rep. 2013; 10(2): 169-86.

[213]   Frick M, Jiménez-Levi E. 2013 Report on Tuberculosis Research Funding Trends, 2005-2012. 2013.

[214]   Pantoja A, Fitzpatrick C, Vassall A, Weyer K, Floyd K. Xpert MTB/RIF for diagnosis of tuberculosis and drug-resistant tuberculosis: a cost and affordability analysis. Eur Respir J. 2013; 42(3): 708-20.

[215]   Villemagne B, Crauste C, Flipo M, Baulard AR, Déprez B, Willand N. Tuberculosis: the drug development pipeline at a glance. Eur J Med Chem. 2012; 51: 1-16.

[216]   Zumla A, Nahid P, Cole ST. Advances in the development of new tuberculosis drugs and treatment regimens. Nat Rev Drug Discov. 2013; 12(5): 388-404.

[217]   Martinez-Jimenez F, Papadatos G, Yang L, Wallace IM, Kumar V, Pieper U, *et al*. Target Prediction for an Open Access Set of Compounds Active against *Mycobacterium tuberculosis*. PLoS Comput Biol. 2013; 9(10): e1003253.

[218]   Nuermberger EL, Spigelman MK, Yew WW. Current development and future prospects in chemotherapy of tuberculosis. Respirology. 2010; 15(5): 764-78.

[219]   Ginsberg AM. *Tuberculosis* drug development: progress, challenges, and the road ahead. Tuberculosis (Edinb). 2010; 90(3): 162-7.

[220]   Ibrahim M, Truffot-Pernot C, Andries K, Jarlier V, Veziris N. Sterilizing activity of R207910 (TMC207)-containing regimens in the murine model of tuberculosis. Am J Respir Crit Care Med. 2009; 180(6): 553-7.

[221]   Ma ZK, Lienhardt C, McIlleron H, Nunn AJ, Wang XX. Global tuberculosis drug development pipeline: the need and the reality. Lancet. 2010; 375(9731): 2100-9.

[222]   Makobongo MO, Einck L, Peek RM, Merrell DS. *In vitro* characterization of the anti-bacterial activity of SQ109 against Helicobacter pylori. PLoS One. 2013; 8(7): e68917.

[223]   Koul A, Arnoult E, Lounis N, Guillemont J, Andries K. The challenge of new drug discovery for tuberculosis. Nature. 2011; 469(7331): 483-90.

[224]   Mitchison D, Davies G. The chemotherapy of tuberculosis: past, present and future. Int J Tuberc Lung Dis. 2012; 16(6): 724-32.

[225]   Wallis RS, Kim P, Cole S, Hanna D, Andrade BB, Maeurer M, *et al*. Tuberculosis biomarkers discovery: developments, needs, and challenges. Lancet Infect Dis. 2013; 13(4): 362-72.

[226]   Zhang Z, Lu J, Wang Y, Pang Y, Zhao Y. Prevalence and molecular characterization of fluoroquinolone-resistant *Mycobacterium tuberculosis* isolates in China. Antimicrob Agents Chemother. 2013.

[227]   Smythe W, Merle CS, Rustomjee R, Gninafon M, Lo MB, Bah-Sow O, *et al*. Evaluation of initial and steady-state gatifloxacin pharmacokinetics and dose in pulmonary tuberculosis patients by using monte carlo simulations. Antimicrob Agents Chemother. 2013; 57(9): 4164-71.

[228]   Hu Y, Coates AR, Mitchison DA. Sterilizing activities of fluoroquinolones against rifampin-tolerant populations of *Mycobacterium tuberculosis*. Antimicrob Agents Chemother. 2003; 47(2): 653-7.

[229]   Johnson JL, Hadad DJ, Boom WH, Daley CL, Peloquin CA, Eisenach KD, *et al*. Early and extended early bactericidal activity of levofloxacin, gatifloxacin and moxifloxacin in pulmonary tuberculosis. Int J Tuberc Lung Dis. 2006; 10(6): 605-12.

[230]   Isaeva Y, Bukatina A, Krylova L, Nosova E, Makarova M, Moroz A. Determination of critical concentrations of moxifloxacin and gatifloxacin for drug susceptibility testing of

Mycobacterium tuberculosis in the BACTEC MGIT 960 system. J Antimicrob Chemother. 2013; 68(10): 2274-81.

[231] Spigelman MK. New tuberculosis therapeutics: a growing pipeline. J Infect Dis. 2007; 196 Suppl 1: S28-34.

[232] Drlica K, Zhao X, Kreiswirth B. Minimising moxifloxacin resistance with tuberculosis. Lancet Infect Dis. 2008; 8(5): 273-5.

[233] Zvada SP, Denti P, Sirgel FA, Chigutsa E, Hatherill M, Charalambous S, *et al.* Moxifloxacin population pharmacokinetics and model-based comparison of efficacy between moxifloxacin and ofloxacin in African patients. Antimicrob Agents Chemother. 2013.

[234] Alvirez-Freites EJ, Carter JL, Cynamon MH. *In vitro* and *in vivo* activities of gatifloxacin against *Mycobacterium tuberculosis*. Antimicrob Agents Chemother. 2002; 46(4): 1022-5.

[235] Cole ST, Riccardi G. New tuberculosis drugs on the horizon. Curr Opin Microbiol. 2011; 14(5): 570-6.

[236] Rosenthal IM, Zhang M, Williams KN, Peloquin CA, Tyagi S, Vernon AA, *et al.* Daily dosing of rifapentine cures tuberculosis in three months or less in the murine model. PLoS Med. 2007; 4(12): e344.

[237] Yano T, Kassovska-Bratinova S, Teh JS, Winkler J, Sullivan K, Isaacs A, *et al.* Reduction of clofazimine by mycobacterial type 2 NADH: quinone oxidoreductase: a pathway for the generation of bactericidal levels of reactive oxygen species. J Biol Chem. 2011; 286(12): 10276-87.

[238] Job CK, Yoder L, Jacobson RR, Hastings RC. Skin pigmentation from clofazimine therapy in leprosy patients: a reappraisal. J Am Acad Dermatol. 1990; 23(2 Pt 1): 236-41.

[239] Fortún J, Martín-Dávila P, Navas E, Pérez-Elías MJ, Cobo J, Tato M, *et al.* Linezolid for the treatment of multidrug-resistant tuberculosis. J Antimicrob Chemother. 2005; 56(1): 180-5.

[240] Koh WJ, Kang YR, Jeon K, Kwon OJ, Lyu J, Kim WS, *et al.* Daily 300 mg dose of linezolid for multidrug-resistant and extensively drug-resistant tuberculosis: updated analysis of 51 patients. J Antimicrob Chemother. 2012; 67(6): 1503-7.

[241] Lee M, Lee J, Carroll MW, Choi H, Min S, Song T, *et al.* Linezolid for treatment of chronic extensively drug-resistant tuberculosis. N Engl J Med. 2012; 367(16): 1508-18.

[242] Sotgiu G, Centis R, D'Ambrosio L, Alffenaar JW, Anger HA, Caminero JA, *et al.* Efficacy, safety and tolerability of linezolid containing regimens in treating MDR-TB and XDR-TB: systematic review and meta-analysis. Eur Respir J. 2012; 40(6): 1430-42.

[243] Hugonnet JE, Blanchard JS. Irreversible inhibition of the *Mycobacterium tuberculosis* beta-lactamase by clavulanate. Biochemistry. 2007; 46(43): 11998-2004.

[244] Hugonnet JE, Tremblay LW, Boshoff HI, Barry CE, Blanchard JS. Meropenem-clavulanate is effective against extensively drug-resistant *Mycobacterium tuberculosis*. Science. 2009; 323(5918): 1215-8.

[245] Kumar P, Arora K, Lloyd JR, Lee IY, Nair V, Fischer E, *et al.* Meropenem inhibits D,D-carboxypeptidase activity in *Mycobacterium tuberculosis*. Mol Microbiol. 2012; 86(2): 367-81.

[246] Pavan FR, Poelhsitz GV, do Nascimento FB, Leite SR, Batista AA, Deflon VM, *et al.* Ruthenium (II) phosphine/picolinate complexes as antimycobacterial agents. Eur J Med Chem. 2010; 45(2): 598-601.

[247]   Oliveira CG, Maia PI, Souza PC, Pavan FR, Leite CQ, Viana RB, *et al.* Manganese(II) complexes with thiosemicarbazones as potential anti-*Mycobacterium tuberculosis* agents. J Inorg Biochem. 2013.

[248]   Pavan FR, Maia PID, Leite SRA, Deflon VM, Batista AA, Sato DN, *et al.* Thiosemicarbazones, semicarbazones, dithiocarbazates and hydrazide/hydrazones: Anti-*Mycobacterium tuberculosis* activity and cytotoxicity. Eur J Med Chem. 2010; 45(5): 1898-905.

[249]   Carmo AM, Silva FM, Machado PA, Fontes AP, Pavan FR, Leite CQ, *et al.* Synthesis of 4-aminoquinoline analogues and their platinum(II) complexes as new antileishmanial and antitubercular agents. Biomed Pharmacother. 2011; 65(3): 204-9.

[250]   Kondreddi RR, Jiricek J, Rao SP, Lakshminarayana SB, Camacho LR, Rao R, *et al.* Design, Synthesis, and Biological Evaluation of Indole-2-carboxamides: A Promising Class of Antituberculosis Agents. J Med Chem. 2013.

[251]   Lin PL, Dartois V, Johnston PJ, Janssen C, Via L, Goodwin MB, *et al.* Metronidazole prevents reactivation of latent *Mycobacterium tuberculosis* infection in macaques. Proc Natl Acad Sci USA. 2012; 109(35): 14188-93.

[252]   Pethe K, Bifani P, Jang J, Kang S, Park S, Ahn S, *et al.* Discovery of Q203, a potent clinical candidate for the treatment of tuberculosis. Nat Med. 2013; 19(9): 1157-60.

[253]   Menendez C, Rodriguez F, Ribeiro AL, Zara F, Frongia C, Lobjois V, *et al.* Synthesis and evaluation of α-ketotriazoles and α,β-diketotriazoles as inhibitors of *Mycobacterium tuberculosis*. Eur J Med Chem. 2013; 69: 167-73.

[254]   Matviiuk T, Rodriguez F, Saffon N, Mallet-Ladeira S, Gorichko M, de Jesus Lopes Ribeiro AL, *et al.* Design, chemical synthesis of 3-(9H-fluoren-9-yl)pyrrolidine-2,5-dione derivatives and biological activity against enoyl-ACP reductase (InhA) and *Mycobacterium tuberculosis*. Eur J Med Chem. 2013; 70C: 37-48.

[255]   Jones D. Tuberculosis success. Nat Rev Drug Discov. 2013; 12(3): 175-6.

[256]   Matteelli A, Carvalho AC, Dooley KE, Kritski A. TMC207: the first compound of a new class of potent anti-tuberculosis drugs. Future Microbiol. 2010; 5(6): 849-58.

[257]   Sacks LV, Behrman RE. Developing new drugs for the treatment of drug-resistant tuberculosis: a regulatory perspective. Tuberculosis (Edinb). 2008; 88 Suppl 1: S93-100.

[258]   Barry CE. Unorthodox approach to the development of a new antituberculosis therapy. N Engl J Med. 2009; 360(23): 2466-7.

[259]   Lounis N, Guillemont J, Veziris N, Koul A, Jarlier V, Andries K. [R207910 (TMC207): a new antibiotic for the treatment of tuberculosis]. Med Mal Infect. 2010; 40(7): 383-90.

[260]   Cole ST, Alzari PM. Microbiology. TB--a new target, a new drug. Science. 2005; 307(5707): 214-5.

[261]   Ashraf H. A new weapon against TB? Drug Discov Today. 2005; 10(4): 230-1.

[262]   Petrella S, Cambau E, Chauffour A, Andries K, Jarlier V, Sougakoff W. Genetic basis for natural and acquired resistance to the diarylquinoline R207910 in mycobacteria. Antimicrob Agents Chemother. 2006; 50(8): 2853-6.

[263]   Rivers EC, Mancera RL. New anti-tuberculosis drugs in clinical trials with novel mechanisms of action. Drug Discov Today. 2008; 13(23-24): 1090-8.

[264]   Chan B, Khadem TM, Brown J. A review of tuberculosis: Focus on bedaquiline. Am J Health Syst Pharm. 2013; 70(22): 1984-94.

[265]   Palomino JC, Martin A. TMC207 becomes bedaquiline, a new anti-TB drug. Future Microbiol. 2013; 8(9): 1071-80.

[266] Diacon AH, Pym A, Grobusch M, Patientia R, Rustomjee R, Page-Shipp L, *et al.* The diarylquinoline TMC207 for multidrug-resistant tuberculosis. N Engl J Med. 2009; 360(23): 2397-405.

[267] Zhang T, Li SY, Williams KN, Andries K, Nuermberger EL. Short-course chemotherapy with TMC207 and rifapentine in a murine model of latent tuberculosis infection. Am J Respir Crit Care Med. 2011; 184(6): 732-7.

[268] Rubinstein E, Keynan Y. Quinolones for mycobacterial infections. Int J Antimicrob Agents. 2013; 42(1): 1-4.

[269] Tasneen R, Li SY, Peloquin CA, Taylor D, Williams KN, Andries K, *et al.* Sterilizing activity of novel TMC207- and PA-824-containing regimens in a murine model of tuberculosis. Antimicrob Agents Chemother. 2011; 55(12): 5485-92.

[270] Rubin EJ. Toward a new therapy for tuberculosis. N Engl J Med. 2005; 352(9): 933-4.

[271] Koul A, Dendouga N, Vergauwen K, Molenberghs B, Vranckx L, Willebrords R, *et al.* Diarylquinolines target subunit c of mycobacterial ATP synthase. Nat Chem Biol. 2007; 3(6): 323-4.

[272] Dhillon J, Andries K, Phillips PP, Mitchison DA. Bactericidal activity of the diarylquinoline TMC207 against *Mycobacterium tuberculosis* outside and within cells. Tuberculosis (Edinb). 2010; 90(5): 301-5.

[273] Haagsma AC, Podasca I, Koul A, Andries K, Guillemont J, Lill H, *et al.* Probing the interaction of the diarylquinoline TMC207 with its target mycobacterial ATP synthase. PLoS One. 2011; 6(8): e23575.

[274] Haagsma AC, Abdillahi-Ibrahim R, Wagner MJ, Krab K, Vergauwen K, Guillemont J, *et al.* Selectivity of TMC207 towards mycobacterial ATP synthase compared with that towards the eukaryotic homologue. Antimicrob Agents Chemother. 2009; 53(3): 1290-2.

[275] Singh R, Manjunatha U, Boshoff HI, Ha YH, Niyomrattanakit P, Ledwidge R, *et al.* PA-824 kills nonreplicating *Mycobacterium tuberculosis* by intracellular NO release. Science. 2008; 322(5906): 1392-5.

[276] Diacon AH, Dawson R, von Groote-Bidlingmaier F, Symons G, Venter A, Donald PR, *et al.* 14-day bactericidal activity of PA-824, bedaquiline, pyrazinamide, and moxifloxacin combinations: a randomised trial. Lancet. 2012; 380(9846): 986-93.

[277] Stover CK, Warrener P, VanDevanter DR, Sherman DR, Arain TM, Langhorne MH, *et al.* A small-molecule nitroimidazopyran drug candidate for the treatment of tuberculosis. Nature. 2000; 405(6789): 962-6.

[278] Nuermberger E, Rosenthal I, Tyagi S, Williams KN, Almeida D, Peloquin CA, *et al.* Combination chemotherapy with the nitroimidazopyran PA-824 and first-line drugs in a murine model of tuberculosis. Antimicrob Agents Chemother. 2006; 50(8): 2621-5.

[279] Tyagi S, Nuermberger E, Yoshimatsu T, Williams K, Rosenthal I, Lounis N, *et al.* Bactericidal activity of the nitroimidazopyran PA-824 in a murine model of tuberculosis. Antimicrob Agents Chemother. 2005; 49(6): 2289-93.

[280] Tasneen R, Tyagi S, Williams K, Grosset J, Nuermberger E. Enhanced bactericidal activity of rifampin and/or pyrazinamide when combined with PA-824 in a murine model of tuberculosis. Antimicrob Agents Chemother. 2008; 52(10): 3664-8.

[281] Manjunatha U, Boshoff HI, Barry CE. The mechanism of action of PA-824: Novel insights from transcriptional profiling. Commun Integr Biol. 2009; 2(3): 215-8.

[282]   Ahmad Z, Peloquin CA, Singh RP, Derendorf H, Tyagi S, Ginsberg A, *et al*. PA-824 exhibits time-dependent activity in a murine model of tuberculosis. Antimicrob Agents Chemother. 2011; 55(1): 239-45.

[283]   Grosset JH, Singer TG, Bishai WR. New drugs for the treatment of tuberculosis: hope and reality. Int J Tuberc Lung Dis. 2012; 16(8): 1005-14.

[284]   Somasundaram S, Anand RS, Venkatesan P, Paramasivan CN. Bactericidal activity of PA-824 against *Mycobacterium tuberculosis* under anaerobic conditions and computational analysis of its novel analogues against mutant Ddn receptor. BMC Microbiol. 2013; 13(1): 218.

[285]   Winter H, Egizi E, Erondu N, Ginsberg A, Rouse DJ, Severynse-Stevens D, *et al*. Evaluation of pharmacokinetic interaction between PA-824 and midazolam in healthy adult subjects. Antimicrob Agents Chemother. 2013; 57(8): 3699-703.

[286]   Mukherjee T, Boshoff H. Nitroimidazoles for the treatment of TB: past, present and future. Future Med Chem. 2011; 3(11): 1427-54.

[287]   Matsumoto M, Hashizume H, Tomishige T, Kawasaki M, Tsubouchi H, Sasaki H, *et al*. OPC-67683, a nitro-dihydro-imidazooxazole derivative with promising action against tuberculosis *in vitro* and in mice. PLoS Med. 2006; 3(11): e466.

[288]   Zhang Q, Liu Y, Tang S, Sha W, Xiao H. Clinical Benefit of Delamanid (OPC-67683) in the Treatment of Multidrug-Resistant Tuberculosis Patients in China. Cell Biochem Biophys. 2013; 67(3): 957-63.

[289]   Ginsberg AM. Drugs in development for tuberculosis. Drugs. 2010; 70(17): 2201-14.

[290]   Saliu OY, Crismale C, Schwander SK, Wallis RS. Bactericidal activity of OPC-67683 against drug-tolerant *Mycobacterium tuberculosis*. J Antimicrob Chemother. 2007; 60(5): 994-8.

[291]   Crunkhorn S. Trial watch: Novel antimicrobial fights TB resistance. Nat Rev Drug Discov. 2012; 11(8): 590.

[292]   Lee RE, Protopopova M, Crooks E, Slayden RA, Terrot M, Barry CE. Combinatorial lead optimization of [1,2]-diamines based on ethambutol as potential antituberculosis preclinical candidates. J Comb Chem. 2003; 5(2): 172-87.

[293]   Protopopova M, Hanrahan C, Nikonenko B, Samala R, Chen P, Gearhart J, *et al*. Identification of a new antitubercular drug candidate, SQ109, from a combinatorial library of 1,2-ethylenediamines. J Antimicrob Chemother. 2005; 56(5): 968-74.

[294]   Nikonenko BV, Protopopova M, Samala R, Einck L, Nacy CA. Drug therapy of experimental tuberculosis (TB): improved outcome by combining SQ109, a new diamine antibiotic, with existing TB drugs. Antimicrob Agents Chemother. 2007; 51(4): 1563-5.

[295]   Tahlan K, Wilson R, Kastrinsky DB, Arora K, Nair V, Fischer E, *et al*. SQ109 targets MmpL3, a membrane transporter of trehalose monomycolate involved in mycolic acid donation to the cell wall core of *Mycobacterium tuberculosis*. Antimicrob Agents Chemother. 2012; 56(4): 1797-809.

[296]   Meng Q, Luo H, Liu Y, Li W, Zhang W, Yao Q. Synthesis and evaluation of carbamate prodrugs of SQ109 as antituberculosis agents. Bioorg Med Chem Lett. 2009; 19(10): 2808-10.

[297]   Chen P, Gearhart J, Protopopova M, Einck L, Nacy CA. Synergistic interactions of SQ109, a new ethylene diamine, with front-line antitubercular drugs *in vitro*. J Antimicrob Chemother. 2006; 58(2): 332-7.

[298] Reddy VM, Dubuisson T, Einck L, Wallis RS, Jakubiec W, Ladukto L, *et al.* SQ109 and PNU-100480 interact to kill *Mycobacterium tuberculosis in vitro.* J Antimicrob Chemother. 2012; 67(5): 1163-6.

[299] Jia L, Tomaszewski JE, Hanrahan C, Coward L, Noker P, Gorman G, *et al.* Pharmacodynamics and pharmacokinetics of SQ109, a new diamine-based antitubercular drug. Br J Pharmacol. 2005; 144(1): 80-7.

[300] Jia L, Coward L, Gorman GS, Noker PE, Tomaszewski JE. Pharmacoproteomic effects of isoniazid, ethambutol, and N-geranyl-N'-(2-adamantyl)ethane-1,2-diamine (SQ109) on *Mycobacterium tuberculosis* H37Rv. J Pharmacol Exp Ther. 2005; 315(2): 905-11.

[301] Wallis RS, Jakubiec W, Mitton-Fry M, Ladutko L, Campbell S, Paige D, *et al.* Rapid evaluation in whole blood culture of regimens for XDR-TB containing PNU-100480 (sutezolid), TMC207, PA-824, SQ109, and pyrazinamide. PLoS One. 2012; 7(1): e30479.

[302] Deidda D, Lampis G, Fioravanti R, Biava M, Porretta GC, Zanetti S, *et al.* Bactericidal activities of the pyrrole derivative BM212 against multidrug-resistant and intramacrophagic *Mycobacterium tuberculosis* strains. Antimicrob Agents Chemother. 1998; 42(11): 3035-7.

CHAPTER 2

Therapeutic Limitations due to Antibiotic Drug Resistance: Road to Alternate Therapies

Ashima Kushwaha Bhardwaj[*], Kittappa Vinothkumar, Neha Rajpara, Priyabrata Mohanty and Braj Mohan Ram Narayan Singh Kutar

Department of Human Health and Diseases, Indian Institute of Advanced Research, Koba Institutional Area, Gandhinagar 382 007, Gujarat, India

Abstract: The antibiotics are destined for obsolescence as microbes would find a way to deal with them either by innate or by acquired genes. It is truly said that the power of bacteria should never be underestimated. There is a constant race between the humans for design and use of new drugs and the acquisition of genes by bacteria to render these novel drugs harmless. Situation has worsened with the indiscriminate use of antibiotics in human and animal health, agriculture, aquaculture and poultry. There have been reports of extremely drug resistant (XDR), totally drug resistant (TDR) bacteria and superbugs that have complicated the treatment of infectious diseases. Methicillin–resistant *Staphylococcus aureus* (MRSA) and vancomycin-resistant *S. aureus* (VRSA) recognized as the bane of hospitals are some of the most dreaded bugs. This chapter discusses various mechanisms of multiple drug resistance (MDR) in bacteria and the limitations of antibacterial chemotherapy due to MDR. Various innate and acquired mechanisms of drug resistance like integrons, SXT elements, efflux pumps and quinolone resistance mechanisms are described in details. Some of the important databases related to these genetic factors have also been described here. The possibility of attacking the virulence of bacteria rather than the bug itself in order to circumvent the crisis of MDR has been discussed. It further highlights some of the novel strategies such as efflux pump inhibition and quorum sensing inhibition as anti-virulence strategies. It is advocated that this never-ending war with bacteria would probably require multifaceted approach combining antibacterial, antivirulent regimes in addition to the constant search for novel drug targets and newer drugs by the pharmaceutical companies. Success of these strategies would involve cumulative and strenuous efforts from public, policy makers, research community, clinicians and pharmaceutical companies.

Keywords: Databases, efflux pumps, government policies, inhibitors, integrons, multidrug resistance, phage therapy, plasmids, quinolone resistance, quorum sensing, SXT elements, virulence, vaccines.

*Corresponding Author Ashima Kushwaha Bhardwaj: Department of Human Health and Diseases, Indian Institute of Advanced Research, Koba Institutional Area, Gandhinagar 382 007, Gujarat, India; Tel: +91-079-30514235; Fax: +91-079-30514110; Email: ashima.bhardwaj@gmail.com

Atta-ur-Rahman / M. Iqbal Choudhary (Eds.)

INTRODUCTION

This chapter highlights the causes and implications of antimicrobial resistance. This text is documented at a time when the crisis due to resistant bacteria looms large in front of mankind and Centers for Diseases Control and Prevention (CDC), World Health Organization (WHO) have seriously recognized the impending catastrophe and The Lancet Infectious Diseases launches a Commission, entitled *Antibiotic resistance – the need for global solutions* [1-3]. Antimicrobial resistance is a global concern and has serious social, economic and clinical consequences. When any microorganism like bacterium, fungus, virus or parasite becomes resistant to an antimicrobial drug to which it was originally sensitive, that organism is said to display antimicrobial resistance. In case of a pathogen that may cause disease to humans, plants or animals, this property of drug resistance often renders the drug ineffective and leads to treatment failure. The problem is compounded when such organisms acquire resistance to a large array of antibiotics/antimicrobials/drugs which is known as multidrug resistance (MDR). This seriously hampers the treatment of diseases caused by these invincible microbes. In recent times, with indiscriminate use of antibiotics in human health, poultry, agriculture and aquaculture, lots of pathogens have accumulated a large battery of genes responsible for conferring these bugs resistance to almost all the drugs used clinically. This has spawned another generation of microbes that are extensively drug resistant (XDR) or totally drug resistant (TDR) and therefore, untreatable by all first-line and second-line drugs. For example, tuberculosis bacterium has been reported in all the three forms, MDR, XDR and TDR. According to WHO report, there were 6,30,000 (52.5%) cases of MDR-TB in 2011 out of a total of 12 million cases of TB (tuberculosis). XDR-TB has been reported from 84 countries and TDR-TB from countries like Iran, India, Italy and South Africa. These superbugs fail to respond to antimicrobial treatments resulting in higher treatment costs, prolonged hospital stay and high case fatality rates. Many ailments such as tuberculosis, malaria, influenza, diarrhoea, gonorrhea and nosocomial infections can no longer be vanquished due to the problem of antimicrobial resistance. Therefore, it becomes imperative to understand various factors that have led to the problem of antimicrobial resistance and assess different alternatives in the scenario of failed antibiotics. In this chapter, the focus will be on antibiotic resistance mechanisms exhibited by bacteria and alternative strategies that could be ventured in case of ineffective antibiotics [1-3].

ANTIBIOTIC RESISTANCE

Development of antimicrobial resistance is a natural phenomenon that every organism undergoes for evolutionary fitness. Greater is the number and generations of antimicrobials, natural or manmade, faster is the development of new resistance mechanisms in a pathogen to counteract these drugs. Many bacteria including clinically significant pathogens have been reported to display MDR. Some of these pathogens are: *Mycobacterium tuberculosis* (*M. tuberculosis*), *Pseudomonas aeruginosa* (*P. aeruginosa*), *Klebsiella pneumoniae* (*K. pneumoniae*), *Escherichia coli* (*E. coli*), methicillin-resistant *Staphylococcus aureus* (MRSA), *Shigella dysenteriae* (*S. dysenteriae*) and *Vibrio cholerae* (*V. cholerae*). These organisms are found in hospitals as a source of nosocomial infections and they are also prevalent in communities leading to community-acquired infections. Antibacterial resistance gets aggravated due to a wide variety of genetic and non-genetic (like social, political, clinical malpractice) factors. Accordingly, to overcome this problem, multiple interventions are required at various levels.

GENETIC FACTORS/MECHANISMS GOVERNING MDR IN BACTERIA

Antibacterials kill or retard the bacteria by targeting the cellular processes or structures in bacteria which differ greatly from that of their host counterparts. The antimicrobial compounds that kill bacteria are called bactericidal while the others that merely retard the growth of bacteria are called bacteriostatic compounds. These drugs interfere with the vital housekeeping processes such as cell wall synthesis, protein, DNA and RNA synthesis or inhibiting the key enzymes of metabolic pathways [4]. To counteract these drugs, bacteria evolve different mechanisms and employ large battery of genes to affect these mechanisms. These resistance mechanisms could be intrinsic/innate (chromosome-borne) or acquired (borne on mobile genetic elements {MGE}). Though innate resistance allows a bacterium to adapt to the changing environment, it gets restricted to that particular bacterium and only gets transferred to the progeny by a process called vertical gene transfer. In contrast to this, the acquired resistance leads to the resistance genes being disseminated quickly within different bacteria crossing the species and genera barriers. This process is carried out by horizontal gene transfer (HGT) and could be mediated through different vehicles like plasmids, integrons, transposons and mechanisms of transduction, conjugation and transformation. The other mechanisms through which bacteria mediate resistance to antibiotics are: chromosomal mutations at the antibiotic target sites, restricting the access of the antibiotics through porins and efflux pumps, enzymatically inactivating the antibiotics, modifying or protecting the antibiotic target and by hindering the activation of antibiotic [4-6]. Often, a bacterium counteracts an antibiotic by synergistic action of more than one of the above mentioned resistance mechanisms [7-10]. For example, resistance of *P. aeruginosa* to ticarcillin has been attributed to overexpression of outer membrane protein OprM, production of β-lactamase and overexpression of AmpC cephalosporinase [7]. Similarly, resistance to tetracycline is often a result of synergy between the efflux pumps (encoded by *tetA* to *tetG*, *tetK*, *tetL*), oxidation of tetracycline and cytoplasmic proteins (encoded by *tetM, tetO, tetQ*) that confer protection to ribosomes from tetracycline [5]. In many cases, acquisition of a single gene/single mutation can offer protection against many different classes of antibiotics. For example, the efflux pumps with specificity for many different antibiotics can lead to resistance for all these antibiotics on overexpression or mutations. Similarly, the enzyme rRNA methylase (encoded by *ermA*, *ermB*, *ermF*, *ermG*) methylates an adenine on 23S rRNA that lies within a region that binds to three classes of antibiotics; macrolides, lincosamides and streptogramins. Therefore, a single gene of this methylase confers resistance against these three structurally distinct classes of antibiotics [5].

It can be envisaged that the source of antibiotic resistance genes could be the bacteria that produce antibiotics. In such producers, these resistance genes provide protection to bacteria from the antibiotics produced by them. Another possible source of these resistance genes could be the organisms naturally resistant to some of the antibiotics. For example, *Lactobacillus* species do not use D-Ala-D-Ala dipeptide as part of their muramyl dipeptide and therefore, they are naturally refractory to the glycopeptide antibiotic vancomycin. Vancomycin prevents crosslinking of peptidoglycan by binding to the D-Ala-D-Ala of the muramyl peptide. Resistance to vancomycin arises due to replacement of this peptide with D-Ala-D-lactate, a dipeptide that does not bind to vancomycin [5].

Bacteria possess an exquisite ability to adapt rapidly to the changing environments and this property is mediated by a large number of genetic elements that contribute to the genome plasticity. In the ensuing sections, two mobile genetic elements for MDR, integrons and SXT elements, are discussed in detail. Subsequently, efflux pumps have been explained as a general mechanism for MDR.

Integrons

Study of drug resistance mechanisms and their dissemination became important since discovery of MDR bacteria during mid 1950s [11]. In 1970s, in many cases, MDR was found to be associated with transmissible plasmids and/or with transposons [12, 13]. Integrons were discovered later in 1980s [14] and these mobile genetic elements harbouring antibiotic resistance gene cassettes are now known in clinical as well as agricultural and environmental samples [15-17]. The term chromosomal integron (CI) was introduced in late 1990s with the discovery of *V. cholerae* super integron [18]. CIs were found to be sedentary in nature and they were not involved in resistance phenotype. The evolutionary history of CI suggested that these elements helped in adaptation along with the change in environment as well as it was the main source of mobile integron's backbone and antibiotic resistance gene cassettes [19].

Structure of Integrons

Integron is a very common tool for antibiotic resistance gene capture and dissemination. It is the platform to acquire open reading frames (ORFs) by site-specific recombination and convert them to functional forms by their expression [19, 20]. Most of the integrons have three key components: 1) an Integrase (*intI*) belonging to tyrosine recombinase family; 2) a promoter (Pc) that directs the expression of the captured genes and 3) a primary recombination site (*attI*).

Additionally, all gene cassettes that incorporate in the integron share some specific characteristics at 3' end of the gene which are mostly imperfect repeats called *attC* (also called 59- base element) [19, 20].

Integrases

Integrases belong to site-specific recombinases known as tyrosine recombinases. Tyrosine recombinase includes a wide variety of enzymes that use a tyrosine residue as the nucleophile in their strand exchange reactions [21, 22]. It is involved in integration and excision or inversion of gene cassettes. The catalytic domain of integrase contains conserved amino acids Arg(R)-His (H)-Arg(R) and the nucleophilic tyrosine, Tyr (Y) [22, 23].

Promoter

Cassettes are generally promoterless but few reports revealed that some of the gene cassettes have their own promoter. For example, *cmlA* cassettes have both promoter and translational attenuation signals, *V. cholerae qnrVC* genes have their own internal promoter and the *qacE* cassettes have a weak promoter [24-26]. The expression of majority of promoterless cassettes is hence dependent on proximity of an external promoter located either in the integrase gene or on *attI* site [27-29].

Primary Recombination Site (attI) and 59-Base Element (attC)

Integrase recognizes and recombines two types of sites that have different structures, the *attI* type (non-palindromic) of site found in the integrase gene and *attC*/59-base elements (palindromic) found on the gene cassettes. The *attI* and *attC* sequences are complex attachment sites that include the crossover site and additional binding sites and integrase monomers act as accessory factors at these additional sites [30-32]. The *attI* sites are located at the end of the 5' conserved region (5'CS) of integrons and their sequences vary considerably. The *attC* sites share a common set of characteristics that enable them to be identified despite the diversity of their sequences and sizes [30, 33]. They are characterized by a palindrome of variable length and sequence between the RYYYAAC (R= Purines; Y= Pyrimidine) inverse core site and the GTTRRRY core site [33]. The size of these recombination sites vary in length from 57 to 141 bp [34]. Mostly gene cassettes are found integrated in variable region of integrons or they can exist as covalently closed circular intermediates. The integrase recognizes *attC* and *attI* sites. In the event of integration *attI×attC* recombination occurs and that allows expression of genes that are downstream to the promoter. In excision, *attC×attC* recombination occurs [20, 35].

Types of Integrons

Two types of integrons are mobile integrons and chromosomal integrons.

Mobile Integrons (MI)

Integrons associated with mobile DNA elements and primarily involved in the spread of antibiotic resistance genes correspond to the mobile integrons [20]. The bacteria of same species or different species use these elements as natural genetic vehicles to transfer a wide array of genes including antibiotic resistance genes. More than 130 different antibiotic resistance cassettes have been identified in MIs [16, 36]. These cassettes have resistance genes for the majority of antibiotic classes like β-lactams, aminoglycosides, chloramphenicol, trimethoprim, streptomycin, quinolones, rifampin, erythromycin and antiseptics of the quarternary ammonium compound family [16, 19, 36]. Five classes of MIs have been well defined to date based on integrase sequences with ~40-58% identities [19, 20]. In this chapter, only three integron classes (class 1, 2 and 3) have been described.

Class 1 integrons are the most widespread and well characterized. They are widely distributed in animal and human clinical strains of Gram–negative bacteria [37, 38] and also in some of the Gram–positive bacteria [39-42]. Class 1 integrons consist of two conserved segments (CS) at 5′- and 3′ ends, separated by a variable region that usually comprises of one or more gene cassettes (Fig. **1**). The 5′CS region contains the integrase gene (*intI1*), the integration site (*attI1*) and a promoter region (Pc) that allows expression of any number of gene cassettes inserted at the *attI1* site in a suitable orientation. The 3′CS region usually comprises of *qacEΔ1* encoding resistance to quaternary ammonium compounds and *sul1* encoding resistance to sulphonamides [34, 43]. Class 1 integrons are embedded within larger transposon Tn 21 [12].

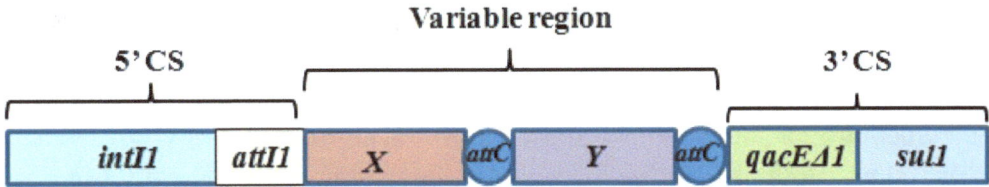

Fig. (1). Structure of a class 1 integron. Integrons consist of a gene *intI1* encoding a site-specific recombinase called "integrase" belonging to tyrosine-recombinase family and a recombination site *attI1* into which the exogenous gene cassettes (X and Y) harbouring the recombination site *attC* are inserted through site-specific recombination. In the 5'conserved sequences (5'CS), a promoter Pc located within *intI1* drives transcription of the captured genes. *qacEΔ1* and *sul1* are conserved regions in 3'conserved sequences (3'CS) which contribute resistance to ethidium bromide and sulfonamides.

Class 2 integrons are associated with Tn7 transposons. They have been found in several species of Gram-negative bacteria isolated from human, animal and environmental sources [37, 44]. Class 2 integrons have also been shown to carry three resistance gene cassettes, *dfrA1, sat1* and *aadA1*, that confer resistance to trimethoprim, streptothricin and streptomycin/spectinomycin, respectively [45]. The gene encoding class 2 integrase contains a nonsense mutation in codon 179 (ochre 179) and thereby it yields a truncated, non-functional protein which can be recovered by a single mutation. Mutation of the ochre179 codon to glutamic acid encoding codon produces an integrase with full recombinase activity [45]. It is not clear whether the cassette recombination in different Tn7 derivatives is due to natural suppression of the ochre 179 codon producing an active integrase or due to trans-acting recombination activity of other integrase which recognizes and recombines the *attI2* site [45, 46]. In addition, functional class 2 integrases have been reported in some instances [47-49]. In one case, class 2 integron was associated with four non-antibiotic resistance gene cassettes while in second case, class 2 integron carried *dfrA14* and a novel lipoprotein signal peptidase gene cassettes [47, 48]. In a recent report, a functional class 2 integron carrying *dfrA14* and three novel gene cassettes with unknown functions was found in 38 clinical isolates of *Proteus mirabilis* [49].

Class 3 integron was first reported in *Serratia marcescens* strain in 1995 [50] and characterized later in 2002 [51]. The configuration of the three potentially definitive features of the class 3 integrons, the *intI3* gene, the adjacent *attI3* recombination site and the P_c promoter that directs transcription of the cassettes was similar to that found in class 1 integron module. The *IntI3* integrase was active and able to recognize and recombine known types of *IntI*-specific recombination sites, the *attI3* site in the integron and different cassette-associated 59-base sites. Both integration of circularized cassettes into the *attI3* site and excision of integrated cassettes were catalyzed by *IntI3* [51]. Class 3 integron with its genes encoding blaGES-1 and OXA/AAC(6')-Ib responsible for the β-lactam and aminoglycoside resistance have been reported [50, 52].

Chromosomal Integrons (CIs)

Chromosomal Integrons or super-integrons (SIs) are located on the chromosomes of large number of bacteria [18, 53-55]. SIs are distinguished from conventional integrons by their size, placement of promoters, chromosomal location, and the nature of gene cassettes they carry [54]. It has been proposed that MDR integrons arose from SIs by the entrapment of *intI* genes and their related *attI* sites on MGEs such as transposons. The gene cassette reservoirs of SIs provide a source of gene cassettes that are recruited by multi-resistant integrons [56].

CIs have been found in bacteria belonging to families such as *Vibrionaceae*, *Pseudoalteromonas*, *Xanthomonadaceae*, *Alteromonadaceae*, *Pseudomonadaceae* and *Spirochaetales* [19, 20]. All of them share general characteristics like they are large (>20 gene cassettes and upto 200) and have homology between the *attC* sites of their endogenous cassettes. The first SI was discovered in *V. cholerae* chromosome II in a clustered region spanning 126 kb. It harbored 214 ORFs out of which the functions for 179 cassettes have not been assigned [56].

The difference between MIs and CIs is as follows [56]:

1.   MIs contain <20 gene cassettes while SIs/CIs contains >20 gene cassettes.

2.   In MIs, the cassettes typically code for antibiotic resistance genes whereas those of SIs are mainly unknown functions.

3.   MIs are associated with mobile elements while the SIs coevolved with their host genomes which strongly suggest that SIs are sedentary.

4.   The *attC* sites of the gene cassettes of MIs are highly variable in length and sequence while the *attC* sites of CI gene cassettes are closely related and species-specific.

5.   Finally, there is evidence that not all of the gene cassettes but only few associated with CIs are significantly expressed.

Gene Cassettes

As described in the earlier section, more than 130 gene cassettes in MIs are known for antibiotic resistance genes [20]. For example, resistance to chloramphenicol is due to acetylation of the antibiotic (*catB* gene) and for the aminoglycosides, due to modification of antibiotic by acetylation (*aacA* and *aacC* genes) and adenylation (*aadA* and *aadB* genes). The β-lactamases encode three distinct families; class A (*blaP* genes), class B metallo β-lactamase (*bla$_{IMP}$* genes) and class D (*oxa* genes) which inactivate the β-lactam drugs. The *dfrA* and *dfrB* genes code for dihydrofolate reductase conferring trimethoprim resistance. Apart from antibiotic resistance genes, many unknown ORFs have also been reported and these ORFs are assigned letters in the order of their identification like *orfA*, *orfC* and *orfD* [34].

In contrast to MIs, CIs contain highly diverse cassettes, mostly of unknown functions. In 2007, 1677 cassettes were identified by the analysis of Vibrionales genome [57]. Among these, 75% of the cassette pool corresponded to accessory genes of unknown functions. Remaining 25% of the cassettes contained genes like phage-related proteins, toxin-antitoxin (TA) systems, acetyltransferases, DNA modification systems, virulence and experimentally confirmed restriction modification systems, lipases, dNTP pyrophosphohydrolases, polysaccharide biosynthesis and sulphate–binding proteins [58-60]. CIs also carry several resistance gene arrays. Many *dfr* cassettes in different environmental isolates of *V. splendidus* have been found while *catB9*, *carb7*, *carb9* (encoding carbenicillin resistance) and *qnr* (encoding resistance to quinolones) cassettes have been identified in *V. cholerae* CI [56, 61-64]. Altogether, CIs are involved not only in acquisition of antibiotic resistance genes but also widely in the adaptation of bacteria in different environments [20, 35].

Toxin- Antitoxin (TA) Genes

The gene content of SI can be ~3% of the bacterial genome content [54, 65]. The cassette array of SI implies either existence of selective pressure to maintain the gene cassettes or mechanisms that promote their persistence in the absence of selection [20]. These addiction modules are selfish genetic elements. Two classes of addiction modules are known *i.e.* toxin/antitoxin (TA) and restriction methylation systems (RMS) [66-68]. TA loci are commonly found on plasmids or within prophages where they have been found to enhance plasmid and phage maintenance by preventing the multiplication of plasmid-free or phage-free progeny in bacterial populations. TA system consists of two ORFs and is organized as an operon. One ORF codes for stable toxin while the other codes for unstable antitoxin. Disruption in expression of TA system leads to the accumulation of free toxin due to loss of antitoxin neutralizing activity and inhibits the multiplication of bacterial growth (devoid of plasmids/ prophages). The TA systems have been proposed to stabilize chromosomal regions by preventing the accidental deletions, when located in unstable segments like MGEs. There are reports of SIs containing the TA cassettes. Thirteen TA cassettes have been reported in the *V. choerae* N16961 SI [54, 69, 70]. Functional analysis of TA cassettes in SI was also carried out in other groups of Vibrios like *V. vulnificus, V. metschnikovii* and *V. fischeri* [70-72]. Similarly, another addiction module RMS consists of long half-life restriction enzymes and comparatively short half-life modification methylases which maintain plasmid stability by post segregational killing [67]. The RMS acquired by bacterium begins to depend on this system for its survival, as the methylase protects the host genome along with RMS cassettes by methylating the specific sequences that could be recognized and cleaved by restriction enzyme. Loss or disruption of expression of RMS systems results in cell death. Thus even in the absence of antibiotic exposure, the resistance conferring gene cassettes linked with this RMS system will be maintained [67]. *Xanthomonads* and *Pseudomonads* SIs contained

RMS systems which may stabilize the cassette array in the absence of selection [70, 73].

SXT Element

SXT element (deriving its name due to encoded resistance to sulfa and trimethoprim), an Integrative and Conjugative Element (ICE), is a conjugative, self-transmissible integrating element that shows similarity to conjugative transposons. It is an important vehicle for spreading of antibiotic resistance in bacteria like *V. cholerae, Providencia alcalifaciens* and *P. rettgeri* [74, 75]. ICEs are a group of MGEs that contain programmes to determine their excision and integration and play important role in genome flexibility of numerous Gram-positive and Gram-negative bacteria [76]. These elements can integrate into the bacterial genomes, replicate as part of host chromosome, get excised and then disseminate to new host genomes by conjugation (Fig. **2**). ICEs help bacteria to adapt to new ecological conditions, to colonize in new niches, to survive in stress conditions like antibiotic exposure and play a very important role in reshaping bacterial genomes [77]. SXT element is also known as constin (conjugable, self-transmissible, integrating element) that helps in bacterial adaptation, evolution and expansion [78]. This MGE harbors a diverse array of genes such as antibiotic resistance genes, genes for complex degradation pathways for toxic compounds and genes for tolerance to heavy metals. Unlike plasmids, SXT elements are not capable of autonomous replication, so they mingle into the host chromosome for their replication and get transferred intracellularly and intercellularly [79]. ICEs combine within them, the properties of plasmids as well as phages. They are transferred to another bacterium through conjugation like a plasmid. Similar to phages, they have the property of integrating into the host genomes and getting excised under certain circumstances. SXT was identified for the first time in *V. cholerae* O139 serotype of MO10 isolated from Madras, India in 1992, where it was responsible for epidemic condition like the one caused by O1 serotype of *V. cholerae* [74]. Because this element was identified in *V. cholerae* MO10, the name was given SXT^{MO10} [74, 80] and it was found to encode resistance property for chloramphenicol, streptomycin, sulfamethoxazole and trimethoprim [74]. Apart from this report, SXT element was also reported in non-O1, non-O139 strains isolated before 1992 from Varanasi [81]. These strains were resistant to co-trimoxazole, trimethoprim, streptomycin, furazolidone and ampicillin. The presence of SXT^{MO10} was observed in other O139 serotypes isolated earlier, whereas this element was not present in O1 serotype of *V. cholerae* [82]. *V. cholerae* O1 El Tor that reappeared dominantly by 1994 in Indian subcontinent showed resistance property for the four antibiotics characteristic of O139 isolate, where the corresponding genes were transferred through ICE. This element was designated as SXT^{ET} [80, 83, 84]. Since 1994, the *V. cholerae* O1 strains carrying SXT element have been reported from various geographic locations like Bangladesh, Mozambique, Laos and India [82, 84-87]. Concurrent with emergence of SXT-harboring O1 strains, the *V. cholerae* O139 strains have been reported with antibiotic resistance profiles different from the earlier O139 strains. These recent O139 strains showed resistance to streptomycin but were found to be sensitive to trimethoprim and sulfamethoxazole [88-90]. Those ICE elements which belong to the same ICE family usually share the same integration site and augment intra-species variability. There are various hot regions in bacterial genome that provide a dramatic illustration of how ICEs generate intra-species diversity at particular locus and inter-genus locus variability [79]. The recombinase and insertion sequences facilitate ICE evolution by acquisition and dissemination of genomic islands due to the effect of variable conditions [91]. Though the SXT element was discovered in 1992 and sequenced, the putative ORFs are still not eloquently characterized [92]. SXT^{MO10}, SXT^{ET}, SXT^{HN1}, SXT^{KN14}, SXT^{MCV09} and SXT^{LAOS} are the known SXT elements which bear different antibiotic resistance genes (http://db-mml.situ.edu.cn/ICEberg).

Origin of SXT Element

Deciphering the evolutionary history of SXT element is much difficult because there may be many recombination processes that seem to have taken place in past, between plasmid, phages and other ICEs. As there is great diversity among ICEs (total reported till date 460), it seems that they do not come from common ancestor but arose independently. DNA sequence-based study of SXT element revealed that this element of approximately 100 kb was composed of genes that could have been derived from plasmids, bacteriophages and many additional diverse unknown sources. The comparison between % GC content of SXT^{MO10} element (47.1%) and *V. cholerae* genome (47.6%) showed almost similar value indicating that SXT element could have been derived from *V. cholerae* genome though it also contained several regions with significantly different GC content [84, 92]. This again indicated that SXT has captured its gene content from varied sources. For example, an insertion with GC content of 42% observed in the transfer region showed sequence similarity to Ti plasmid from *Agrobacterium tumifaciens* [92].

Structure of SXT Elements

Typically, the SXT elements show modular organization and harbor three modules responsible for their maintenance, dissemination and regulation [77]. Maintenance module consists of *Int* gene encoding a recombinase that catalyses recombination between *attP* site on SXT and an *attB* site on the target bacterial chromosome. Recombination occurs through an extra chromosomal circular intermediate of SXT generating two junctions *attL* and *attR* (Fig. **2a**). The intermediate can only express its function on being integrated into the chromosomal DNA. SXT also encodes a protein Xis required for excision of this element from the host genome [93]. The recombinases could most often be tyrosine recombinases like in integrons and could sometimes be serine recombinases like in Tn5397 from *Clostridium difficile* [94]. Apart from *Int, Xis, attB* and *attP*, ICEs may also contain additional mechanisms to ensure their stability through bacterial generations even in the absence of factors favoring their selection. For the dissemination of ICE, they encode proteins that promote conjugation between the donor and the recipient bacteria. Conjugative transfer is initiated at a *cis*-acting 299 bp locus called the Origin of transfer (OriT) that is nicked by a putative relaxase called TraI to produce single-stranded DNA. This DNA gets translocated to the recipient bacterium through a mating pore [95]. This single-stranded DNA gets converted into double-stranded DNA in the host, re-circularized and finally gets recombined/integrated into the host genome [95]. The transfer of ICE elements therefore could be mostly in the form of single-stranded DNA and also sometimes in the form of double-stranded DNA like in the case of pSAM2 from *Streptomyces ambofaciens* [96]. Regulation of ICE mobility could be induced by various environmental or stress factors that promote their dissemination to new host providing these hosts the ability to survive these stress conditions.

Factors Responsible for Maintenance, Acquisition and Dissemination of SXT Element

As mentioned in earlier sections, the SXT element basically requires three functionally conserved key genetic components: integration and excision component, conjugation component and regulation component. This conserved backbone can acquire other genes through insertion sequences, transposons and recombinases. The integration of SXT element in bacterial chromosome is site-specific unlike the other conjugative transposons that can integrate into many different sites in the bacterial genome. Integration and excision at 5'end of *prfC* region encoding peptide chain releasing factor 3 involved in termination of translation, occurs through non-replicative circular intermediate [97]. The SXT-encoded recombinase Int is mainly responsible for integration and excision from chromosome and is activated by SetC and SetD but Int alone does not promote efficient excision (Fig. **2b**). SetC and SetD, two loci of SXT element, which are similar to master activators of flagellar transcription FlhC and FlhD, are required for *int* expression by regulating host promoter [79, 92]. A repressor molecule SetR from *V. cholerae* SXT, homologous to lambda repressor cI, controls the dissemination of SXT DNA. ICE loss frequency increased when *mosT* and *mosA* genes were deleted [95]. MosT and MosA toxin-antitoxin proteins promote the maintenance of SXT element [98-100]. Although, SXT element's low frequency loss occur even in the absence of *mosT* and *mosA* genes, it suggests that SXT element may encode additional factors to promote its conservation [101]. As described above, conjugative transfer of SXT element is dependent on SXT relaxase TraI that binds covalently to well conserved SXT *oriT* present between *s003* and *rumB* [102]. During SOS responses, repression by SetR is lifted leading to dissemination of SXT element to a new host [77]. Mitomycin C treatment of cells harboring SXT elements has been shown to induce transfer of this element 400-folds [103]. Hence, the DNA damaging agents Mitomycin C and quinolone antibiotics promote the spread of SXT and equivalent ICEs [103]. *prfC* region, the major integration module of *V. cholerae* and other γ-proteobacteria, is also responsible for integration of closely related ICEs including R391, R997 and pMERPH. In the absence of *prfC* region, SXT can preferentially integrate in others alternative sites, such as the 5' end of *pntB* which encodes a pyrimidine nucleotide transhydrogenase [79, 104, 105]. The Recombination Directionality Factor (RDF)-like factor which is encoded by novel SXT Xis (excisionase) facilitates more prominently excision of SXT element [77, 79].

Fig. (2). Horizontal gene transfer in bacterial population containing SXT element. a. Donor bacterium transferring chromosomal ICE SXT element to recipient bacterium by conjugation. **b.** Circular intermediate of SXT element contain conjugative machinery, UV repair DNA polymerase genes (*rumA*, *rumB*), regulatory genes (*int*, *setC*, *setD*, *setR*). Between *rumA* and *rumB*, antibiotic resistance genes *sulII*, *strA*, *strB*, *dfr18* are located. This circular intermediate gets integrated at *prfC* (encoding peptide chain releasing factor 3) region of chromosomal DNA in bacterium; **c.** Effect of SOS response on SXT regulation and expression: SOS response in bacterial cell mediates auto-proteolysis of setR due to activation of recombinase A. This in turn activates *setC* and *setD* leading to increased expression of integrase gene *int* (responsible for integration and excision).

SXT/R391Family

Till date, a total of 28 ICE families have been defined based firstly on integrase similarity and secondarily on core structure synteny [106]. SXT/R391 is the biggest and most widespread of these 28 families and has SXT and R391 elements as its original members. Some other previously identified families also included Tn916, Tn4371, CTnDOT/ERL and ICE6013 [106]. R391 was reported from a clinical isolate of *P. rettgeri* in South Africa in 1972 where it encoded resistance to mercury and kanamycin [107]. The mechanisms of R391 and SXT integration into the 5' end of *prfC* gene and their excision were found to be similar [104]. Nucleotide sequence analysis of 99.5 kb SXT and 89 kb R391 revealed close similarity between these elements which shared about 65 kb of DNA. This conserved sequence included the machinery for mobility of these elements including the genes for conjugative transfer, integration, excision and regulation of these events [75]. The SXT/R391 family was then defined by Burrus *et al.* in 2006 where they proposed that any ICE that encodes an integrase gene closely related to *int*SXT and that integrates into *prfC* be considered part of the SXT/R391 family of ICEs [85]. In addition the *tra* genes, which encode the ICE conjugation apparatus, are also a defining feature of this family of ICEs. The ICE*Vfl*Ind1 of this family was reported to facilitate excision of genomic islands including some pathogenicity islands from three species of Vibrios and their conjugative transfer by recognition of a similar OriT in these islands as that of the SXT/R391 family [108]. This finding has again emphasized the importance of ICEs in genome plasticity/evolution. These ICEs have five hotspots (HS1-HS5) for DNA insertion and four minimal gene set modules: *int-xis* (integration and excision module); *mob* (DNA mobilization and processing module); *mfp* (mating pair formation module); *reg* (regulation module) which are required for integrity of these elements [101]. On the basis of acquisition of another member, SXT/R391 family was divided in two groups S and R. The S group SXT/R391 limits the acquisition of another S group but did not limit the acquisition of R group SXT/R391 ICE [109]. The TraG and entry exclusion protein Eex are inner-membrane proteins that promote exclusion activity of SXT/R391 ICEs [109].

Efflux Pumps

Efflux pumps are one of the major determinants of MDR in various pathogenic microorganisms. They play variety of important biological roles across all kingdoms of life from prokaryotes to eukaryotes with functions ranging from simple transport to secretion of a diverse range of secondary metabolites as a defense against herbivores and microbial pathogens in plants [110]. They also play a vital role in bacterial survival and pathogenicity. Based on sequence similarity with known transporters, it has been estimated that 15–20% of *E. coli* or *Saccharomyces cerevisiae* genome codes for these type of proteins [111]. The size of genomes have been found to be directly proportional to the number of efflux pump genes harbored by them indicating that these proteins are crucial for cell survival [112-114].

Efflux pumps are universal transport systems present both in antibiotic susceptible and resistant bacterial strains. Efflux pump-encoding genes could be present in the chromosome or could reside on MGEs like plasmids, transposons and integrons, which allow faster dissemination of these genes in the bacterial population [6, 15, 115-117]. These pumps enable microbes to extrude structurally diverse antimicrobials, facilitating their survival in toxic environments. Efflux pumps also have important physiological functions like bile tolerance in enteric bacteria, colonization, invasion and survival in host [113, 115, 118, 119]. Efflux as a mechanism of antibiotic resistance was first described against tetracyclines but now numerous efflux pumps have been discovered and fully characterized in terms of their structure and degree of resistance they confer towards variety of substrates [113, 115, 120-124]. Some of the efflux pumps like TetA and CmlA are specific for the antibiotics tetracycline and chloramphenicol respectively, but a large number of pumps like MexAB-OprM, NorA and BmrA can recognize and efflux out a diverse array of structurally unrelated compounds [6]. The latter type are called MDR pumps [115]. Efflux pumps confer relatively low to moderate degree of drug resistance (1- to 64-fold increase in minimum inhibitory concentration {MIC}) that makes their clinical relevance debatable [125-127]. However, different types of efflux pumps in synergy with other known drug resistance mechanisms like quinolone resistance proteins, β-lactamases and mutations in topoisomerase genes, contribute immensely towards MDR leading to clinically significant MIC values [8, 10]. These pumps have also been shown to play vital role in the antibiotic resistance displayed by biofilms [128]. Efflux is a dynamic process and regulation of efflux is still not completely understood. These efflux pumps genes are regulated by a master operon which overexpresses efflux pump genes but in turn also downregulates porin activity. Chromosomally encoded local and global regulatory proteins controlling the expression of MDR pumps have been studied extensively in bacteria [111].

Classification and Structure of Efflux Pumps

Efflux pumps usually consist of a monocomponent protein with several transmembrane spanning domains. However, in Gram-negative bacteria, which are protected by an outer membrane, efflux transporters can be organized as multicomponent systems [129]. These efflux pumps could either be primary transporters that utilize energy derived from ATP hydrolysis, or they could be secondary transporters that utilize proton motive force (PMF) [111]. These efflux pump genes are classified based on sequence homology and utilization of energy [6, 115]. There are essentially five different families of efflux pump proteins in bacteria; ABC (ATP-binding cassette) transporters, SMR (small multidrug resistance) pumps of the drug/metabolite transporters (DMT) superfamily, MFS (major facilitator superfamily), RND (resistance nodulation division) family exclusive to Gram-negative bacteria and MATE (multidrug and toxic compound extrusion) pumps of multidrug/oligosaccharidyl-lipid/polysaccharide flippases (MOP) superfamily. The characteristics of each pump are described below.

ABC Transporters

The ABC-type efflux pumps are symporters that transport a diverse array of substrates where extrusion occurs by energy derived from ATP hydrolysis. In these transport proteins, a transport channel is made by two transmembrane domains (TMDs) that are composed of alpha helical membrane spanning regions [130]. These TMDs show variability in different ABC pumps. TMDs work in conjunction with two highly conserved nucleotide-binding domains (NBDs) which bind to ATP and hydrolyse it to produce energy facilitating the transport process [130]. NBDs are comprised of Walker A and B motifs characteristic of all the ATP-binding proteins. They also carry within them a signature motif (LSGGQ) unique to the transporter family of ATP-binding proteins. The Vga (E) variant protein in *Staphylococcus* spp. conferring resistance to pleuromutilins, lincosamides and streptogramin A and LmrA in *Lactobacillus* spp. are members of this family of transport proteins [6, 131]. Though the role of ABC pumps in drug resistance in eukaryotes has been deciphered (P-glycoprotein), their role still remains dubious in prokaryotes in terms of MDR. They have been shown to play a major role in the MDR of cancer cells [6].

MFS Pumps

MFS comprises a diverse family of secondary transporters. These pumps could be uniporters mediating transport of their substrates without parallel ion movement, symporters that carry out transport with concomitant movement of ions in the same direction as the substrate or they could be antiporters where the substrate transport is coupled with the movement of ions in the opposite direction [132]. MFS pumps comprise of 250-400 amino acid residues spanning 12-14 transmembrane segments (TMS) [133]. These pumps play an active role in antibiotics export and belong to drug/ proton antiporters (DHA) superfamily which is subsequently divided into three major sub-families *i.e.* DHA1, 2 and 3 [134]. While DHA1 and 2 are widely distributed in prokaryotes and eukaryotes transporting a large array of drugs, DHA3 are exclusively found in bacteria and are specifically involved in antibiotic transport. DHA3 pumps have been shown to transport macrolides and tetracycline and have been reported from Gram-positive as well as Gram-negative bacteria. NorA of *S. aureus*, PmrA of *Streptococcus pneumoniae* and EmeA of *Enterococcus faecalis* are some of the well studied MFS pumps [135-137].

SMR Pumps

SMR family of pumps are prokaryotic transport systems consisting of homodimeric or heterodimeric structures having 100-120 amino acid residues with four transmembrane α-helices [138, 139]. Energy in the form of PMF provides the driving force for drug transport. There are very few reports of members of this family of transporters conferring resistance to antibiotics. EmrE of *E. coli* [140] and AbeS of *Acinetobacter baumannii* [141] are members of this family of transporter proteins.

RND Pumps

Efflux pumps of this class have been shown to play a significant role in conferring MDR in Gram-negative bacteria [129]. They are proton antiporters that use the proton gradient across the membrane to power efflux exchanging one proton for one drug molecule. They have tripartite organization where the efflux pump in cytoplasmic membrane works in conjunction with a periplasmic adapter protein and an outer membrane channel. This allows any drug/substrate of these pumps to be expelled directly outside the cell rather than in the periplasmic space. MexAB-OprM of *P. aeruginosa* and AcrAB-TolC of *E. coli* are the most studied transporters of this family of efflux pumps where MexB and AcrB are the RND pumps, OprM and TolC are the outer membrane proteins and MexA and AcrA are the periplasmic adapter proteins. Some of these RND pumps such as AcrB display wide substrate specificity and efflux out not only the antibiotics but also dyes, detergents and solvents. The genes encoding the RND efflux pumps are organized as well regulated operons and the outer membrane proteins may or may not be co-located with the other genes in the operons [113].

MATE Pumps

MATE family of efflux pumps includes functionally characterized multidrug efflux systems. The prototype member was NorM from *V. parahaemolyticus* [142]. Subsequently, several homologues from other closely related bacteria were reported that function by a drug:Na^+/H^+ antiport mechanism. These include a putative ethionine resistance protein of *S. cerevisiae*, a cationic drug efflux pump from *Arabidopsis thaliana* and the DNA damage-inducible protein F (DinF) of *E. coli* [121]. These proteins are ~450 amino acid residues long and exhibit 10-12 putative TMS. They arose by an internal gene duplication event from a primordial 6 TMS-encoding genetic element. The family is conserved in bacteria, archaea and all eukaryotic kingdoms and includes hundreds of functionally uncharacterized but sequenced homologues [143]. MATE family proteins exhibit similar topological features as MFS but form a distinct group due to relatively low degree of homology at the level of amino acid residues. NorM from *E. coli* and *V. cholerae*, YdhE from *E. coli* and VFH and VFD from *V. fluvialis* are some of the examples of MATE pumps [115, 142, 144, 145]. These are the most recently identified group of efflux pumps assessed for their role in multidrug resistance. They transport fluoroquinolones, aminoglycosides, and cationic dyes.

Regulation of Efflux Pump Expression

Complex regulatory operons/mechanisms control the expression of proteins that are responsible for influx and efflux of the drugs thus maintaining the intracellular concentration of these compounds. The *mar* (multiple antibiotic resistance) locus in *E. coli* is known to accumulate mutations leading to the acquisition of MAR phenotype. While the *marR* gene encodes a repressor for this operon and accumulates mutations, the *marA* gene product is known to activate a plethora of genes related to antibiotic resistance and oxidative stress. MarA regulator controls the expression of porins and efflux pumps and the expression of this regulator is in turn controlled by some antibiotics. For example, imipenem that is not a substrate of an efflux pump in *Enterobacter aerogenes* results in expression of the gene encoding *marA* regulator and alters the permeability of the membrane for some other antibiotics leading to increased resistance towards chloramphenicol, quinolones and tetarcyclines [146]. Therefore, even though *marRA* does not encode a multidrug efflux system/porin, the *marRAB* locus confers resistance to compounds like tetracycline, chloramphenicol, fluoroquinolones, nalidixic acid and rifampin because it controls the expression of other loci important in mediating drug resistance *e.g.* the porin OmpF and *acrAB* gene for AcrAB efflux pump [121].

Role of Porin and Efflux Pump Mutations in MDR

The bacterial cell envelope acts as a semipermeable membrane composed of porins and efflux pumps. These porins and efflux pumps together help in determining the effective concentration of antibiotics inside a bacterium. Thus, presence of their number determines the membrane permeability and in turn decides the fate of the bacterium *i.e.* antibiotic susceptible or resistant microorganism. Innate resistance to various antibiotics in many microbes like

P. aeruginosa can be attributed to low membrane permeability. Therefore, susceptibility of a bacterium is a direct correlation of mutations affecting the expression and function of porins as well as efflux pumps [134].

Porins are proteins that act as channels for uptake of nutrients and a variety of other compounds including antibiotics. These were first reported from *E. coli* [147]. Mutations in porins could have variable effects on their structure and functions such as complete loss of porins, change in the size of these channels or their conductance and their altered expression. These consequently result in reduced uptake of antibiotics into bacterial cells leading to decrease in cell death. Such porin-related mutations have been shown to accentuate resistance towards various antibiotics. Loss of OmpF porin from *E. coli* was shown to confer resistance towards β-lactams and subsequently role of porins in MDR was established in other bacterial species [148]. Loss of a porin could be due to deletion in its gene, a point mutation resulting in translation termination, an insertion element disrupting the porin gene and mutations in the regulatory genes or the promoter regions [149, 150]. As described above, mutations may affect the expression of porins, but some of the mutations could also alter the function of porin channels without affecting their expression. For example, a mutation Asp116Ala in the putative antibiotic-binding site of OmpU porin in *V. cholerae* was shown to reduce uptake of cephalosporins and increase the bacterial resistance towards these drugs [151]. Apart from the antibiotic-binding site, the scaffold provided by other parts of porin also plays a vital role in its function. The imipenem binding sites of OprD porin of *P. aeruginosa* requires the intact scaffold provided by loops 2 and 3 [152], while regulation of porin size is achieved by external loops 5, 7 and 8 [153].

As described above, similar to porins, efflux pumps are also the major determinants of antibiotic concentration inside a bacterium. Therefore, mutations in these efflux pumps would affect the resistance status of the host bacterium. These mutations could be localized in the structural genes, their promoter regions or in the genes encoding regulatory proteins [154, 155]. The clinical isolates of *P. aeruginosa* obtained from cystic fibrosis patients were found to have mutations in the MexY structural gene. The resulting amino acid change increased the efflux activity of this RND pump leading to resistance towards many antibiotics that were the substrates for MexXY pump [154].

AN INTERESTING EXAMPLE OF CONTRIBUTION OF DIFFERENT MECHANISMS: RESISTANCE TO QUINOLONES

Resistance mechanisms for different classes of antibiotics vary. β-lactamases inactivate the β-lactam group of antibiotics by hydrolyzing the lactam ring. Aminoglycosides are inactivated by the enzymatic modification of the antibiotics by phosphoryl, adenyl, or acetyl groups. Chloramphenicol is rendered ineffective by the modifying enzyme chloramphenicol acetyl transferase that adds an acetyl group to the antibiotic [5]. Apart from these mechanisms specific for a particular class of antibiotics, all the antibiotics can also be made ineffective by combination of several other general mechanisms such as mutations in porins or efflux pumps. In this section, quinolone class of antibiotics has been discussed in details *vis-à-vis* their structure and different drug resistance mechanisms that operate in synergy to decide the quinolone resistance phenotype.

The emergence of drug resistance, since the introduction of antibiotics had made the humans to continuously seek for new antibiotics which overcome the evolving pathogens. This paved way for the development of various synthetic and semi-synthetic antibiotics with improved efficacy and extended target coverage. Among different synthetic antibiotics like sulfonamides, quinolones and oxazolidinones, quinolones gained popularity because of their wider application, broader spectrum of activity and drug safety [156-158]. In addition, it was hypothesized that resistance would not be mounted against the synthetic compounds which are not seen by bacteria in natural ecosystem. In this section, the focus would be on quinolone class of antibiotics and the bacterial resistance machinery against these widely used synthetic antibiotics.

Quinolones are a class of antibiotics which specifically kill bacteria by inhibiting the synthesis of nucleic acids. The parent compound of quinolones, nalidixic acid, was derived from the antimalarial drug chloroquine in 1962 [159, 160]. Nalidixic acid is composed of naphthyridine ring having ethyl and methyl group attached to its N1 and C7 position respectively along with keto and carboxyl group attached to its C4 and C3 positions respectively (Fig. **3**). Though it had narrow spectrum antibacterial activity, it was widely used for urinary tract infections and diarrhoea until the introduction of broad spectrum fluoroquinolones [161, 162]. Fluoroquinolones were derived from nalidixic acid by the introduction of a fluorine atom at C6 position of naphthyridine ring and also replacing the N8 by a carbon atom (Fig. **3**) [163].

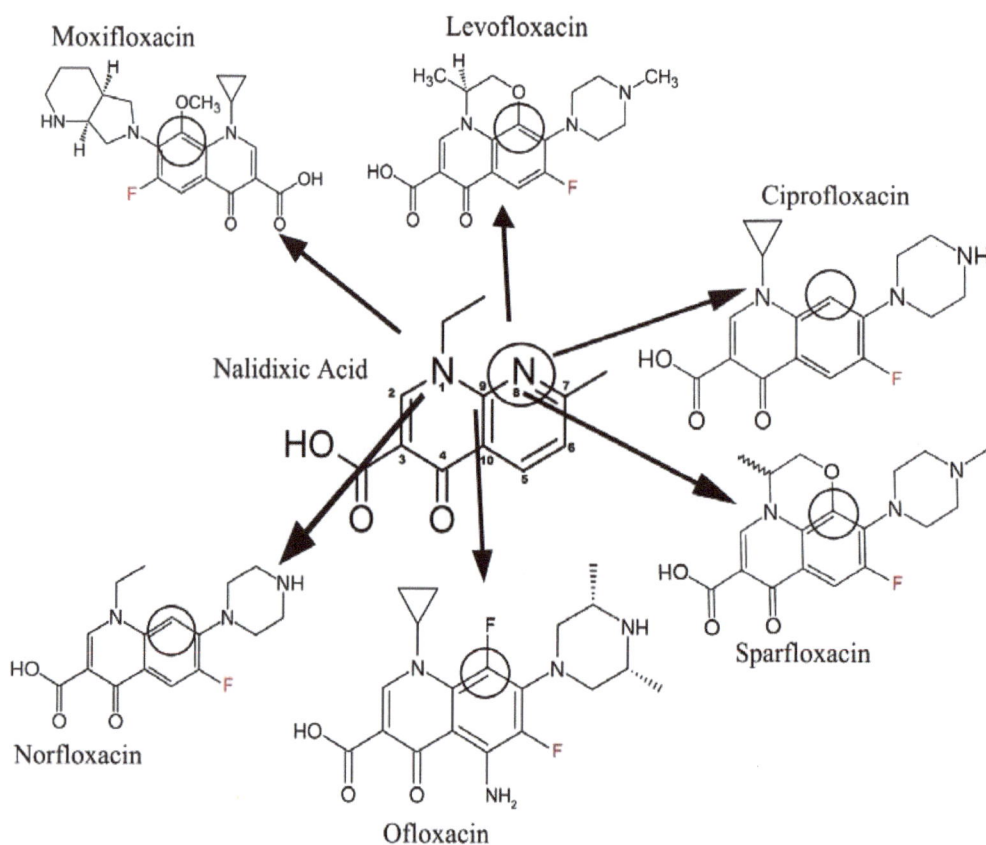

Fig. (**3**). **Structures of nalidixic acid and some of the fluoroquinolones.** Derivation of fluoroquinolones from parent quinolone (nalidixic acid) by the addition of a fluorine atom (shown in red) at C6 position of naphthyridine ring and by replacing N8 by a carbon atom (shown inside circles)

All the available quinolones are grouped into four generations based on their spectrum of activity [159, 164]. The first generation quinolones like nalidixic acid and cinoxacin were active against aerobic Gram-negative bacteria, but showed little activity against aerobic Gram-positive bacteria or anaerobes. The second generation quinolones include fluoroquinolones such as norfloxacin, ciprofloxacin, ofloxacin, lomefloxacin and levofloxacin which showed broader Gram-negative spectrum and moderately increased Gram-positive spectrum. Piperazine moiety at C7 position of quinolone nucleus is the general feature of second generation quinolones which increased activity against *P. aeruginosa*. Sparfloxacin, gatifloxacin and grepafloxacin fall under third generation quinolones that showed greater potency against Gram-positive organisms. A superior coverage against pneumococci and anaerobes were achieved by fourth generation quinolones like trovofloxacin, moxifloxacin, gemifloxacin and garenoxin [159, 160, 164]. Although many of the quinolone derivatives were removed from the market because of some safety concerns, remaining drugs which are proved as safe, gained widespread use due to its favorable pharmacokinetics and broad antimicrobial spectra [159].

Quinolone Targets and Their Action

Quinolones target two enzymes DNA gyrase and topoisomerase IV which are essential for the vital activities of bacterial cell like DNA replication, transcription, recombination and repair. DNA gyrase is a special type II topoisomerse which is present in prokaryotes only and it introduces negative supercoiling rather than removing it [165]. During replication and transcription, the double stranded DNA are separated by helicase action that causes a reduction in linking number which in turn results in positive supercoiling in front of the replication fork. DNA gyrase removes the positive supercoiling ahead of the replication fork by introducing negative supercoiling and thereby renders an uninterrupted movement of replication fork. The topoisomerase IV enzyme is known for unlinking of daughter chromosomes after replication (decatenation). DNA gyrase is a tetrameric protein having two A (GyrA) and two B (Gyr B) subunits which wrap DNA into a positive supercoil. The active site of the enzyme consists of tyrosine, which breaks the phospodiester bond of a duplex DNA and forms phospho-tyrosine bond through its hydroxyl group. The other end of the DNA is also held by the enzyme to form a protein bridge. Another region of DNA is passed through the nick created by DNA gyrase and then the nick would be resealed [162, 165]. Both DNA gyrase and topoisomerase IV create double strand break and allow double strand passage and they require ATP for this action. The main difference in the action of these two enzymes is that gyrase wraps DNA around itself while topoisomerase IV does not which may lead to the functional differences [162].

It was evidenced that quinolones form a ternary complex with topoisomerase enzymes and DNA and cease the enzyme activity. This complex is called as cleaved complex as it contains broken DNA. As discussed above, type II topoisomerase enzymes cause a double strand break and allow the passage of another duplex through the nick. But the reversible binding of quinolones with the DNA-enzyme binary complex allows the enzyme to generate the double strand break only and not the passage of another duplex [166, 167]. Quinolones were found to interact with both the DNA and the enzyme in the cleaved complex. The drugs, with the help of aromatic rings stack against the DNA bases (-1 and + 1 base pairs) at the site of cleavage and thus cause a misalignment of DNA at both the sides of the break which eventually prevents the religation of the cleaved DNA. Similarly, helix-4 of the GyrA or ParC which harbors quinolone resistance determining region (QRDR) of the enzymes seems to interact with drug [168-173].

Though binding of quinolones to the enzyme-DNA complex leads to inhibition of nucleic acid synthesis, it does not cause lethality to the cells. The binding of quinolones just causes a bacteriostatic action as the formation of cleaved complex is reversible. The lethality to the cell is caused as a result of chromosome fragmentation and cell death induced by ROS [174]. The chromosome fragmentation occurs in two ways, one is protein synthesis-dependent as it involves proteases or nucleases in releasing DNA breaks from the cleaved complex and the other is protein synthesis-independent where quinolones facilitate the dissociation of gyrase subunits and release the double strand break [175-177]. The former pathway can be inhibited by chloroamphenicol and so the first generation quinolones like nalidixic acid fail to kill the cells in presence of chloroamphenicol whereas second generation quinolones like ciprofloxacin are not influenced by it [162, 174, 178]. The chromosome fragmentation eventually triggers the accumulation of highly toxic ROS which amplifies the lethal action of the drug ultimately causing the cell death [179-181].

Quinolone Resistance Mechanisms

Development of resistance towards quinolones started right with the introduction of first generation quinolone, nalidixic acid in 1962. The increased use of this drug led to the increased development of resistance [182]. Earlier it was believed that target mutations and efflux pumps were the possible mechanisms of quinolone resistance. Later that belief was disproved due to discovery of various molecular factors like target-protecting proteins, quinolone-modifying enzymes and efflux pumps [182, 183]. Quinolone resistance could be mediated by either chromosome-borne or plasmid-borne genetic elements. The chromosome-borne genetic factors involve, (i) mutations in the DNA gyrase (*gyrA* and *gyrB*) and (or) topoisomerase IV (*parC* and *parE*) genes, (ii) chromosomal efflux pumps genes and (iii) chromosomal quinolone resistance (*qnr*) genes. The plasmid-mediated quinolone resistance (PMQR) has also been described with three mechanisms, (i) a quinolone-resistance/topoisomerase-protection mechanisms encoded by the *qnr* genes, (ii) a ciprofloxacin-modifying enzyme encoded by *aac(6')-Ib-cr* gene [184]; and (iii) plasmid borne-efflux pumps [185, 186]. These PMQRs are transferable traits and also play a main role in quinolone resistance. In the following sections, all these mechanisms are discussed in detail.

Mutations in the Topoisomerase Genes

Mutations in the genes of topoisomerase enzymes are the main cause of quinolone resistance. Such spontaneous mutations occur as a result of replication error in a bacterium, at rates as high as 1 in 10^6 to 1 in 10^9 [187]. A mutant bacterium having alteration in topoisomerase enzymes could withstand antibiotic stress and evolves as a resistant bug. Mutations tend to cluster in regions called the QRDRs of subunits of DNA gyrase or topoisomerase IV which results in reduced drug affinity of those enzymes [161, 182, 188, 189]. Mutations in *gyrA, gyrB, parC* and *parE* genes have variable effects on MICs in different species of bacteria. In Gram-negative bacteria, high level quinolone resistance is mainly due to the mutations in the genes encoding gyrase subunits, *gyrA* and *gyrB* (mainly in *gyrA*), whereas mutations in genes encoding topoisomerase IV subunits *parC* and *parE* are prevalent in Gram-positive bacteria [183]. Mutations conferring resistance typically occur in stepwise manner. Generally, the initial mutation occurs in *gyrA* (in case of Gram-negative bacteria) or *parC* (in case of Gram-positive bacteria) genes [161, 162]. The first mutation helps to select the bacteria in quinolone stress by reducing the susceptibility of topoisomerase to the drug and allows accumulation of more mutations in the subunits of same or other target enzyme. The accumulation of multiple mutations in the drug target facilitates the development of high-level resistance to quinolones in bacteria [161, 162, 182, 190]. The type of bacterial species and the kind of quinolone used determine the order in which mutations occur and the quantum of change in MIC [191]. Clinical failure of quinolones can occur as a result of many such bacterial mutations. The mutations at amino acid positions 83 and 87 of GyrA and positions 80 and 84 of ParC have been reported as a cause for reduced susceptibility of bacteria towards quinolones [9, 87, 162, 174, 192, 193]. The substitution of hydrophilic amino acid (serine) by hydrophobic residues (leucine or isoleucine), or substitution of acidic residue (aspartic acid) by basic amino acid (asparagine) or substitution of negatively charged amino acid (glutamic acid) by positively charged residue (lysine) are the well documented substitutions which reduce the susceptibility of the target enzymes to quinolones. These residues are known to interact with the drug at quinolone binding pocket (QBP), the region where quinolones interact with both QRDR of enzyme and cleaved DNA [194]. The alteration in the residues of QRDR of topoisomerase enzymes causes a conformational change in QBP, which eventually prevents the binding of drug in the pocket [194].

Generally, these mutations occur as a replication error prior to the antibiotic exposure and at the time of antibiotic pressure, it helps the cells to resist the drug beyond the concentration required to kill wild type cells. The wild type cells fail to form colony at or above MIC. The selective enrichment of resistant mutants occurs only above MIC and the concentration where the colony recovery of mutants ceases is called mutant prevention concentration (MPC). Additional mutation is required for the bacteria to withstand the concentration beyond MPC, which is a rare phenomenon. So the drug concentration range which favors the selection of mutants, between MIC and MPC is called Mutant selection window [195]. As described above, the resistance conferring mutations occur in stepwise manner and at each step of acquisition of mutations, the values of MICs and

MPCs increase [196, 197]. In other words, selection window increases at each step of mutation acquisition. Hence, mutant selection window is important to optimize antimicrobial dose regimens and to avoid the emergence of resistant mutants [195].

Efflux Pumps (Chromosome- and Plasmid-Borne)

The second resistance mechanism involves expression/over expression of efflux pumps that transport quinolones and other antibiotics out of the cell. Efflux pumps are ubiquitous and are encoded either by chromosomal genes or by genes associated with mobile genetic elements. These genes are responsible for intrinsic resistance under constitutive expression and cause low to moderate level of quinolone drug resistance under induced or activated conditions [161]. Mutations that occur in the regulatory elements of efflux pumps lead to overexpression of pumps which ultimately causes increased efflux activity [198-201]. Quinolone-specific efflux pumps have been reported and characterized (like SmrA, PmrA, NorA, NorM, PmpM, AcrB, VcrM, VcmA, BmrA, MepA, VCH and VFH) from different bacterial species [115, 145, 161, 202]. The MATE family efflux pumps like NorM, VCH, VFH are known to effectively efflux out hydrophilic quinolones like norfloxacin, ciprofloxacin and ofloxacin and not the hydrophobic quinolones such as sparfloxacin, nalidixic acid and moxifloxacin [145, 190, 202]. Resistance due to efflux pumps causes only low to moderate level of resistance but they favor the emergence of resistance mutants by rendering the surviving ability to the cells at suboptimal concentration of antibiotics [125, 161,190].

Two plasmid-mediated quinolone transporters (OqxAB and QepA) have been described [117, 186, 203-206]. The presence of *qepA* in *Enterobacteriaceae* and *Vibrionaceae* was reported from different parts of the globe [203, 207-209]. QepA is a 511-amino acid protein belonging to MFS transporters and shown to efflux out mainly norfloxacin, ciprofloxacin, nalidixic acid and also other compounds like erythromycin, acriflavine and ethidium bromide. The RND family pumps OqxAB confer resistance to Olaquindox (a quinoxaline derivative), nalidixic acid and ciprofloxacin [204-206, 210, 211].

Qnr Genes (Chromosome- and Plasmid-Borne)

Qnr proteins belong to pentapeptide repeat family and are capable of protecting DNA gyrase from quinolone action. These proteins are characterized by five semi-conserved tandem repeat motifs represented by [Ser, Thr, Ala or Val] [Asp or Asn] [Leu or Phe] [Ser, Thr or Arg] [Gly] [210-212]. Qnr proteins consist of two domains of pentapeptide repeats separated by a single amino acid, usually glycine [211, 212]. Qnr acts by protecting DNA gyrase and topoisomerase IV from quinolones by binding to the enzyme prior to the binding of DNA [213]. These proteins mimic the structure of DNA and they compete with the DNA for enzyme binding. As Qnr occupies the DNA binding site of the enzyme, it prevents the binding of DNA to the enzyme and hence the number of enzyme-DNA complexes, the target of quinolone is reduced. As a result of this, the formation of cleaved complex is minimized and eventually cells are protected from the lethal action of quinolones [214, 215]. Several *qnr* genes have been widely reported from *Enterobacteriaceae* and *Vibrionaceae* families and *Vibrionaceae* family was found to be a possible reservoir for Qnr-like quinolone resistance determinants [216]. So far, five families of *qnr (qnrA, qnrB, qnrC, qnrD* and *qnrS)* have been reported in plasmids among the bacterial species [210, 211]. Both *qnrA* and *qnrS* genes encode 218-amino acid proteins and exist as seven and nine alleles respectively. The *qnrC* gene encodes 221-amino acid protein whereas *qnrD* encodes 214-amino acid peptide and the allelic forms of these two genes were not reported so far. The 214-amino acid protein encoding *qnrB* genes are found to exist in seventy three allelic forms [http://www.lahey.org/qnrStudies/] [210, 211, 217].

Genes for pentapeptide repeat proteins with sequence similarity to plasmid-borne Qnr proteins have been reported on the chromosomes of both Gram-positive and Gram-negative bacteria [211]. The chromosome borne *qnr*-like genes were largely reported in *Vibrionaceae* family (*V. vulnificus*, *V. fisheri* and *Photobacterium profundum*) [216, 218, 219]. *qnrVC1* isolated from *V. cholerae* O1 from a cholera epidemic in Brazil was found as gene cassette in chromosomal class 1 integron [25]. The origin of these *qnr* genes is likely to be the chromosomes of aquatic environmental organisms. Accumulation of quinolones in the environment enriched the organisms having *qnr* genes and that acted as a reservoir from where other pathogenic organisms acquired these genes [210, 211]. A recent study has shown that the *qnrVC5* gene of chromosomal origin was associated with a transferrable plasmid from a clinical isolates of *V. fluvialis* [9]. This study showed that these genes are of chromosomal origin and circulating among the bacterial community through plasmids. Qnr proteins are found to have functional similarity with other well-studied pentapeptide repeat proteins like MfpA and McbG having amino acid identity 18.9% and 19.6% respectively with that of QnrA. The organisms producing the microcin B17, a topoisomerase poison, also produce McbG to protect its own DNA gyrase from the toxic effect of microcin B17 [220, 221]. So it is evident that the pentapeptide repeat proteins are generally evolved for protecting topoisomerases from the naturally occurring toxins that inhibit those enzymes and also evolved to protect the enzymes from other topoisomerase inhibiting agents like quinolones. Though higher-level *qnr*-mediated resistance has not been reported, they could help the isolates to attain clinical breakpoint of resistance in combination with the other mechanisms [8, 9, 193, 222].

Ciprofloxacin Modifying Enzyme (AAC (6')-Ib-Cr)

AAC(6')-Ib-cr, a variant aminoglycoside acetyl transferase, capable of reducing ciprofloxacin activity in addition to modifying aminoglycosides, is carried on plasmids and more prevalent than Qnr proteins [184]. This enzyme has acquired the ability to inactivate quinolones (ciprofloxacin and norfloxacin) by N-acetylating the amino nitrogen on its piperazinyl group. Two amino acid changes (Trp102Arg and Asp179Tyr) rendered the ability of the enzyme to additionally inactivate quinolones apart from aminoglycosides. The effect on MIC by AAC (6')-Ib-cr is less than that conferred by Qnr protein and the drug spectrum covered by this enzyme is also small (ciprofloxacin and norfloxacin only).

It is reasonably well documented that quinolone resistance in pathogenic bacteria through intrinsic and acquired traits causes a major health problem. The synergistic action of all these chromosomal and plasmid-borne factors helps the pathogen acquire higher-level resistance towards quinolones, as described by many researchers [8, 222-224].

OTHER FACTORS RESPONSIBLE FOR MDR

There are many other social/clinical/policy-related factors that lead to the emergence and dissemination of antibiotic resistant bacteria at a particular geographical location. These include the indiscriminate use of antibiotics, poor surveillance systems for various epidemics/pandemics, absence of comprehensive and coordinated response by government in case of spread of a serious infection, lack of preparedness in terms of efficient diagnostics, prevention and therapeutic tools [3]. In addition to this, the pharmaceutical companies have lost interest in the development of new antibiotics as this research is no longer lucrative. As anti-infective drugs are taken for shorter times till the infection persists, the companies refrain from investments on these pharmacologically active agents as compared to blockbuster drugs for lowering the cholesterol levels, for hypertension, diabetes *etc.* which are taken for prolonged periods and mostly lifelong. Accordingly, the government funding in this area has also been diminishing. There has been a drastic cutdown on antibiotic discovery programmes [225]. This amounts to the use of same old antibiotics in clinics and hospitals leading to development of bacterial resistance against them.

ANTIBIOTICS INDUCE SOS RESPONSE LEADING TO THE EVOLUTION OF ANTIBIOTIC RESISTANCE MECHANISMS

Before we embark on our journey to understand various strategies to combat MDR bacteria, it must be understood that the challenge of a bacterial cell with an antibiotic is similar to an SOS response. A bacterium will resort to a series of changes to overcome the effect of a drug that challenges its existence. Any type of horizontal gene transfer through conjugation, transformation and transduction or any type of antibiotic challenge induces SOS response through events mediated by single-stranded DNA, RecA protein and LexA repressor [35]. The LexA repressor has been shown to bind the promoter of the integrase of an integron. RecA activation leads to autoproteolysis of LexA repressor that keeps the SOS regulon in the repressed state under normal conditions. During SOS, this repressor gets inactivated leading to the expression of a diverse array of genes that were repressed by LexA. Integrases are one such genes that gets activated during SOS leading to the expression of gene cassettes harbored by integrons [35]. Similar to the integrons, the activation of SXT, their excision, integration or dissemination events are triggered during SOS response. The expression of SXT integrase requires two transcriptional activators, setC and setD which are in turn controlled by the repressor setR rather than LexA. During SOS response, when single-stranded DNA is bound to recA, setR concentrations are depleted which results in the activation of SXT integrases and formation of hybrid ICE elements [226]. This clearly shows that SOS response leads to reshaping of the bacterial genomes through integrons as well as ICE elements. The direct regulation of SOS response by antibiotics itself has also been described [227]. The regulation of expression of *qnrB2* (a quinolone resistance determinant) through SOS response is induced by ciprofloxacin in LexA/RecA-dependent manner. Even sub-inhibitory concentration of ciprofloxacin was found to cleave LexA repressor so that it was prevented from binding on the LexA binding site present in the promoter region of *qnrB2* gene [227].

DATABASES OR TOOLS RELATED TO ANTIBIOTIC RESISTANCE MECHANISMS

As described in earlier sections, genes related to various mechanisms and factors responsible for drug resistance have been compiled by various workers for easy referencing. Compilation of data in form of databases is freely available on web. These databases and tools help a researcher to share the knowledge and to systematically analyze their data in easier way. The databases encompassing various genetic elements especially integrons, ICEs, efflux pumps and quinolone resistance mechanisms have been described below.

INTEGRALL (http://integrall.bio.ua.pt)

It is a database and search engine for integrons, integrases and gene cassettes found in integrons. It is a web-based platform developed by microbiologists and computer scientists. Initially in the year of 2009, the database contained more than 4800 integron sequences out of which ~70% corresponded to uncultured bacteria and 27% belonged to γ-proteobacteria. Remaining 3% constituted integron sequences from ά-, β-, δ- and ε-Proteobacteria, Actinobacteria, Firmicutes, Cyanobacteria *etc*. Thus, though integrons have a broad host range, higher occurrence of integrons has been reported in γ-proteobacteria. The database provides a public genetic repository for integron sequence data, their nomenclature, genetic contexts and molecular arrangements [228]. As of 31st December 2013, the database consists of 6777 entries of integrons, 1498 integrase genes, 8522 gene cassettes from 119 genera and 250 species.

Annotation of Cassette and Integron Data (ACID) (http://integron.biochem. dal.ca/ACID/login.php)

It compiles and annotates integron-integrase genes and non-coding cassettes-associated *attC* recombination sites and all publicly available sequence information regarding these genetic elements. Manually curated open access database information was used for automated detection, annotation of integrons and their gene cassettes. ACID enables future sequence data to be incorporated easily. This database allows its users to annotate and save their data. They can also send the data to curators for its addition to the main database. In the first version of ACID, 5622 gene cassettes and 471 integrase sequences have been documented and new sequences are continuously updated [229].

Repository of Antibiotic Resistance Cassettes (RAC) (http://www2.chi.unsw. edu.au/rac)

Archive of gene cassettes which include alternative gene names are made available by RAC databases. Information regarding gene cassettes help to determine new gene cassettes. The automatic annotation engine allows users to easily and accurately access and annotate cassette arrays in bacterial DNA sequences. It also provides a process for assignment of unique name for newly sequenced antibiotic resistance cassettes in mobile resistance integrons consistent with existing nomenclature systems [230]. RAC now has a conglomeration of 387 antibiotic resistance gene cassettes.

Integron Analysis and Cassette Identification (XXR) (http://mobyle.pasteur. fr/cgi-bin/portal.py?forms=xxr)

The program detects the *attC* sites of integron gene cassette arrays. The software utilises the data from previously known sequences of integrons to predict putative cassette structures [70].

Antibiotic Resistance Genes Database (ARDB) (http://ardb.cbcb.umd.edu)

The database consolidates most of the publicly available antibiotic resistance genes and provides a reliable annotation with rich information, resistance profile, mechanism of action, ontology, Clusters of Orthologus Groups of proteins (COG) and Conserved Domain Database (CDD) annotation [231]. It also provides external links to sequence and protein databases. The information provided by the database can be used for further identification of the resistance genes of newly sequenced genes, genomes or metagenomes. As of 31st December 2013, ARDB contains a total of 23,137 genes, 380 types of gene cassettes for 249 antibiotics from 1737 species and 267 genera. It also contains pre-annotated 2881 vectors/plasmids and 632 genomes conferring resistance to various antibiotics.

ICEberg (http://db-mml.sjtu.edu.cn/ICEberg/)

On 13th August 2011, this database was mainly dedicated to ICEs which incorporated in bacterial genomes. This is a PostgreSQL-based database; that facilitates resourceful knowledge for ICEs like their integrative conjugative machinery, putative ORFs, antibiotic drug resistance gene cassettes and virulence determinants [106]. ICEberg provides information about predicted as well as experimentally proved ICE-related data. As of 31st December 2013, the database has a collection of 460 ICEs.

Insertion Sequence [IS] Finder (www-is.biotoul.fr)

This is another database dedicated to Insertion Sequences [IS], a type of short DNA sequences that act as transposable genetic elements [232]. IS finder is the tool for IS elements which are found in various mobile genetic elements like bacteriophages, conjugative transposons, integrons, unit transposons, composite transposons and insertion sequences (ISs). IS finder allows researchers to have coherent nomenclature for IS. It also includes detailed information about the IS of the repository like its DNA sequences, ORFs, end sequences, target sites of these elements, their origin, distribution and bibliography. It also imparts knowledge about the updated comprehensive grasping and the phylogeny of ISs [232]. The latest updated database constitutes 4115 insertion sequences.

Pathogenicity Islands Database (PAIDB) (http://www.gem.re.kr/paidb)

PAIDB is a comprehensive database for all those reported genetic elements whose products are essential to the process of disease development [233]. These PAIs horizontally transfer among microbes and contribute to the evolution of pathogenicity. This database provides convenient graphical presentation for name, host strain, function, insertion site and associated GenBank accessions which are helpful for phylogenetic as well as bioinformatic analysis. The latest version of PAIDB (31st December, 2013) has 112 kinds of PAIs, 889 GenBank accessions, 2681 virulence genes and total 7842 ORFs from 497 pathogenic strains. Also it has 743 PAI-like regions from 115 pathogenic strains having atleast one PAI-like region and 259 PAI-like regions from 77 non-pathogenic organisms with unconfirmed pathogenicity.

A Classification of Mobile Genetic Elements (ACLAME) (http://aclame.ulb.ac.be)

ACLAME is a database which provides classification and collection of Mobile Genetic Elements (gene sequences and proteins) from phages, transposons and plasmids. This database was first released in 2004. At that time, database classified 5069 MGE-associated proteins from 119 DNA bacteriophages into over 400 functional families. This database is publicly accessible in which TRIBE-MCL, a graph-theory-based Markov clustering algorithm was used to classify MGEs and proteins. Different evolutionary database versions like 0.1, 0.2, 0.3 and 0.4 have been released, in which 0.4 is the latest version which contains 122154 proteins from 2326 MGEs of 811 host organisms. Proteins have been clustered into families that are as follows; Prophages with 6822 clusters, Plasmids with 18228 clusters, Viruses and prophages with 16057 clusters and Viruses with 11503 clusters with a total of 32919 clusters. Evolutionary Cohesive Modules (ECMs) were generated for phages, which share replication, lysis/lysogeny, DNA packaging, and head and tail morphogenesis with reticulate relationship. These ECMs, helpful in studying phylogenicity, are stored in the ACLAME database [234]. They are accessible on the web site through the MGE viewer, following the link 'ECM'. The advance 0.4 version of ACLAME database is now running under the PostgreSQL relational database management system (RDBMS) version 8.3 (http://www.postgresql.org) [235].

Type-2 Toxin-Antitoxin Loci Database (TADB) (http://bioinfo-mml.sjtu.edu.cn/TADB/)

It is a comprehensive database for type 2 toxin-antitoxin loci distributed in bacterial and archaeal genomes. This database contains unique compilation of both predicted and experimentally supported Type 2 TA gene pairs identified within 1240 prokaryotic genomes and details of over 240 directly relevant scientific publications [236]. TADB provides a web-interface, allowing users to view an entire genome's TA loci repertoire within the context of the whole replicon and to access individual pages dedicated to each TA locus pair, toxin and antitoxin as required. TADB allows researchers to gain insight into the cognate TA proteins that are either hypothesized or proven to play vital role in stabilization of horizontally acquired genetic elements. As of 31st December, 2013, 6757 TA loci found in 750 genomes have been organized into the 44 toxin-antitoxin domain pair groupings.

Transporter Classification Database (TCDB) (http://www.tcdb.org)

TCDB is an online, curated repository of comprehensive database containing sequences, classification, structural, functional and evolutionary information about transporters from various living organisms. Originally in 2006, the database was a congregative repository for factual information compiled from >10 000 references with ~3000 representative transporters and putative transporters classified into >400 families. The database categorizes transporters as Enzyme Nomenclature on Recommendations of the Nomenclature Committee of the International Union of Biochemistry and Molecular Biology [237]. As efflux pumps are integral part of transporters, TCDB can be considered as a conglomerate of all known and putative efflux pumps. The database offers several different methods for accessing the data including step-by-step access to hierarchical classification, sequence information or TC (Transporter Classification) number and full-text searching. The database is based on functional ontology algorithm that facilitates powerful query searches and yields valuable data in a quick and easy way. The TCDB website also provides several tools specifically designed for analyzing the unique characteristics of transport proteins. TCDB is not only a repository of curated information about classifying newly identified membrane proteins; it also serves as a genome transporter annotation tool. As of 31st December, 2013, it contains over 10000 published references of about 5600 unique protein sequences which are classified into over 600 transporter families based on the TC system.

Databases Available for Quinolone Resistance Genes

Since the discovery of first PMQR resistance gene *qnrA1* in 1998, a considerable number of *qnr* genes and other PMQR genes have been discovered and reported in last decade. The *qnr* genes reported from several parts of the globe lacked a standard nomenclature or numbering system which created a chaos. In order to avoid the ambiguity and to systematically name the *qnr* genes of varying sequences, Jacoby *et al.*, attempted to frame the criteria based on which the genes could be classified [217]. They have created a database where all the newly found *qnr* alleles can be verified and numbered accordingly (http://www.lahey.org/qnr Studies/). It is having a collection of 71 alleles of QnrB as of 31st, December, 2013. Similarly, in order to find the *qnr* genes in a fragmented nucleotide sequence of metagenomic data set, a tool/software was developed by Systems Biology and Bioinformatics group of University of Gothenburg, Sweden [238] (http://bioinformatics.math.chalmers.se/qnr/index.html). They have developed this tool in order to understand the role of environment as reservoir of these kinds of genes and to focus on their routes of transfer.

STRATEGIES TO COMBAT THE PROBLEM OF MDR

From the above discussion, it might appear that the antibiotics are no longer the magic bullets that they were once thought to be. It also leads to an apprehension in community that we are at the end of antibiotic era. As described in the sections above, bacteria employ various tactics to keep them alive in the varying environments. An insight into these mechanisms can lead to the development of various strategies to circumvent the problem of MDR. The strategies could be antibacterial meant to kill the bacterium itself (whether antibiotic resistant or antibiotic susceptible) or they could be antivirulent. In antivirulent regimes, instead of attacking the vital life processes of bacteria (antibacterial), it is aimed to target the virulence factors elaborated by bacteria. This results in control of the pathogenicity caused by these bugs. In the subsequent sections, the antibacterial, antivirulent and other general strategies are discussed in light of their use in combating the diseases caused by MDR pathogens.

Antibacterial Therapies

Some of the antibacterial therapies have been reviewed that target transcriptional regulators, toxin-receptor binding or replication initiation in the bacterial cell [225, 239]. Kibdelomycin, a novel inhibitor of type IIA topoisomerase of *S. aureus* has been proposed to control the bacteria as well as its drug resistance. This antibiotic is produced by a new member of the genus *Kibdelosporangium* and found to inhibit the ATPase activity of topoisomerase enzymes [240]. NXL 101, an inhibitor of topoisomerase IV was found to be effective against Gram-negative bacteria with mutations in the gyrase enzyme [225]. A large number of loci and protein-coding genes have been identified as drug targets to control bacterial growth [241, 242]. Some of the other antibacterial therapies would be described in the ensuing sections.

Phage Therapy

Phage therapy has been used to cure a large number of bacterial infections such as cholera, typhoid and plague [239, 243, 244]. MDR strains, where most of the antibiotics fail to work, could be killed by the phages. Phages kill the pathogenic bacteria reducing the toxin load that leads to the control of disease transmission. Especially interesting in this case are superficial infections easily accessible for phages. These infections include infected wounds in case of diabetes and burns. Either single phage drugs or phage cocktails could be used in such cases. The bottleneck in phage therapy is to find the phages that could treat the variant strains of the same pathogen like *S. aureus* and the apprehension that the phage resistant strains may emerge in due course of time. Phage therapy in humans is still a debatable issue for the fear of toxicity of phage-based drugs. Most of the phage therapy research has therefore been carried out in veterinary medicine and funding for its human application has been limited A phage enzyme used for dissolving anthrax bacteria has been shown to be effective in animal experiments [245]. A phage enzyme has also been used to dissolve *Listeria monocytogenes* in a highly specific manner in order to keep cheese rinds free of the bacteria. This bacterium spreads through contaminated vegetables and dairy products and is harmful as it also multiplies in the refrigerator [245]. A phage preparation for *Xanthomonas campestris* infections in tomatoes is available for purchase in the US. Inspite of many bottlenecks described above, there have been some success stories of phage therapy in human trials [243]. The phages were reported to be effective in treating children with dysentery in Georgia in 1963. The phase I and phase II clinical trials for safety and efficacy of phages were reported in 2005 and 2009 respectively. In 2009 trial, phages were shown to be effective in treating chronic drug-resistant ear infections of *P. aeruginosa* [243].

Phage therapy has its own advantages and disadvantages, which are described below [245].

Advantages

a.   Phages are highly specific for the bacterium they infect and therefore, they do not interfere with the growth of other microbiota and thus do not cause selection of antibiotic resistance traits in them. This means that the therapy would have no side effects like diarrhoea or secondary infections which are common during antibiotic treatments.

b.   Phages are generally innocuous to humans and animals and therefore, they can also be used for combating harmful bacteria in fattening animals and food.

c.   Bacteria that become resistant to one kind of phage do not acquire resistance to the other type of phage and therefore, are not invincible.

d.   Since nature is full of phages, it is easier to find new phages as compared to finding new antiobiotics.

e.   Phages could provide an inexhaustible supply of reagents that can rapidly evolve and can be genetically modified to meet the challenges of antibiotic resistant bacteria.

f.   As described above, phage products like lysins can also be used to treat bacteria.

g.   Phage therapy is effective for antibiotic resistant as well as sensitive bacteria.

Disadvantages

a.   There is a paucity of data to support phage therapy in humans though it has been extensively tried in case of animals.

b.   Resistance of bacteria to phages could again be a problem in successful phage therapy.

c.   Phages could prove ineffective in case of infections caused by the bacteria that take refuge inside the human cells and therefore may be inaccessible to the phages that are larger in size as compared to the small drug molecules.

d.   Phages injected in the bloodstream are recognized by human immune system as foreign and this elicits immune responses against these phages followed by their disposal outside the human body. Humoral and cellular immune responses generated against therapeutic phages could therefore compromise their efficacy.

e.   Administration of therapeutic phages is more difficult than administration of antibiotics. Hence it requires special skills and training for the physicians.

f.   A lot of research still needs to be done to assess the shelf life of phages.

Vaccines

Vaccination is another antibacterial strategy that would control bacteria irrespective of their resistance to antibiotics. Vaccination interrupts transmission of the causative organism and the communities may develop herd immunity. Vaccines could also be antivirulent for example passive immunization in case of diphtheria. Here, the antibodies neutralise the diphtheria toxin and save the patients. In case of tetanus, the antibodies bind to and neutralize the circulating tetanus toxin leading to the survival of patient. Similarly, for prevention of cholera, oral cholera vaccines are used. In case of *V. cholerae*, the cholera toxin (CT), flagella, fimbriae and lipopolysaccharides have been shown to be the antigens involved in protective immunity. Though cholera pathogenicity has been attributed to CT, the protective immune responses have been shown to be antibacterial rather than antitoxic [246, 247]. The vaccine formulations for this pathogen involved recombinant B subunit killed whole cell (rBS-WC) vaccine and the live attenuated CVD 103-HgR vaccine. One of the vaccines recommended by WHO is Dukoral which consists of mixture of virulent *V. cholerae* cells belonging to both the classical and El Tor biotype and an inactive B subunit of cholera toxin. Whole cell killed bivalent vaccines mOrvac and Shanchol have resulted from a technology transfer from Sweden to India (Shantha Biotech, Hyderabad) and Vietnam (National Institute of Hygiene and Epidemiology, Hanoi). These vaccines are comprised of whole cell killed *V. cholerae* serogroups O1 and O139, and do not contain recombinant B subunit, due to which they do not need to be reconstituted in a buffer solution [248]. A vaccine not only limits the total number of cases but could also offer additional benefit of lowering the resistant bacteria. Pneumococcal conjugate vaccine has been shown to be highly effective in controlling resistant *Streptococcus pneumonia*e [249, 250]. Vaccine for *Haemophilus influenzae* has been successful in treating meningitis. Therefore, vaccination could prove to be an effective tool to contain the infections caused by MDR bacteria thus not only facilitating the containment and emergence of infections but also making organ transplantations and cancer chemotherapy more successful and safe.

Antivirulent Therapies-New Horizons

Quorum Sensing Inhibition (QSI)

Quorum sensing (QS) is a process that bacteria employ for ensuring that they are present in sufficient numbers to elicit a biological response to any external stimulus. QS involves generation of signal molecules upto certain threshold concentration and their recognition by the receptors in bacterial cell. This signal transduction leads to the expression of a diverse array of genes that are utilized by bacterium for various processes like biofilm formation, virulence, spore formation, evasion of host defenses, swarming and motility, to name a few [251]. QS has been studied in many bacteria including *V. fischeri*, *V. harveyi*, *V. cholerae*, *S. aureus*, *P. aeruginosa* and *E. coli*. The signal molecules produced during QS are called autoinducers (AIs) and there are many types of QS systems known in microorganisms based on the kind of AI employed in each [251, 252]. For Autoinducer type 1 (AI-1) system, N-acyl homoserine lactone (AHL) class of molecules act as signal molecules. These molecules are composed of a homoserine lactone (HSL) ring with an acyl chain that varies in the chain length, the degree of saturation and the number of oxygen substitutions. Though AHLs with small fatty acid chains can freely diffuse through the bacterial cell membrane, AHLs with long fatty acid side chains require efflux pumps to permeate outside the cell. AI-2 system was discovered in marine bioluminescent bacteria *V. harveyi*. It utilizes a receptor kinase network and the signal molecule made up of complex, multi-ringed, cyclical furanosyl molecules containing a boron atom. These interconvertible furanosyl molecules are derived from spontaneous cyclisation of DPD (S-4, 5-dihydroxy-2, 3-pentanedione) due to high reactivity of its 2, 3-dicarbonyl motif. Bacteria use AI-2 signals from other bacterial species to hijack their signal system and AI-2 is therefore considered as a mode for inter-species communication while AI-1 is used as intra-species communication. AI-3 is composed of two component receptor kinase intracellular signaling complex where the signal molecule is probably similar to catecholamines. AI-3 is also involved in interspecies and inter-kingdom communication [253]. QS in Gram-positive bacteria utilizes short cyclical autoinducing peptides (AIPs) as signal molecules. These AIPs are synthesized as propeptides that are further modified before being transported out of the bacterial cell by transport systems [254]. *S. aureus* is divided into four specificity groups based on the identity of AIP [255]. This system is referred to as accessory gene regulator system (agr) in *Staphylococci* and as *Enterococcus faecalis* regulator system (frs) in *Enterococci* [256, 257]. *Agr* locus consists of two operons, RNAII and RNAIII. While RNAII constitutes *agrA* to *agrD* genes involved in the synthesis of AIP system, the transcribed product of RNAIII functions as regulatory RNA sequence controlling genes of the virulome. Apart from these four QS systems described above, other systems are also known to act in synergy with these systems and utilize the signal molecules like diketopiperazines (DKPs) and quinolone signals (PQS) in *P. aeruginosa* [251, 253]. In *V. cholerae*, the CAI-1 (Cholerae Auto Inducer-1) system comprising of (S)-3-hydroxytridecan-4-one, acts in synergy with AI-2 pathway [258].

QSIs, also called quorum quenchers (QQ) are attractive alternatives for inhibiting QS and its related processes to control not only the MDR bacteria but also different strains and serogroups of the pathogens [259-262]. QSIs do not threaten bacteria with life-or-death situation and therefore do not suffer from the problem of resistance of bacteria against them. QSI also offers the advantage of high specificity as QS is only found in bacterium and not in the human host. These inhibitors could either be natural or man-made and manifest their activity by interfering with any of the processes involved in QS. These could be:

a.   Generation of the signal molecule/AI.

b.   Activity of the AI.

c.   Detection of AI by its receptor.

The QS systems and QSIs have been extensively reviewed and can be referred for more details [251, 253, 259-268]. Furanones are one of the most well studied QSIs. The natural compound (5Z)-4-bromo-5-(bromomethylene)-3-butyl-2(5H)-furanone also called furanone 1 has been shown to inhibit swarming and biofilm formation in *E. coli* at concentrations non-inhibitory to planktonic growth [269]. AHL as well as AI-2 based QS systems are inhibited by furanones as these compounds are structural mimics of QS signals (lactones and tetrahydrofuran rings) in both these QS systems [269]. The enzymes AHL lactonase, AHL-acylase and paraoxonases (PONs) degrade the QS signals by either hydrolyzing the lactone ring of AHL, by hydrolyzing the amide bond of AHLs producing the fatty acid component and the homoserine lactone respectively. Small molecule like triclosan inhibits enoyl-ACP reductase required for synthesis of an intermediate in AHL biosynthesis [270]. Another molecule closantel inhibits histidine kinase sensor [271]. Some compounds have been designed that are analogues of the signals generated during AI-1 or AI-2 [272, 273]. They compete with native signals for binding to the receptor thus inhibiting QS. For example, library of HSL analogues has been screened for AHL inhibitors and the QSI compounds found by this method inhibited the expression of Green Fluorescent Protein (GFP) by 50% [274, 275]. Boronic acids and DPD analogues have been used as AI-2 antagonists [276-279]. Garlic extract was used as QSI in a first human clinical trial with 26 cystic fibrosis patients. The extract was shown to improve the lung function, weight and symptom score [280]. A recent study has shown that a sulfur-rich compound from garlic extract called ajoene is involved in QSI [281]. Synthetic peptides, antibodies and antibiotics have also been used in several cases as QSIs. Synthetic AIP targeting all four AIP-types of *S. aureus* were designed as universal inhibitors [282]. As described above, as RNAIII product plays a regulatory role in mediating quorum sensing and biofilm formation in staphylococci, an RNAIII-inhibiting peptide was shown to inhibit the *agr*-mediated biofilm formation in drug resistant *S. epidermidis* thus acting as a QSI [283]. Antibodies generated against QS signals can also be used as QSIs as they would block the QS signal and its activity. Antibodies against AI-1 signal molecules have been shown to disrupt QS and render protection in mice against lethal lung infection by *P. aeruginosa* [284]. Many antibiotics like macrolides, ceftazidime, ciprofloxacin, azithromycin have been used to inhibit QS in *P. aeruginosa* [285, 286]. This indicated that antibiotics also interfere with the process of QS and biofilm formation thus directly influencing bacterial virulence.

The advantage of QSI is that they do not kill the pathogen directly but act in synergy with the antibiotics and host immune system to control the bacterial virulence. QSIs have been shown to be useful in controlling plant pathogens, nematodes and pulmonary infection in mice models [251]. Apart from controlling the virulence of the bacteria, they offer additional advantages like softening of the bacterial biofilms to make them susceptible to antibiotics and the host immune system.

For anti-virulence strategies, one could also think of using inhibitors of the toxin receptor as a therapeutic agent [239]. Also, molecules like virstatin have been tested for controlling the virulence and intestinal colonization of *V. cholerae* [287]. Virstatin acts by inhibiting the transcriptional regulator ToxT and downregulates the expression of cholera toxin and toxin corregulated pilus.

Efflux Pump Inhibition

Efflux of antibiotics to decrease the intracellular concentration of these drugs by efflux pumps has been a major determinant of drug resistance exhibited by the bacteria. Efflux pump inhibition has been pursued as a promising approach to restore the efficacy of those antibiotics that are substrates for the efflux pumps [6, 288, 289]. EPIs have been used as adjuvants in antibiotic therapy and also as diagnostic tools for detection of antibiotic resistance due to the efflux pumps. As these pumps have been shown to be crucial for bacterial survival, virulence and pathogenicity, EPIs could be used to control the bacterial virulence [113, 115]. A variety of EPIs have been derived from natural sources, screening of libraries of chemical compounds and secondary evaluation of current therapeutics [288, 289]. For achieving inhibition of efflux pumps, the strategies devised have been described below along with the examples of EPIs that have been designed based on that strategy:

Designing New Antibiotics or Modification of the Existing Antibiotics in Such a Way that they are Refractory to Recognition by Efflux Pumps

Glycylcyclines and ketolides have lower affinity for the efflux pumps. Tigecycline bypasses MFS pumps specific for tetracycline [290]. Telithromycin bypasses MefA/E and AcrAB systems [291]. Levofloxacin, moxifloxacin and gatifloxacin are not affected by NorA and PmrA efflux pumps [6].

Interfering with the Assembly/Functioning of the Efflux Pumps

In case of tripartite efflux pumps like RND pumps, blocking the outer membrane channel can lead to the inhibition of pump activity [292, 293].

Interfering with the Regulatory Steps in the Expression of the Efflux Pump Genes so that Expression of the Efflux Pumps Declines

The membrane permeability of a bacterial cell is often under complex regulatory mechanisms that control the expression of the porins and the efflux pumps simultaneously to achieve certain standards of permeability. These regulators termed as Mar regulators can be targeted to control the efflux pump expression.

For example, MarA regulator that controls the membrane permeability in *E. aerogenes* regulates the expression of both the porins as well as AcrAB-TolC efflux pump, and can be affected by imipenem. Though this antibiotic is not a substrate for this efflux pump, in the presence of this drug, the bacterium becomes resistant to quinolones, tetracycline and chloramphenicol thus leading to cross resistance [146]. Mutations in Mar regulator often causes resistance to many classes of antibiotics [294]. Interference with these regulatory steps therefore could be used to decrease the expression of efflux pumps thus restoring the antibiotic activity.

Blocking the Energy Required by the Efflux Pumps to Operate

Energy decouplers can be used as a general mechanism to dissipate the energy gradients driving the efflux pumps [288, 295]. As most of the efflux pumps utilize the PMF as their energy source, any compound that dissipates this PMF will act as an inhibitor of the efflux pump [295, 296]. Examples include Carbonyl Cyanide m-ChloroPhenyl-hydrazone (CCCP), valinomycin and dinitrophenol (DNP). However, these compounds do not directly bind the efflux pumps to cause their inhibition. They dissipate the PMF by modifying the trans-membrane electrochemical potential. This class of molecules have not been used clinically or patented due to cytotoxicity issues [297].

Competitive/Non-Competitive Inhibition of Efflux Pumps

These inhibitors are beneficial in many ways clinically as they not only circumvent the problem of bacterial resistance to antibiotics by inhibiting efflux pumps, they also reverse the acquired resistance associated with the overexpression of efflux pumps and suppress the emergence of mutations leading to resistance [295, 297-300]. Example of competitive inhibitor is MC-207, 110 (Phenylalanine Arginyl β-Naphthylamide/PAβN). This compound has been shown to decrease the frequency of the emergence of highly levofloxacin resistant *P. aeruginosa* strains and reduced the intrinsic resistance of the bug to levofloxacin 8-folds [301-303]. MC-207, 110 is a competitive inhibitor of the efflux pumps and acts by binding to the same pocket or at a site closer to the antibiotic substrate binding site [295, 300]. The compound has not only restored the activity of levofloxacin but has also been found to potentiate the activity of other antibiotics like oxazolidinones, chloramphenicol, rifampicin, macroliodes/ ketolides [289, 304]. Also, it has been shown to be effective not only for *P. aeruginosa*, but also for *K. pneumoniae, C. jejuni, E. coli, S. typhimurium* and *E. aerogenes* [296, 302, 305-307]. To summarise, PAβN appears to be a promising inhibitor with a broad host as well as antibiotic range and an effective mode of efflux pump inhibition. The derivatives of PAβN have been produced by substitution of amino acid or use of D-amino acids [302, 308-310]. As their toxicity has limited their clinical applications, to circumvent this problem, MC-04, 124 compound has been designed with lesser toxicity and higher stability [311].

Blocking the Efflux Pump Protein or Gene

This falls under the category of biological inhibition of efflux pumps. Efflux pumps could be deactivated with the means of specific antibodies [293]. A monoclonal antibody was synthesized and used to block the E2 loop of the extracellular domain of OprM pump of MexAB-OprM tripartite pump in *P. aeruginosa*. This antibody/its variant without Fc domain/ humanized antibody were administered with the antibiotic, and an increase in the efficacy of this antibiotic was observed. These formulations could also contain a pharmaceutically acceptable carrier along with the antibiotic and the antibody and could be used to inhibit the OprM subunit in both MexAB-OprM and MexXY-OprM.

Alternatively, the genes encoding these pumps or their regulators could be blocked using antisense strategies. The antisense approach has been shown to work for AcrAB efflux pump in *E. coli* and has also been patented [312, 313]. These antisense oligonucleotides hybridise with nucleic acids encoding efflux pump AcrB or with nucleic acids regulating the expression of an efflux pump (*marA, rob* or *soxS*). Other EPIs included ribozymes directed against the above mentioned genes or antibodies to the efflux pump or proteins that regulate the expression of this efflux pump.

Both QSIs and EPIs can be used as adjuvants with the antibiotics to increase their efficacy [6, 251]. Still, caution needs to be exercised in using these reagents for controlling bacterial virulence as they suffer from some disadvantages. For example, emergence of resistance to QSIs or EPIs cannot be ruled out [6, 251]. QSIs based on lactone rings like AHL-analogues could present the problem of low stability due to the degradation of lactone ring by lactonases [314].

Other General Strategies

To successfully circumvent the problem of MDR, awareness and concerted efforts are required from the community, clinicians, pharmaceutical industry, governments and scientists. Some of the general strategies to be employed by them are described below:

- Improved water, sanitation and hygiene could help to control the water- and food-borne infections. Continuous surveillance is very critical to determine the prevailing patterns of antibiotic resistance in a given geographical location and thus to assess which of the antibiotics are still active. It is also important to continuously monitor the changes in the antibiotic sensitivity patterns in that location to keep pace with the ever changing pathogens [3].

- Representative strains with MDR phenotypes should be studied carefully in the laboratories to understand the kind of resistance mechanisms adopted by bacteria.

- In addition, we need to improve the existing antibiotics and develop new antibiotics which are inevitably costlier than the already existing drugs. The situation of funding in the area of antibiotic research and development needs to be improved to provide incentives to big and small pharmaceutical companies and research labs for carrying out research in this field.

- One of the other interventions for reversing antibiotic resistance is to relieve the antibiotic pressure in the ecological niches of bacteria like environmental water in case of *V. cholerae* and animal reservoirs in case of *Campylobacter jejuni*. This way, the bacteria would shed the extra genetic baggage that it required to deal with these antibiotics. Appropriate policies should be devised to stop the indiscriminate use of antibiotics after consultation of government agencies, pharmaceutical industries, researchers and clinicians. It should be seen that the antibiotics used in animals are different from those used in humans. In addition to this, the use of antimicrobials in the case of upper respiratory tract infections or other infections of viral origin should be discouraged as should be the empirical therapy and broad spectrum antimicrobials-based therapy [315].

- Novel drug targets combined with new drugs, efficient diagnostic techniques and vaccine could provide a new hope to curb these pathogens [315].

- In this era, use of bioinformatics tools like *in silico* target identification, design of small drug molecules, and docking studies to predict their binding to target could aid in achieving this aim faster. Some companies like Intercell are employing anti-genome technology to identify new targets for vaccines and drugs. Projects have been initiated to identify novel targets in *S. aureus, S. pneumoniae* and *S. pyogenes* [315]. The advent of technologies based on genomics, proteomics, combinatorial chemistry and high throughput screening could lead to success stories inspite of the large funds required for them.

- The governments should realize the seriousness of impending disaster due to MDR bacteria and urgency of the situation due to their limitations in controlling the diseases caused by MDR bacteria [315]. Accordingly, the new policies should be made to deal with this problem. For example, American Society of Microbiology (ASM) set up a task force on antimicrobial resistance in 1995, The CDC published their "Guidelines for the Evaluation of Surveillance Systems" in 1998 and CDC also issued a Public Health Action Plan to combat Antimicrobial resistance in June 2000. The Infectious Diseases Society of America produced a shocking report in 2004 to draw the attention of the government towards the problem of MDR and to draw the attention of dwindling funds in research and development of new anti-infective agents by pharmaceutical industries. The report was titled "Bad Bugs, No Drugs: As Antibiotic Discovery Stagnates------- A Public Health Crisis Brews". Similarly, the UK Department of Health issued an "Antimicrobial Resistance Strategy and Action Plan' in 2000. An efficient surveillance system has been set up in Europe by the name of European Antimicrobial Resistance Surveillance System (EARSS) (http://www.rivm.nl/earss). In India, national policy has been made for containment of antimicrobial resistance by Directorate General of Health Services (2011) when the superbug carrying New Delhi metallo-beta lactamase was reported in a Swedish patient of Indian origin. A task force was constituted to work on various aspects related to national surveillance system for antibiotic resistance, enhancing regulatory provisions for use of antibiotics in human, veterinary and industrial use, to enhance the rational use of antibiotics and strengthen the diagnostic methods for antimicrobial resistance monitoring. Health ministry has also approved an antimicrobial resistance programme that will be monitored and reviewed by The National Centre for Disease Control (NCDC). Global Antibiotic Resistance Partnership (GARP) develops different policy proposals on antibiotic resistance for low-and middle-income countries. Phase 1 of GARP has been initiated in India, Kenya, South Africa and Vietnam. In addition to this endeavour, in August 2012, the annual conference of Clinical Infectious Disease Society was held at Chennai, India. In this meeting of medical societies of India which also had many national and international representatives, a roadmap was made to tackle the problem of antimicrobial resistance in India. The document resulting from the discussions held at this meeting was named "Chennai Declaration". The recommendations made in Chennai Declaration would be considered by Indian Ministry of Health for formulating a national antibiotic policy.

CONCLUDING REMARKS

Considering the resilience of bacteria, it is imminent that other strategies and avenues apart from antibiotics be explored to control the MDR bacteria. As described in the section above, a multifaceted approach is perhaps required to vanquish these bugs. To conclude this chapter, the statement by Dr. Joshua Lederberg seems appropriate to describe the current situation.

The future of microbes and mankind will probably unfold as episodes of a suspense thriller that could be entitled "Our wits *versus* their genes"

ACKNOWLEDGEMENTS

The laboratory is supported by the grants from the Department of Biotechnology (DBT), Ministry of Science and Technology, Government of India (No. BT/PR/11634/INF/22/104/2008), Gujarat State Biotechnology Mission (GSBTM), Department of Science and Technology, Government of Gujarat (No. GSBTM/MD/PROJECTS/SSA/1535/2013-14) and Indian Council of Medical Research, New Delhi, India (No. the grant AMR/49/11-ECDI). N.R. is a recipient of Senior Research Fellowship from Indian Council of Medical Research, New Delhi, India and K.V. is a recipient of Junior Research Fellowship from the GSBTM grant mentioned above. P. M. is a recipient of ICMR senior research fellowship (No. F/815/2011-ECD-II) and B. M. R. N. S. K. is a recipient of senior research fellowship from CSIR (No. 09/988/(0003)/2010-EMR-I). The authors thankfully acknowledge The Puri Foundation for Education in India for providing infrastructure facilities.

CONFLICT OF INTEREST

The authors confirm that this chapter contents have no conflict of interest.

DISCLOSURE

Parts of this book chapter have been previously published in two articles by the authors of this chapter. These articles are: Recent Patents on Anti-infective Drug Discovery, Volume: 7; Issue: 1; Pages 73-89 (17); and Recent Patents on Anti-infective Drug Discovery, Volume: 8; Issue: 1; Pages 68-83 (16).

REFERENCES

[1]   Antibiotic resistance: a final warning. Lancet 2013; 382: 1072.
[2]   Antibiotic resistance threats in the United States, 2013. Centers for Diseases Control and Prevention 2013; 11-28.
[3]   Sack DA, Lyke C, McLaughlin C, *et al.*, Antimicrobial resistance in shigellosis, cholera and campylobacteriosis. World Health Organization 2001; 1-20.
[4]   Willey JM, Sherwood L, Woolverton CJ, *et al.*, 7th. Prescott, Harley, and Klein's microbiology. McGraw-Hill Higher Education 2008; 835-58.
[5]   Salyers AA, Whitt DD, 2nd. Bacterial pathogenesis: a molecular approach. ASM Press 2002; 168-84.

[6]   Bhardwaj AK, Mohanty P. Bacterial efflux pumps involved in multidrug resistance and their inhibitors: rejuvinating the antimicrobial chemotherapy. Recent Pat Antiinfect Drug Discov 2012; 7: 73-89.

[7]   Cavallo JD, Plesiat P, Couetdic G, *et al*. Mechanisms of beta-lactam resistance in *Pseudomonas aeruginosa*: prevalence of OprM-overproducing strains in a French multicentre study (1997). J Antimicrob Chemother 2002; 50: 1039-43.

[8]   Baranwal S, Dey K, Ramamurthy T, *et al*. Role of active efflux in association with target gene mutations in fluoroquinolone resistance in clinical isolates of *Vibrio cholerae*. Antimicrob Agents Chemother 2002; 46: 2676-8.

[9]   Singh R, Rajpara N, Tak J, *et al*. Clinical isolates of *Vibrio fluvialis* from Kolkata, India, obtained during 2006: plasmids, the *qnr* gene and a mutation in gyrase A as mechanisms of multidrug resistance. J Med Microbiol 2012; 61: 369-74.

[10]   Pazhani GP, Chakraborty S, Fujihara K, *et al*. QRDR mutations, efflux system & antimicrobial resistance genes in enterotoxigenic *Escherichia coli* isolated from an outbreak of diarrhoea in Ahmedabad, India. Indian J Med Res 2011; 134: 214-23.

[11]   Mitsuhashi S, Harada K, Hashimoto H, *et al*. On the drug-resistance of enteric bacteria. 4. Drug-resistance of *Shigella* prevalent in Japan. Jpn J Exp Med 1961; 31: 47-52.

[12]   Liebert CA, Hall RM, Summers AO. Transposon Tn21, flagship of the floating genome. Microbiol Mol Biol Rev 1999; 63: 507-22.

[13]   Coppo A, Colombo M, Pazzani C, *et al*. *Vibrio cholerae* in the horn of Africa: epidemiology, plasmids, tetracycline resistance gene amplification, and comparison between O1 and non-O1 strains. Am J Trop Med Hyg 1995; 53: 351-9.

[14]   Stokes HW, Hall RM. A novel family of potentially mobile DNA elements encoding site-specific gene-integration functions: integrons. Mol Microbiol 1989; 3: 1669-83.

[15]   Rajpara N, Patel A, Tiwari N, *et al*. Mechanism of drug resistance in a clinical isolate of *Vibrio fluvialis*: involvement of multiple plasmids and integrons. Int J Antimicrob Agents 2009; 34: 220-5.

[16]   Partridge SR, Tsafnat G, Coiera E, *et al*. Gene cassettes and cassette arrays in mobile resistance integrons. FEMS Microbiol Rev 2009; 33: 757-84.

[17]   Stokes HW, Nesbo CL, Holley M, *et al*. Class 1 integrons potentially predating the association with tn402-like transposition genes are present in a sediment microbial community. J Bacteriol 2006; 188: 5722-30.

[18]   Mazel D, Dychinco B, Webb VA, *et al*. A distinctive class of integron in the *Vibrio cholerae* genome. Science 1998; 280: 605-8.

[19]   Mazel D. Integrons: agents of bacterial evolution. Nat Rev Microbiol 2006; 4: 608-20.

[20]   Cambray G, Guerout AM, Mazel D. Integrons. Annu Rev Genet 2010; 44: 141-66.

[21]   Esposito D, Scocca JJ. The integrase family of tyrosine recombinases: evolution of a conserved active site domain. Nucleic Acids Res 1997; 25: 3605-14.

[22]   Nunes-Duby SE, Kwon HJ, Tirumalai RS, *et al*. Similarities and differences among 105 members of the Int family of site-specific recombinases. Nucleic Acids Res 1998; 26: 391-406.

[23]   Demarre G, Frumerie C, Gopaul DN, *et al*. Identification of key structural determinants of the IntI1 integron integrase that influence *attC* x *attI1* recombination efficiency. Nucleic Acids Res 2007; 35: 6475-89.

[24] Stokes HW, Hall RM. Sequence analysis of the inducible chloramphenicol resistance determinant in the Tn1696 integron suggests regulation by translational attenuation. Plasmid 1991; 26: 10-9.

[25] da Fonseca EL, Vicente AC. Functional characterization of a Cassette-specific promoter in the class 1 integron-associated *qnrVC1* gene. Antimicrob Agents Chemother 2012; 56: 3392-4.

[26] Guerineau F, Brooks L, Mullineaux P. Expression of the sulfonamide resistance gene from plasmid R46. Plasmid 1990; 23: 35-41.

[27] Levesque C, Brassard S, Lapointe J, *et al.* Diversity and relative strength of tandem promoters for the antibiotic-resistance genes of several integrons. Gene 1994; 142: 49-54.

[28] Collis CM, Hall RM. Expression of antibiotic resistance genes in the integrated cassettes of integrons. Antimicrob Agents Chemother 1995; 39: 155-62.

[29] Jove T, Da Re S, Denis F, *et al.* Inverse correlation between promoter strength and excision activity in class 1 integrons. PLoS Genet 2010; 6: e1000793.

[30] Gravel A, Fournier B, Roy PH. DNA complexes obtained with the integron integrase IntI1 at the attI1 site. Nucleic Acids Res 1998; 26: 4347-55.

[31] Collis CM, Kim MJ, Stokes HW, *et al.* Binding of the purified integron DNA integrase IntI1 to integron- and cassette-associated recombination sites. Mol Microbiol 1998; 29: 477-90.

[32] Collis CM, Hall RM. Comparison of the structure-activity relationships of the integron-associated recombination sites *attI3* and *attI1* reveals common features. Microbiology 2004; 150: 1591-601.

[33] Stokes HW, O'Gorman DB, Recchia GD, *et al.* Structure and function of 59-base element recombination sites associated with mobile gene cassettes. Mol Microbiol 1997; 26: 731-45.

[34] Recchia GD, Hall RM. Gene cassettes: a new class of mobile element. Microbiology 1995; 141 (Pt 12): 3015-27.

[35] Baharoglu Z, Garriss G, Mazel D. Multiple pathways of genome plasticity leading to development of antibiotic resistance. Antibiotics 2013; 2: 288-315.

[36] Fluit AC, Schmitz FJ. Resistance integrons and super-integrons. Clin Microbiol Infect 2004; 10: 272-88.

[37] Goldstein C, Lee MD, Sanchez S, *et al.* Incidence of class 1 and 2 integrases in clinical and commensal bacteria from livestock, companion animals, and exotics. Antimicrob Agents Chemother 2001; 45: 723-6.

[38] Labbate M, Case RJ, Stokes HW. The integron/gene cassette system: an active player in bacterial adaptation. Methods Mol Biol 2009; 532: 103-25.

[39] Martin C, Timm J, Rauzier J, *et al.* Transposition of an antibiotic resistance element in mycobacteria. Nature 1990; 345: 739-43.

[40] Nandi S, Maurer JJ, Hofacre C, *et al.* Gram-positive bacteria are a major reservoir of Class 1 antibiotic resistance integrons in poultry litter. Proc Natl Acad Sci USA 2004; 101: 7118-22.

[41] Nesvera J, Hochmannova J, Patek M. An integron of class 1 is present on the plasmid pCG4 from gram-positive bacterium *Corynebacterium glutamicum*. FEMS Microbiol Lett 1998; 169: 391-5.

[42] Shi L, Zheng M, Xiao Z, *et al.* Unnoticed spread of class 1 integrons in gram-positive clinical strains isolated in Guangzhou, China. Microbiol Immunol 2006; 50: 463-7.

[43]   Rouch DA, Cram DS, DiBerardino D, *et al.* Efflux-mediated antiseptic resistance gene *qacA* from *Staphylococcus aureus*: common ancestry with tetracycline- and sugar-transport proteins. Mol Microbiol 1990; 4: 2051-62.

[44]   Uyaguari MI, Scott GI, Norman RS. Abundance of class 1-3 integrons in South Carolina estuarine ecosystems under high and low levels of anthropogenic influence. Mar Pollut Bull 2013; 76: 77-84.

[45]   Hansson K, Sundstrom L, Pelletier A, *et al.* IntI2 integron integrase in Tn7. J Bacteriol 2002; 184: 1712-21.

[46]   Collis CM, Kim MJ, Stokes HW, *et al.* Integron-encoded IntI integrases preferentially recognize the adjacent cognate attI site in recombination with a 59-be site. Mol Microbiol 2002; 46: 1415-27.

[47]   Barlow RS, Gobius KS. Diverse class 2 integrons in bacteria from beef cattle sources. J Antimicrob Chemother 2006; 58: 1133-8.

[48]   Marquez C, Labbate M, Ingold AJ, *et al.* Recovery of a functional class 2 integron from an *Escherichia coli* strain mediating a urinary tract infection. Antimicrob Agents Chemother 2008; 52: 4153-4.

[49]   Wei Q, Hu Q, Li S, *et al.* A novel functional class 2 integron in clinical *Proteus mirabilis* isolates. J Antimicrob Chemother 2014; 69: 973-6.

[50]   Arakawa Y, Murakami M, Suzuki K, *et al.* A novel integron-like element carrying the metallo-beta-lactamase gene *blaIMP*. Antimicrob Agents Chemother 1995; 39: 1612-5.

[51]   Collis CM, Kim MJ, Partridge SR, *et al.* Characterization of the class 3 integron and the site-specific recombination system it determines. J Bacteriol 2002; 184: 3017-26.

[52]   Correia M, Boavida F, Grosso F, *et al.* Molecular characterization of a new class 3 integron in *Klebsiella pneumoniae*. Antimicrob Agents Chemother 2003; 47: 2838-43.

[53]   Clark CA, Purins L, Kaewrakon P, *et al.* The *Vibrio cholerae* O1 chromosomal integron. Microbiology 2000; 146 (Pt 10): 2605-12.

[54]   Heidelberg JF, Eisen JA, Nelson WC, *et al.* DNA sequence of both chromosomes of the cholera pathogen *Vibrio cholerae*. Nature 2000; 406: 477-83.

[55]   Drouin F, Melancon J, Roy PH. The IntI-like tyrosine recombinase of *Shewanella oneidensis* is active as an integron integrase. J Bacteriol 2002; 184: 1811-5.

[56]   Rowe-Magnus DA, Guerout AM, Mazel D. Bacterial resistance evolution by recruitment of super-integron gene cassettes. Mol Microbiol 2002; 43: 1657-69.

[57]   Boucher Y, Labbate M, Koenig JE, *et al.* Integrons: mobilizable platforms that promote genetic diversity in bacteria. Trends Microbiol 2007; 15: 301-9.

[58]   Nield BS, Willows RD, Torda AE, *et al.* New enzymes from environmental cassette arrays: functional attributes of a phosphotransferase and an RNA-methyltransferase. Protein Sci 2004; 13: 1651-9.

[59]   Robinson A, Wu PS, Harrop SJ, *et al.* Integron-associated mobile gene cassettes code for folded proteins: the structure of Bal32a, a new member of the adaptable alpha+beta barrel family. J Mol Biol 2005; 346: 1229-41.

[60]   Smith AB, Siebeling RJ. Identification of genetic loci required for capsular expression in *Vibrio vulnificus*. Infect Immun 2003; 71: 1091-7.

[61]   Fonseca EL, Dos Santos Freitas F, Vieira VV, *et al.* New *qnr* gene cassettes associated with superintegron repeats in *Vibrio cholerae* O1. Emerg Infect Dis 2008; 14: 1129-31.

[62]   Le Roux F, Zouine M, Chakroun N, *et al.* Genome sequence of *Vibrio splendidus*: an abundant planctonic marine species with a large genotypic diversity. Environ Microbiol 2009; 11: 1959-70.

[63]   Melano R, Petroni A, Garutti A, *et al.* New carbenicillin-hydrolyzing beta-lactamase (CARB-7) from *Vibrio cholerae* non-O1, non-O139 strains encoded by the VCR region of the *V. cholerae* genome. Antimicrob Agents Chemother 2002; 46: 2162-8.

[64]   Petroni A, Melano RG, Saka HA, *et al.* CARB-9, a carbenicillinase encoded in the VCR region of *Vibrio cholerae* non-O1, non-O139 belongs to a family of cassette-encoded beta-lactamases. Antimicrob Agents Chemother 2004; 48: 4042-6.

[65]   Chen CY, Wu KM, Chang YC, *et al.* Comparative genome analysis of *Vibrio vulnificus*, a marine pathogen. Genome Res 2003; 13: 2577-87.

[66]   Gerdes K, Gultyaev AP, Franch T, *et al.* Antisense RNA-regulated programmed cell death. Annu Rev Genet 1997; 31: 1-31.

[67]   Kobayashi I. Behavior of restriction-modification systems as selfish mobile elements and their impact on genome evolution. Nucleic Acids Res 2001; 29: 3742-56.

[68]   Van Melderen L, Saavedra De Bast M. Bacterial toxin-antitoxin systems: more than selfish entities? PLoS Genet 2009; 5: e1000437.

[69]   Pandey DP, Gerdes K. Toxin-antitoxin loci are highly abundant in free-living but lost from host-associated prokaryotes. Nucleic Acids Res 2005; 33: 966-76.

[70]   Rowe-Magnus DA, Guerout AM, Biskri L, *et al.* Comparative analysis of superintegrons: engineering extensive genetic diversity in the *Vibrionaceae*. Genome Res 2003; 13: 428-42.

[71]   Szekeres S, Dauti M, Wilde C, *et al.* Chromosomal toxin-antitoxin loci can diminish large-scale genome reductions in the absence of selection. Mol Microbiol 2007; 63: 1588-605.

[72]   Christensen-Dalsgaard M, Gerdes K. Two *higBA* loci in the *Vibrio cholerae* superintegron encode mRNA cleaving enzymes and can stabilize plasmids. Mol Microbiol 2006; 62: 397-411.

[73]   Vaisvila R, Morgan RD, Posfai J, *et al.* Discovery and distribution of super-integrons among pseudomonads. Mol Microbiol 2001; 42: 587-601.

[74]   Waldor MK, Tschape H, Mekalanos JJ. A new type of conjugative transposon encodes resistance to sulfamethoxazole, trimethoprim, and streptomycin in *Vibrio cholerae* O139. J Bacteriol 1996; 178: 4157-65.

[75]   Beaber JW, Burrus V, Hochhut B, *et al.* Comparison of SXT and R391, two conjugative integrating elements: definition of a genetic backbone for the mobilization of resistance determinants. Cell Mol Life Sci 2002; 59: 2065-70.

[76]   Ceccarelli D, Spagnoletti M, Bacciu D, *et al.* ICEVchInd5 is prevalent in epidemic *Vibrio cholerae* O1 El Tor strains isolated in India. Int J Med Microbiol 2011; 301: 318-24.

[77]   Burrus V, Waldor MK. Shaping bacterial genomes with integrative and conjugative elements. Res Microbiol 2004; 155: 376-86.

[78]   Osborn AM, Boltner D. When phage, plasmids, and transposons collide: genomic islands, and conjugative- and mobilizable-transposons as a mosaic continuum. Plasmid 2002; 48: 202-12.

[79]   Burrus V, Waldor MK. Control of SXT integration and excision. J Bacteriol 2003; 185: 5045-54.

[80]   Hochhut B, Lotfi Y, Mazel D, *et al.* Molecular analysis of antibiotic resistance gene clusters in *Vibrio cholerae* O139 and O1 SXT constins. Antimicrob Agents Chemother 2001; 45: 2991-3000.

[81]   Mohapatra H, Mohapatra SS, Mantri CK, *et al. Vibrio cholerae* non-O1, non-O139 strains isolated before 1992 from Varanasi, India are multiple drug resistant, contain *intSXT*, *dfr18* and *aadA5* genes. Environ Microbiol 2008; 10: 866-73

[82]   Amita, Chowdhury SR, Thungapathra M, *et al.* Class I integrons and SXT elements in El Tor strains isolated before and after 1992 *Vibrio cholerae* O139 outbreak, Calcutta, India. Emerg Infect Dis 2003; 9: 500-2.

[83]   Alam M, Hasan NA, Sadique A, *et al.* Seasonal cholera caused by *Vibrio cholerae* serogroups O1 and O139 in the coastal aquatic environment of Bangladesh. Appl Environ Microbiol 2006; 72: 4096-104.

[84]   Toma C, Nakasone N, Song T, *et al. Vibrio cholerae* SXT element, Laos. Emerg Infect Dis 2005; 11: 346-7.

[85]   Burrus V, Marrero J, Waldor MK. The current ICE age: biology and evolution of SXT-related integrating conjugative elements. Plasmid 2006; 55: 173-83

[86]   Dalsgaard A, Forslund A, Sandvang D, *et al. Vibrio cholerae* O1 outbreak isolates in Mozambique and South Africa in 1998 are multiple-drug resistant, contain the SXT element and the *aadA2* gene located on class 1 integrons. J Antimicrob Chemother 2001; 48: 827-38.

[87]   Kutar BM, Rajpara N, Upadhyay H, *et al.* Clinical isolates of *Vibrio cholerae* O1 El Tor Ogawa of 2009 from Kolkata, India: preponderance of SXT element and presence of Haitian *ctxB* variant. PLoS One 2013; 8: e56477.

[88]   Mitra R, Basu A, Dutta D, *et al.* Resurgence of *Vibrio cholerae* O139 Bengal with altered antibiogram in Calcutta, India. Lancet 1996; 348: 1181.

[89]   Sinha S, Chakraborty R, De K, *et al.* Escalating association of *Vibrio cholerae* O139 with cholera outbreaks in India. J Clin Microbiol 2002; 40: 2635-7.

[90]   Yam WC, Yuen KY, Wong SS, *et al. Vibrio cholerae* O139 susceptible to vibriostatic agent 0/129 and co-trimoxazole. Lancet 1994; 344: 404-5.

[91]   Schubert S, Dufke S, Sorsa J, *et al.* A novel integrative and conjugative element (ICE) of *Escherichia coli*: the putative progenitor of the Yersinia high-pathogenicity island. Mol Microbiol 2004; 51: 837-48.

[92]   Beaber JW, Hochhut B, Waldor MK. Genomic and functional analyses of SXT, an integrating antibiotic resistance gene transfer element derived from *Vibrio cholerae*. J Bacteriol 2002; 184: 4259-69.

[93]   Lewis JA, Hatfull GF. Control of directionality in integrase-mediated recombination: examination of recombination directionality factors (RDFs) including Xis and Cox proteins. Nucleic Acids Res 2001; 29: 2205-16.

[94]   Wang H, Roberts AP, Lyras D, *et al.* Characterization of the ends and target sites of the novel conjugative transposon Tn5397 from *Clostridium difficile*: excision and circularization is mediated by the large resolvase, TndX. J Bacteriol 2000; 182: 3775-83.

[95]   Wozniak RA, Fouts DE, Spagnoletti M, *et al.* Comparative ICE genomics: insights into the evolution of the SXT/R391 family of ICEs. PLoS Genet 2009; 5: e1000786.

[96]   Grohmann E, Muth G, Espinosa M. Conjugative plasmid transfer in gram-positive bacteria. Microbiol Mol Biol Rev 2003; 67: 277-301.

[97]   Hochhut B, Waldor MK. Site-specific integration of the conjugal *Vibrio cholerae* SXT element into *prfC*. Mol Microbiol 1999; 32: 99-110.

[98]   Van Melderen L, Saavedra De Bast M. Bacterial toxin-antitoxin systems: more than selfish entities? PLoS Genet 2009; 5: e1000437.

[99]   Magnuson RD. Hypothetical functions of toxin-antitoxin systems. J Bacteriol 2007; 189: 6089-92.

[100]   Hayes F. Toxins-antitoxins: plasmid maintenance, programmed cell death, and cell cycle arrest. Science 2003; 301: 1496-9.

[101]   Wozniak RA, Waldor MK. Integrative and conjugative elements: mosaic mobile genetic elements enabling dynamic lateral gene flow. Nat Rev Microbiol 2010; 8: 552-63

[102]   Ceccarelli D, Daccord A, Rene M, *et al.* Identification of the origin of transfer (oriT) and a new gene required for mobilization of the SXT/R391 family of integrating conjugative elements. J Bacteriol 2008; 190: 5328-38.

[103]   Beaber JW, Hochhut B, Waldor MK. SOS response promotes horizontal dissemination of antibiotic resistance genes. Nature 2004; 427: 72-4.

[104]   Hochhut B, Beaber JW, Woodgate R, *et al.* Formation of chromosomal tandem arrays of the SXT element and R391, two conjugative chromosomally integrating elements that share an attachment site. J Bacteriol 2001; 183: 1124-32.

[105]   Pembroke JT, MacMahon C, McGrath B. The role of conjugative transposons in the *Enterobacteriaceae*. Cell Mol Life Sci 2002; 59: 2055-64.

[106]   Bi D, Xu Z, Harrison EM, *et al.* ICEberg: a web-based resource for integrative and conjugative elements found in Bacteria. Nucleic Acids Res 2012; 40: D621-6.

[107]   Coetzee JN, Datta N, Hedges RW. R factors from *Proteus rettgeri*. J Gen Microbiol 1972; 72: 543-52.

[108]   Daccord A, Ceccarelli D, Burrus V. Integrating conjugative elements of the SXT/R391 family trigger the excision and drive the mobilization of a new class of Vibrio genomic islands. Mol Microbiol 2010; 78: 576-88.

[109]   Marrero J, Waldor MK. The SXT/R391 family of integrative conjugative elements is composed of two exclusion groups. J Bacteriol 2007; 189: 3302-5.

[110]   Van Bambeke F, Glupczynski Y, Plesiat P, *et al.* Antibiotic efflux pumps in prokaryotic cells: occurrence, impact on resistance and strategies for the future of antimicrobial therapy. J Antimicrob Chemother 2003; 51: 1055-65.

[111]   Poole K. Efflux-mediated resistance to fluoroquinolones in gram-negative bacteria. Antimicrob Agents Chemother 2000; 44: 2233-41.

[112]   Lehtinen J, Lilius EM. Promethazine renders *Escherichia coli* susceptible to penicillin G: real-time measurement of bacterial susceptibility by fluoro-luminometry. Int J Antimicrob Agents 2007; 30: 44-51.

[113]   Piddock LJ. Multidrug-resistance efflux pumps - not just for resistance. Nat Rev Microbiol 2006; 4: 629-36.

[114]   Ren Q, Paulsen IT. Comparative analyses of fundamental differences in membrane transport capabilities in prokaryotes and eukaryotes. PLoS Comput Biol 2005; 1: e27.

[115]   Piddock LJ. Clinically relevant chromosomally encoded multidrug resistance efflux pumps in bacteria. Clin Microbiol Rev 2006; 19: 382-402.

[116]   Butaye P, Cloeckaert A, Schwarz S. Mobile genes coding for efflux-mediated antimicrobial resistance in Gram-positive and Gram-negative bacteria. Int J Antimicrob Agents 2003; 22: 205-10.

[117]   Zhao J, Chen Z, Chen S, *et al.* Prevalence and dissemination of *oqxAB* in *Escherichia coli* isolates from animals, farmworkers, and the environment. Antimicrob Agents Chemother 2010; 54: 4219-24.

[118] Bina JE, Mekalanos JJ. *Vibrio cholerae tolC* is required for bile resistance and colonization. Infect Immun 2001; 69: 4681-5.

[119] Bina XR, Provenzano D, Nguyen N, *et al. Vibrio cholerae* RND family efflux systems are required for antimicrobial resistance, optimal virulence factor production, and colonization of the infant mouse small intestine. Infect Immun 2008; 76: 3595-605.

[120] McMurry L, Petrucci RE, Jr., Levy SB. Active efflux of tetracycline encoded by four genetically different tetracycline resistance determinants in *Escherichia coli*. Proc Natl Acad Sci USA 1980; 77: 3974-7.

[121] Poole K. Efflux-mediated antimicrobial resistance. J Antimicrob Chemother 2005; 56: 20-51.

[122] Borges-Walmsley MI, McKeegan KS, Walmsley AR. Structure and function of efflux pumps that confer resistance to drugs. Biochem J 2003; 376: 313-38.

[123] Higgins MK, Bokma E, Koronakis E, *et al.* Structure of the periplasmic component of a bacterial drug efflux pump. Proc Natl Acad Sci USA 2004; 101: 9994-9.

[124] He X, Szewczyk P, Karyakin A, *et al.* Structure of a cation-bound multidrug and toxic compound extrusion transporter. Nature 2010; 467: 991-4.

[125] Lomovskaya O, Lee A, Hoshino K, *et al.* Use of a genetic approach to evaluate the consequences of inhibition of efflux pumps in *Pseudomonas aeruginosa*. Antimicrob Agents Chemother 1999; 43: 1340-6.

[126] Mazzariol A, Cornaglia G, Nikaido H. Contributions of the AmpC beta-lactamase and the AcrAB multidrug efflux system in intrinsic resistance of *Escherichia coli* K-12 to beta-lactams. Antimicrob Agents Chemother 2000; 44: 1387-90.

[127] Lynch IJ, Martinez FJ. Clinical relevance of macrolide-resistant *Streptococcus pneumoniae* for community-acquired pneumonia. Clin Infect Dis 2002; 34 Suppl 1: S27-46.

[128] Askoura M, Mottawea W, Abujamel T, *et al.* Efflux pump inhibitors (EPIs) as new antimicrobial agents against *Pseudomonas aeruginosa*. Libyan J Med 2011; 6:

[129] Nikaido H. Multidrug resistance in bacteria. Annu Rev Biochem 2009; 78: 119-46.

[130] Moussatova A, Kandt C, O'Mara ML, *et al.* ATP-binding cassette transporters in *Escherichia coli*. Biochim Biophys Acta 2008; 1778: 1757-71.

[131] Li J, Li B, Wendlandt S, *et al.* Identification of a novel *vga(E)* gene variant that confers resistance to pleuromutilins, lincosamides and streptogramin A antibiotics in staphylococci of porcine origin. J Antimicrob Chemother. 2014; 69: 919-23.

[132] Marger MD, Saier MH, Jr. A major superfamily of transmembrane facilitators that catalyse uniport, symport and antiport. Trends Biochem Sci 1993; 18: 13-20.

[133] Paulsen IT, Skurray RA. Topology, structure and evolution of two families of proteins involved in antibiotic and antiseptic resistance in eukaryotes and prokaryotes--an analysis. Gene 1993; 124: 1-11.

[134] Fernandez L, Hancock RE. Adaptive and mutational resistance: role of porins and efflux pumps in drug resistance. Clin Microbiol Rev 2012; 25: 661-81.

[135] Yoshida H, Bogaki M, Nakamura S, *et al.* Nucleotide sequence and characterization of the *Staphylococcus aureus norA* gene, which confers resistance to quinolones. J Bacteriol 1990; 172: 6942-9.

[136] Gill MJ, Brenwald NP, Wise R. Identification of an efflux pump gene, *pmrA*, associated with fluoroquinolone resistance in *Streptococcus pneumoniae*. Antimicrob Agents Chemother 1999; 43: 187-9.

[137]   Lee EW, Chen J, Huda MN, *et al.* Functional cloning and expression of *emeA*, and characterization of EmeA, a multidrug efflux pump from *Enterococcus faecalis*. Biol Pharm Bull 2003; 26: 266-70.

[138]   Chung YJ, Saier MH, Jr. SMR-type multidrug resistance pumps. Curr Opin Drug Discov Devel 2001; 4: 237-45.

[139]   Bay DC, Rommens KL, Turner RJ. Small multidrug resistance proteins: a multidrug transporter family that continues to grow. Biochim Biophys Acta 2008; 1778: 1814-38.

[140]   Venkatraman J, Nagana Gowda GA, Balaram P. Structural analysis of synthetic peptide fragments from EmrE, a multidrug resistance protein, in a membrane-mimetic environment. Biochemistry 2002; 41: 6631-9.

[141]   Srinivasan VB, Rajamohan G, Gebreyes WA. Role of AbeS, a novel efflux pump of the SMR family of transporters, in resistance to antimicrobial agents in *Acinetobacter baumannii*. Antimicrob Agents Chemother 2009; 53: 5312-6.

[142]   Morita Y, Kodama K, Shiota S, *et al.* NorM, a putative multidrug efflux protein, of *Vibrio parahaemolyticus* and its homolog in *Escherichia coli*. Antimicrob Agents Chemother 1998; 42: 1778-82.

[143]   Kuroda T, Tsuchiya T. Multidrug efflux transporters in the MATE family. Biochim Biophys Acta 2009; 1794: 763-8.

[144]   Begum A, Rahman MM, Ogawa W, *et al.* Gene cloning and characterization of four MATE family multidrug efflux pumps from *Vibrio cholerae* non-O1. Microbiol Immunol 2005; 49: 949-57.

[145]   Mohanty P, Patel A, Kushwaha Bhardwaj A. Role of H- and D- MATE-type transporters from multidrug resistant clinical isolates of *Vibrio fluvialis* in conferring fluoroquinolone resistance. PLoS One 2012; 7: e35752.

[146]   Bornet C, Chollet R, Mallea M, *et al.* Imipenem and expression of multidrug efflux pump in *Enterobacter aerogenes*. Biochem Biophys Res Commun 2003; 301: 985-90.

[147]   Nakae T. Identification of the outer membrane protein of *E. coli* that produces transmembrane channels in reconstituted vesicle membranes. Biochem Biophys Res Commun 1976; 71: 877-84.

[148]   Harder KJ, Nikaido H, Matsuhashi M. Mutants of *Escherichia coli* that are resistant to certain beta-lactam compounds lack the *ompF* porin. Antimicrob Agents Chemother 1981; 20: 549-52.

[149]   Sanbongi Y, Shimizu A, Suzuki T, *et al.* Classification of OprD sequence and correlation with antimicrobial activity of carbapenem agents in *Pseudomonas aeruginosa* clinical isolates collected in Japan. Microbiol Immunol 2009; 53: 361-7.

[150]   Kohler T, Michea-Hamzehpour M, Henze U, *et al.* Characterization of MexE-MexF-OprN, a positively regulated multidrug efflux system of *Pseudomonas aeruginosa*. Mol Microbiol 1997; 23: 345-54.

[151]   Pagel M, Simonet V, Li J, *et al.* Phenotypic characterization of pore mutants of the *Vibrio cholerae* porin OmpU. J Bacteriol 2007; 189: 8593-600.

[152]   Ochs MM, Bains M, Hancock RE. Role of putative loops 2 and 3 in imipenem passage through the specific porin OprD of *Pseudomonas aeruginosa*. Antimicrob Agents Chemother 2000; 44: 1983-5.

[153]   Huang H, Jeanteur D, Pattus F, *et al.* Membrane topology and site-specific mutagenesis of *Pseudomonas aeruginosa* porin OprD. Mol Microbiol 1995; 16: 931-41.

[154] Vettoretti L, Plesiat P, Muller C, *et al.* Efflux unbalance in *Pseudomonas aeruginosa* isolates from cystic fibrosis patients. Antimicrob Agents Chemother 2009; 53: 1987-97.

[155] Olliver A, Valle M, Chaslus-Dancla E, *et al.* Overexpression of the multidrug efflux operon *acrEF* by insertional activation with IS1 or IS10 elements in *Salmonella enterica* serovar *typhimurium* DT204 *acrB* mutants selected with fluoroquinolones. Antimicrob Agents Chemother 2005; 49: 289-301.

[156] Walker RC. The fluoroquinolones. Mayo Clin Proc 1999; 74: 1030-7.

[157] Saravanos K, Duff P. The quinolone antibiotics. Obstet Gynecol Clin North Am 1992; 19: 529-37.

[158] Brown SA. Fluoroquinolones in animal health. J Vet Pharmacol Ther 1996; 19: 1-14.

[159] Bolon MK. The newer fluoroquinolones. Med Clin North Am 2011; 95: 793-817.

[160] Andriole VT. The quinolones: past, present, and future. Clin Infect Dis 2005; 41 Suppl 2: S113-9.

[161] Van Bambeke F, Michot JM, Van Eldere J, *et al.* Quinolones in 2005: an update. Clin Microbiol Infect 2005; 11: 256-80.

[162] Drlica K, Zhao X. DNA gyrase, topoisomerase IV, and the 4-quinolones. Microbiol Mol Biol Rev 1997; 61: 377-92.

[163] Ball P. Quinolone generations: natural history or natural selection? J Antimicrob Chemother 2000; 46 Suppl T1: 17-24.

[164] O'Donnell JA, Gelone SP. The newer fluoroquinolones. Infect Dis Clin North Am 2004; 18: 691-716, x.

[165] Watson JD, Baker TA, Bell SP *et al.* Molecular biology of the gene, 5th ed.; Cold Spring Harbour Laboratory Press 2004; pp. 115-22

[166] Shen LL, Kohlbrenner WE, Weigl D, *et al.* Mechanism of quinolone inhibition of DNA gyrase. Appearance of unique norfloxacin binding sites in enzyme-DNA complexes. J Biol Chem 1989; 264: 2973-8.

[167] Kampranis SC, Maxwell A. The DNA gyrase-quinolone complex. ATP hydrolysis and the mechanism of DNA cleavage. J Biol Chem 1998; 273: 22615-26.

[168] Morais Cabral JH, Jackson AP, Smith CV, *et al.* Crystal structure of the breakage-reunion domain of DNA gyrase. Nature 1997; 388: 903-6.

[169] Berger JM, Gamblin SJ, Harrison SC, *et al.* Structure and mechanism of DNA topoisomerase II. Nature 1996; 379: 225-32.

[170] Laponogov I, Sohi MK, Veselkov DA, *et al.* Structural insight into the quinolone-DNA cleavage complex of type IIA topoisomerases. Nat Struct Mol Biol 2009; 16: 667-9.

[171] Laponogov I, Pan XS, Veselkov DA, *et al.* Structural basis of gate-DNA breakage and resealing by type II topoisomerases. PLoS One 2010; 5: e11338.

[172] Bax BD, Chan PF, Eggleston DS, *et al.* Type IIA topoisomerase inhibition by a new class of antibacterial agents. Nature 2010; 466: 935-40.

[173] Wohlkonig A, Chan PF, Fosberry AP, *et al.* Structural basis of quinolone inhibition of type IIA topoisomerases and target-mediated resistance. Nat Struct Mol Biol 2010; 17: 1152-3.

[174] Drlica K, Hiasa H, Kerns R, *et al.* Quinolones: action and resistance updated. Curr Top Med Chem 2009; 9: 981-98.

[175] Malik M, Zhao X, Drlica K. Lethal fragmentation of bacterial chromosomes mediated by DNA gyrase and quinolones. Mol Microbiol 2006; 61: 810-25.

[176]   Ikeda H, Aoki K, Naito A. Illegitimate recombination mediated *in vitro* by DNA gyrase of *Escherichia coli*: structure of recombinant DNA molecules. Proc Natl Acad Sci USA 1982; 79: 3724-8.

[177]   Ikeda H, Kawasaki I, Gellert M. Mechanism of illegitimate recombination: common sites for recombination and cleavage mediated by *E. coli* DNA gyrase. Mol Gen Genet 1984; 196: 546-9.

[178]   Collin F, Karkare S, Maxwell A. Exploiting bacterial DNA gyrase as a drug target: current state and perspectives. Appl Microbiol Biotechnol 2011; 92: 479-97.

[179]   Dwyer DJ, Kohanski MA, Hayete B, *et al*. Gyrase inhibitors induce an oxidative damage cellular death pathway in *Escherichia coli*. Mol Syst Biol 2007; 3: 91.

[180]   Kohanski MA, Dwyer DJ, Collins JJ. How antibiotics kill bacteria: from targets to networks. Nat Rev Microbiol 2010; 8: 423-35.

[181]   Kohanski MA, Dwyer DJ, Hayete B, *et al*. A common mechanism of cellular death induced by bactericidal antibiotics. Cell 2007; 130: 797-810.

[182]   Jacoby GA. Mechanisms of resistance to quinolones. Clin Infect Dis 2005; 41 Suppl 2: S120-6.

[183]   Hernandez A, Sanchez MB, Martinez JL. Quinolone resistance: much more than predicted. Front Microbiol 2011; 2: 22.

[184]   Robicsek A, Strahilevitz J, Jacoby GA, *et al*. Fluoroquinolone-modifying enzyme: a new adaptation of a common aminoglycoside acetyltransferase. Nat Med 2006; 12: 83-8.

[185]   Perichon B, Courvalin P, Galimand M. Transferable resistance to aminoglycosides by methylation of G1405 in 16S rRNA and to hydrophilic fluoroquinolones by QepA-mediated efflux in *Escherichia coli*. Antimicrob Agents Chemother 2007; 51: 2464-9.

[186]   Yamane K, Wachino J, Suzuki S, *et al*. New plasmid-mediated fluoroquinolone efflux pump, QepA, found in an *Escherichia coli* clinical isolate. Antimicrob Agents Chemother 2007; 51: 3354-60.

[187]   Sanders CC. Mechanisms responsible for cross-resistance and dichotomous resistance among the quinolones. Clin Infect Dis 2001; 32 Suppl 1: S1-8.

[188]   Yoshida H, Bogaki M, Nakamura M, *et al*. Quinolone resistance-determining region in the DNA gyrase *gyrA* gene of *Escherichia coli*. Antimicrob Agents Chemother 1990; 34: 1271-2.

[189]   Kakinuma Y, Maeda Y, Mason C, *et al*. Molecular characterisation of the quinolone resistance-determining regions (QRDR) including *gyrA*, *gyrB*, *parC* and *parE* genes in *Streptococcus pneumoniae*. Br J Biomed Sci 2012; 69: 123-5.

[190]   Dougherty TJ, Beaulieu D, Barrett JF. New quinolones and the impact on resistance. Drug Discov Today 2001; 6: 529-36.

[191]   Bearden DT, Danziger LH. Mechanism of action of and resistance to quinolones. Pharmacotherapy 2001; 21: 224S-32S.

[192]   Fu Y, Zhang W, Wang H, *et al*. Specific patterns of *gyrA* mutations determine the resistance difference to ciprofloxacin and levofloxacin in *Klebsiella pneumoniae* and *Escherichia coli*. BMC Infect Dis 2013; 13: 8.

[193]   Chowdhury G, Pazhani GP, Nair GB, *et al*. Transferable plasmid-mediated quinolone resistance in association with extended-spectrum beta-lactamases and fluoroquinolone-acetylating aminoglycoside-6'-N-acetyltransferase in clinical isolates of *Vibrio fluvialis*. Int J Antimicrob Agents 2011; 38: 169-73.

[194] Heddle J, Maxwell A. Quinolone-binding pocket of DNA gyrase: role of GyrB. Antimicrob Agents Chemother 2002; 46: 1805-15.

[195] Drlica K, Zhao X. Mutant selection window hypothesis updated. Clin Infect Dis 2007; 44: 681-8.

[196] Eliopoulos GM, Gardella A, Moellering RC, Jr. *In vitro* activity of ciprofloxacin, a new carboxyquinoline antimicrobial agent. Antimicrob Agents Chemother 1984; 25: 331-5.

[197] Li X, Zhao X, Drlica K. Selection of *Streptococcus pneumoniae* mutants having reduced susceptibility to moxifloxacin and levofloxacin. Antimicrob Agents Chemother 2002; 46: 522-4.

[198] Wang H, Dzink-Fox JL, Chen M, *et al.* Genetic characterization of highly fluoroquinolone-resistant clinical *Escherichia coli* strains from China: role of *acrR* mutations. Antimicrob Agents Chemother 2001; 45: 1515-21.

[199] Cohen SP, McMurry LM, Hooper DC, *et al.* Cross-resistance to fluoroquinolones in multiple-antibiotic-resistant (Mar) *Escherichia coli* selected by tetracycline or chloramphenicol: decreased drug accumulation associated with membrane changes in addition to OmpF reduction. Antimicrob Agents Chemother 1989; 33: 1318-25.

[200] Alekshun MN, Levy SB. Regulation of chromosomally mediated multiple antibiotic resistance: the *mar* regulon. Antimicrob Agents Chemother 1997; 41: 2067-75.

[201] Cohen SP, Yan W, Levy SB. A multidrug resistance regulatory chromosomal locus is widespread among enteric bacteria. J Infect Dis 1993; 168: 484-8.

[202] Morita Y, Kataoka A, Shiota S, *et al.* NorM of *Vibrio parahaemolyticus* is an Na(+)-driven multidrug efflux pump. J Bacteriol 2000; 182: 6694-7.

[203] Cattoir V, Poirel L, Nordmann P. Plasmid-mediated quinolone resistance pump QepA2 in an *Escherichia coli* isolate from France. Antimicrob Agents Chemother 2008; 52: 3801-4.

[204] Hansen LH, Johannesen E, Burmolle M, *et al.* Plasmid-encoded multidrug efflux pump conferring resistance to olaquindox in *Escherichia coli*. Antimicrob Agents Chemother 2004; 48: 3332-7.

[205] Hansen LH, Sorensen SJ, Jorgensen HS, *et al.* The prevalence of the OqxAB multidrug efflux pump amongst olaquindox-resistant *Escherichia coli* in pigs. Microb Drug Resist 2005; 11: 378-82.

[206] Hansen LH, Jensen LB, Sorensen HI, *et al.* Substrate specificity of the OqxAB multidrug resistance pump in *Escherichia coli* and selected enteric bacteria. J Antimicrob Chemother 2007; 60: 145-7.

[207] Kim ES, Jeong JY, Choi SH, *et al.* Plasmid-mediated fluoroquinolone efflux pump gene, *qepA*, in *Escherichia coli* clinical isolates in Korea. Diagn Microbiol Infect Dis 2009; 65: 335-8.

[208] Ma J, Zeng Z, Chen Z, *et al.* High prevalence of plasmid-mediated quinolone resistance determinants *qnr, aac(6')-Ib-cr,* and *qepA* among ceftiofur-resistant *Enterobacteriaceae* isolates from companion and food-producing animals. Antimicrob Agents Chemother 2009; 53: 519-24.

[209] Amin AK, Wareham DW. Plasmid-mediated quinolone resistance genes in *Enterobacteriaceae* isolates associated with community and nosocomial urinary tract infection in East London, UK. Int J Antimicrob Agents 2009; 34: 490-1.

[210] Rodriguez-Martinez JM, Cano ME, Velasco C, *et al.* Plasmid-mediated quinolone resistance: an update. J Infect Chemother 2011; 17: 149-82.

[211] Strahilevitz J, Jacoby GA, Hooper DC, *et al.* Plasmid-mediated quinolone resistance: a multifaceted threat. Clin Microbiol Rev 2009; 22: 664-89.

[212] Vetting MW, Hegde SS, Fajardo JE, *et al.* Pentapeptide repeat proteins. Biochemistry 2006; 45: 1-10.

[213] Tran JH, Jacoby GA. Mechanism of plasmid-mediated quinolone resistance. Proc Natl Acad Sci USA 2002; 99: 5638-42.

[214] Tran JH, Jacoby GA, Hooper DC. Interaction of the plasmid-encoded quinolone resistance protein Qnr with *Escherichia coli* DNA gyrase. Antimicrob Agents Chemother 2005; 49: 118-25.

[215] Tran JH, Jacoby GA, Hooper DC. Interaction of the plasmid-encoded quinolone resistance protein QnrA with *Escherichia coli* topoisomerase IV. Antimicrob Agents Chemother 2005; 49: 3050-2.

[216] Poirel L, Rodriguez-Martinez JM, Mammeri H, *et al.* Origin of plasmid-mediated quinolone resistance determinant QnrA. Antimicrob Agents Chemother 2005; 49: 3523-5.

[217] Jacoby G, Cattoir V, Hooper D, *et al. qnr* Gene nomenclature. Antimicrob Agents Chemother 2008; 52: 2297-9.

[218] Saga T, Kaku M, Onodera Y, *et al. Vibrio parahaemolyticus* chromosomal *qnr* homologue VPA0095: demonstration by transformation with a mutated gene of its potential to reduce quinolone susceptibility in *Escherichia coli*. Antimicrob Agents Chemother 2005; 49: 2144-5.

[219] Kim HB, Wang M, Ahmed S, *et al.* Transferable quinolone resistance in *Vibrio cholerae*. Antimicrob Agents Chemother 2010; 54: 799-803.

[220] Heddle JG, Blance SJ, Zamble DB, *et al.* The antibiotic microcin B17 is a DNA gyrase poison: characterisation of the mode of inhibition. J Mol Biol 2001; 307: 1223-34.

[221] Garrido MC, Herrero M, Kolter R, *et al.* The export of the DNA replication inhibitor Microcin B17 provides immunity for the host cell. Embo J 1988; 7: 1853-62.

[222] Srinivasan VB, Virk RK, Kaundal A, *et al.* Mechanism of drug resistance in clonally related clinical isolates of *Vibrio fluvialis* isolated in Kolkata, India. Antimicrob Agents Chemother 2006; 50: 2428-32.

[223] Rushdy AA, Mabrouk MI, Abu-Sef FA, *et al.* Contribution of different mechanisms to the resistance to fluoroquinolones in clinical isolates of *Salmonella enterica*. Braz J Infect Dis 2013; 17: 431-7.

[224] Zhu JM, Jiang RJ, Kong HS, *et al.* Emergence of novel variants of *gyrA, parC, qnrS* genes in multi-drug resistant *Klebsiella* caused pneumonia. Zhonghua Liu Xing Bing Xue Za Zhi 2013; 34: 61-6.

[225] Gould IM, Bal AM. New antibiotic agents in the pipeline and how they can help overcome microbial resistance. Virulence 2013; 4: 185-91.

[226] Baharoglu Z, Mazel D. *Vibrio cholerae* triggers SOS and mutagenesis in response to a wide range of antibiotics: a route towards multiresistance. Antimicrob Agents Chemother 2011; 55: 2438-41.

[227] Da Re S, Garnier F, Guerin E, *et al.* The SOS response promotes *qnrB* quinolone-resistance determinant expression. EMBO Rep 2009; 10: 929-33.

[228] Moura A, Soares M, Pereira C, *et al.* INTEGRALL: a database and search engine for integrons, integrases and gene cassettes. Bioinformatics 2009; 25: 1096-8.

[229] Joss MJ, Koenig JE, Labbate M, *et al.* ACID: annotation of cassette and integron data. BMC Bioinformatics 2009; 10: 118.

[230] Tsafnat G, Copty J, Partridge SR. RAC: Repository of Antibiotic resistance Cassettes. Database (Oxford) 2011; 2011: bar054.

[231] Liu B, Pop M. ARDB--Antibiotic Resistance Genes Database. Nucleic Acids Res 2009; 37: D443-7.

[232] Siguier P, Perochon J, Lestrade L, *et al.* ISfinder: the reference centre for bacterial insertion sequences. Nucleic Acids Res 2006; 34: D32-6.

[233] Yoon SH, Park YK, Lee S, *et al.* Towards pathogenomics: a web-based resource for pathogenicity islands. Nucleic Acids Res 2007; 35: D395-400.

[234] Lima-Mendez G, Van Helden J, Toussaint A, *et al.* Reticulate representation of evolutionary and functional relationships between phage genomes. Mol Biol Evol 2008; 25: 762-77.

[235] Leplae R, Lima-Mendez G, Toussaint A. ACLAME: a CLAssification of Mobile genetic Elements, update 2010. Nucleic Acids Res 2010; 38: D57-61.

[236] Shao Y, Harrison EM, Bi D, *et al.* TADB: a web-based resource for Type 2 toxin-antitoxin loci in bacteria and archaea. Nucleic Acids Res 2011; 39: D606-11.

[237] Saier MH, Jr., Tran CV, Barabote RD. TCDB: the Transporter Classification Database for membrane transport protein analyses and information. Nucleic Acids Res 2006; 34: D181-6.

[238] Boulund F, Johnning A, Pereira MB, *et al.* A novel method to discover fluoroquinolone antibiotic resistance (*qnr*) genes in fragmented nucleotide sequences. BMC Genomics 2012; 13: 695.

[239] Fazil MH, Singh DV. *Vibrio cholerae* infection, novel drug targets and phage therapy. Future Microbiol 2011; 6: 1199-208

[240] Phillips JW, Goetz MA, Smith SK, *et al.* Discovery of kibdelomycin, a potent new class of bacterial type II topoisomerase inhibitor by chemical-genetic profiling in *Staphylococcus aureus.* Chem Biol 2011; 18: 955-65.

[241] Katara P, Grover A, Kuntal H, *et al. In silico* prediction of drug targets in *Vibrio cholerae.* Protoplasma 2011; 248: 799-804.

[242] Barh D, Kumar A, Misra AN. Genomic Target Database (GTD): a database of potential targets in human pathogenic bacteria. Bioinformation 2010; 4: 50-1.

[243] Keen EC. Phage therapy: concept to cure. Frontiers Microbiol 2012; 3:1-3.

[244] Marcuk LM, Nikiforov VN, Scerbak JF, *et al.* Clinical studies of the use of bacteriophage in the treatment of cholera. Bull World Health Organ 1971; 45: 77-83.

[245] Häusler T, Viruses *vs* superbugs : a solution to the antibiotics crisis? Macmillan 2006; pp. 248-60.

[246] Levine MM, Nalin DR, Craig JP, *et al.* Immunity of cholera in man: relative role of antibacterial *versus* antitoxic immunity. Trans R Soc Trop Med Hyg 1979; 73: 3-9.

[247] Holmgren J, Clemens J, Sack DA, *et al.* New cholera vaccines. Vaccine 1989; 7: 94-6.

[248] Cholera, 2012. Wkly Epidemiol Rec 2013; 88: 321-34.

[249] Stephens DS, Zughaier SM, Whitney CG, *et al.* Incidence of macrolide resistance in *Streptococcus pneumonia*e after introduction of the pneumococcal conjugate vaccine: population-based assessment. Lancet 2005; 365: 855-63.

[250] Kyaw MH, Lynfield R, Schaffner W, *et al.* Effect of introduction of the pneumococcal conjugate vaccine on drug-resistant *Streptococcus pneumoniae.* N Engl J Med 2006; 354: 1455-63.

[251] Bhardwaj AK, Vinothkumar K, Rajpara N. Bacterial quorum sensing inhibitors: attractive alternatives for control of infectious pathogens showing multiple drug resistance. Recent Pat Antiinfect Drug Discov 2013; 8: 68-83.

[252] Williams P. Quorum sensing, communication and cross-kingdom signalling in the bacterial world. Microbiology 2007; 153: 3923-38.

[253] Lowery CA, Dickerson TJ, Janda KD. Interspecies and interkingdom communication mediated by bacterial quorum sensing. Chem Soc Rev 2008; 37: 1337-46.

[254] Jayaraman A, Wood TK. Bacterial quorum sensing: signals, circuits, and implications for biofilms and disease. Annu Rev Biomed Eng 2008; 10: 145-67.

[255] Ji G, Beavis R, Novick RP. Bacterial interference caused by autoinducing peptide variants. Science 1997; 276: 2027-30.

[256] Gov Y, Borovok I, Korem M, *et al.* Quorum sensing in *Staphylococci* is regulated *via* phosphorylation of three conserved histidine residues. J Biol Chem 2004; 279: 14665-72.

[257] Mylonakis E, Engelbert M, Qin X, *et al.* The *Enterococcus faecalis fsrB* gene, a key component of the *fsr* quorum-sensing system, is associated with virulence in the rabbit endophthalmitis model. Infect Immun 2002; 70: 4678-81.

[258] Wei Y, Perez LJ, Ng WL, *et al.* Mechanism of *Vibrio cholerae* autoinducer-1 biosynthesis. ACS Chem Biol 2011; 6: 356-65.

[259] Sintim HO, Smith JA, Wang J, *et al.* Paradigm shift in discovering next-generation anti-infective agents: targeting quorum sensing, c-di-GMP signaling and biofilm formation in bacteria with small molecules. Future Med Chem 2010; 2: 1005-35.

[260] Galloway WR, Hodgkinson JT, Bowden SD, *et al.* Quorum sensing in Gram-negative bacteria: small-molecule modulation of AHL and AI-2 quorum sensing pathways. Chem Rev 2011; 111: 28-67.

[261] Rasmussen TB, Givskov M. Quorum sensing inhibitors: a bargain of effects. Microbiology 2006; 152: 895-904.

[262] Fulghesu L, Giallorenzo C, Savoia D. Evaluation of different compounds as quorum sensing inhibitors in *Pseudomonas aeruginosa*. J Chemother 2007; 19: 388-91.

[263] Asad S, Opal SM. Bench-to-bedside review: Quorum sensing and the role of cell-to-cell communication during invasive bacterial infection. Crit Care 2008; 12: 236.

[264] Williams P, Winzer K, Chan WC, *et al.* Look who's talking: communication and quorum sensing in the bacterial world. Philos Trans R Soc Lond B Biol Sci 2007; 362: 1119-34.

[265] Dong YH, Wang LY, Zhang LH. Quorum-quenching microbial infections: mechanisms and implications. Philos Trans R Soc Lond B Biol Sci 2007; 362: 1201-11.

[266] Miller MB, Bassler BL. Quorum sensing in bacteria. Annu Rev Microbiol 2001; 55: 165-99.

[267] Rutherford ST, Bassler BL. Bacterial quorum sensing: its role in virulence and possibilities for its control. Cold Spring Harb Perspect Med 2012; 2(11).

[268] Pan J, Ren D. Quorum sensing inhibitors: a patent overview. Expert Opin Ther Pat 2009; 19: 1581-601.

[269] Chan YY, Chua KL. The *Burkholderia pseudomallei* BpeAB-OprB efflux pump: expression and impact on quorum sensing and virulence. J Bacteriol 2005; 187: 4707-19.

[270] Hoang TT, Schweizer HP. Characterization of *Pseudomonas aeruginosa* enoyl-acyl carrier protein reductase (FabI): a target for the antimicrobial triclosan and its role in acylated homoserine lactone synthesis. J Bacteriol 1999; 181: 5489-97.

[271] Stephenson K, Yamaguchi Y, Hoch JA. The mechanism of action of inhibitors of bacterial two-component signal transduction systems. J Biol Chem 2000; 275: 38900-4.

[272] Lyon GJ, Mayville P, Muir TW, *et al.* Rational design of a global inhibitor of the virulence response in *Staphylococcus aureus*, based in part on localization of the site of inhibition to the receptor-histidine kinase, AgrC. Proc Natl Acad Sci USA 2000; 97: 13330-5.

[273] Smith KM, Bu Y, Suga H. Induction and inhibition of *Pseudomonas aeruginosa* quorum sensing by synthetic autoinducer analogs. Chem Biol 2003; 10: 81-9.

[274] Suga H, BU Y. Combinatorial libraries of autoinducer analogs, autoinducer agonist and antagonist, and methods of use thereof. US20080027115 (2008).

[275] Suga H, Smith KM. Molecular mechanisms of bacterial quorum sensing as a new drug target. Curr Opin Chem Biol 2003; 7: 586-91.

[276] Guo M, Gamby S, Nakayama S, *et al.* A pro-drug approach for selective modulation of AI-2-mediated bacterial cell-to-cell communication. Sensors (Basel) 2012; 12: 3762-72.

[277] Ganin H, Tang X, Meijler MM. Inhibition of *Pseudomonas aeruginosa* quorum sensing by AI-2 analogs. Bioorg Med Chem Lett 2009; 19: 3941-4.

[278] Li M, Ni N, Chou HT, *et al.* Structure-based discovery and experimental verification of novel AI-2 quorum sensing inhibitors against *Vibrio harveyi*. ChemMedChem 2008; 3: 1242-9.

[279] Lowery CA, Park J, Kaufmann GF, *et al.* An unexpected switch in the modulation of AI-2-based quorum sensing discovered through synthetic 4, 5-dihydroxy-2, 3-pentanedione analogues. J Am Chem Soc 2008; 130: 9200-1.

[280] Smyth AR, Cifelli PM, Ortori CA, *et al.* Garlic as an inhibitor of *Pseudomonas aeruginosa* quorum sensing in cystic fibrosis--a pilot randomized controlled trial. Pediatr Pulmonol 2010; 45: 356-62.

[281] Jakobsen TH, van Gennip M, Phipps RK, *et al.* Ajoene, a sulfur-rich molecule from garlic, inhibits genes controlled by quorum sensing. Antimicrob Agents Chemother 2012; 56: 2314-25.

[282] McDowell P, Affas Z, Reynolds C, *et al.* Structure, activity and evolution of the group I thiolactone peptide quorum-sensing system of *Staphylococcus aureus*. Mol Microbiol 2001; 41: 503-12.

[283] Balaban N, Giacometti A, Cirioni O, *et al.* Use of the quorum-sensing inhibitor RNAIII-inhibiting peptide to prevent biofilm formation *in vivo* by drug-resistant *Staphylococcus epidermidis*. J Infect Dis 2003; 187: 625-30.

[284] Miyairi S, Tateda K, Fuse ET, *et al.* Immunization with 3-oxododecanoyl-L-homoserine lactone-protein conjugate protects mice from lethal *Pseudomonas aeruginosa* lung infection. J Med Microbiol 2006; 55: 1381-7.

[285] Tateda K, Standiford TJ, Pechere JC, *et al.* Regulatory effects of macrolides on bacterial virulence: potential role as quorum-sensing inhibitors. Curr Pharm Des 2004; 10: 3055-65.

[286] Skindersoe ME, Alhede M, Phipps R, *et al.* Effects of antibiotics on quorum sensing in *Pseudomonas aeruginosa*. Antimicrob Agents Chemother 2008; 52: 3648-63.

[287] Hung DT, Shakhnovich EA, Pierson E, *et al.* Small-molecule inhibitor of *Vibrio cholerae* virulence and intestinal colonization. Science 2005; 310: 670-4.

[288] Van Bambeke F, Pages JM, Lee VJ. Inhibitors of bacterial efflux pumps as adjuvants in antibiotic treatments and diagnostic tools for detection of resistance by efflux. Recent Pat Antiinfect Drug Discov 2006; 1: 157-75.

[289]   Zechini B, Versace I. Inhibitors of multidrug resistant efflux systems in bacteria. Recent Pat Antiinfect Drug Discov 2009; 4: 37-50.

[290]   Chopra I. New developments in tetracycline antibiotics: glycylcyclines and tetracycline efflux pump inhibitors. Drug Resist Updat 2002; 5: 119-25.

[291]   Chollet R, Chevalier J, Bryskier A, *et al.* The AcrAB-TolC pump is involved in macrolide resistance but not in telithromycin efflux in *Enterobacter aerogenes* and *Escherichia coli.* Antimicrob Agents Chemother 2004; 48: 3621-4.

[292]   Zgurskaya HI, Nikaido H. Multidrug resistance mechanisms: drug efflux across two membranes. Mol Microbiol 2000; 37: 219-25.

[293]   Yoshihara, E., Inoko, H. Method or agent for inhibiting the function of efflux pump in *Pseudomonas aeruginosa.* US7985410B2 (2011).

[294]   Kern WV, Oethinger M, Jellen-Ritter AS, *et al.* Non-target gene mutations in the development of fluoroquinolone resistance in *Escherichia coli.* Antimicrob Agents Chemother 2000; 44: 814-20.

[295]   Pages JM, Masi M, Barbe J. Inhibitors of efflux pumps in Gram-negative bacteria. Trends Mol Med 2005; 11: 382-9.

[296]   Mallea M, Chevalier J, Eyraud A, *et al.* Inhibitors of antibiotic efflux pump in resistant *Enterobacter aerogenes* strains. Biochem Biophys Res Commun 2002; 293: 1370-3.

[297]   Mahamoud A, Chevalier J, Alibert-Franco S, *et al.* Antibiotic efflux pumps in Gram-negative bacteria: the inhibitor response strategy. J Antimicrob Chemother 2007; 59: 1223-9.

[298]   Marquez B. Bacterial efflux systems and efflux pumps inhibitors. Biochimie 2005; 87: 1137-47.

[299]   Lynch AS. Efflux systems in bacterial pathogens: an opportunity for therapeutic intervention? An industry view. Biochem Pharmacol 2006; 71: 949-56.

[300]   Lomovskaya O, Bostian KA. Practical applications and feasibility of efflux pump inhibitors in the clinic--a vision for applied use. Biochem Pharmacol 2006; 71: 910-8.

[301]   Lomovskaya O, Warren MS, Lee A, *et al.* Identification and characterization of inhibitors of multidrug resistance efflux pumps in *Pseudomonas aeruginosa*: novel agents for combination therapy. Antimicrob Agents Chemother 2001; 45: 105-16.

[302]   Renau TE, Leger R, Flamme EM, *et al.* Inhibitors of efflux pumps in *Pseudomonas aeruginosa* potentiate the activity of the fluoroquinolone antibacterial levofloxacin. J Med Chem 1999; 42: 4928-31.

[303]   Coban AY, Ekinci B, Durupinar B. A multidrug efflux pump inhibitor reduces fluoroquinolone resistance in *Pseudomonas aeruginosa* isolates. Chemotherapy 2004; 50: 22-6.

[304]   Mamelli L, Amoros JP, Pages JM, *et al.* A phenylalanine-arginine beta-naphthylamide sensitive multidrug efflux pump involved in intrinsic and acquired resistance of *Campylobacter* to macrolides. Int J Antimicrob Agents 2003; 22: 237-41.

[305]   Hasdemir UO, Chevalier J, Nordmann P, *et al.* Detection and prevalence of active drug efflux mechanism in various multidrug-resistant *Klebsiella pneumoniae* strains from Turkey. J Clin Microbiol 2004; 42: 2701-6.

[306]   Mazzariol A, Tokue Y, Kanegawa TM, *et al.* High-level fluoroquinolone-resistant clinical isolates of *Escherichia coli* overproduce multidrug efflux protein AcrA. Antimicrob Agents Chemother 2000; 44: 3441-3.

[307]   Baucheron S, Imberechts H, Chaslus-Dancla E, *et al.* The AcrB multidrug transporter plays a major role in high-level fluoroquinolone resistance in *Salmonella enterica* serovar *typhimurium* phage type DT204. Microb Drug Resist 2002; 8: 281-9.

[308]   Renau TE, Leger R, Flamme EM, *et al.* Addressing the stability of C-capped dipeptide efflux pump inhibitors that potentiate the activity of levofloxacin in *Pseudomonas aeruginosa*. Bioorg Med Chem Lett 2001; 11: 663-7.

[309]   Renau TE, Leger R, Yen R, *et al.* Peptidomimetics of efflux pump inhibitors potentiate the activity of levofloxacin in *Pseudomonas aeruginosa*. Bioorg Med Chem Lett 2002; 12: 763-6.

[310]   Renau TE, Leger R, Filonova L, *et al.* Conformationally-restricted analogues of efflux pump inhibitors that potentiate the activity of levofloxacin in *Pseudomonas aeruginosa*. Bioorg Med Chem Lett 2003; 13: 2755-8.

[311]   Watkins WJ, Landaverry Y, Leger R, *et al.* The relationship between physicochemical properties, *in vitro* activity and pharmacokinetic profiles of analogues of diamine-containing efflux pump inhibitors. Bioorg Med Chem Lett 2003; 13: 4241-4.

[312]   Oethinger M, Levy SB. Methods of reducing microbial resistance to drugs. US6346391B1 (2002).

[313]   Oethinger, M., Levy S. B. Methods of screening for compounds that reduce microbial resistance to fluoroquinolones. US8012711B2 (2011).

[314]   Chun CK, Ozer EA, Welsh MJ, *et al.* Inactivation of a *Pseudomonas aeruginosa* quorum-sensing signal by human airway epithelia. Proc Natl Acad Sci USA 2004; 101: 3587-90.

[315]   Finch R, Hunter PA. Antibiotic resistance--action to promote new technologies: report of an EU Intergovernmental Conference held in Birmingham, UK, 12-13 December 2005. J Antimicrob Chemother 2006; 58 Suppl 1: i3-i22.

CHAPTER 3

Applications for Virus Vaccine Vectors in Infectious Disease Research

Kathleen L. Hefferon[*]

Cornell University, Ithaca, NY 14886, USA

Abstract: As basic knowledge regarding the molecular biology of viruses and their interactions with their hosts improves, virus expression vectors increase in sophistication and their applications in the field of medicine broadens. Virus expression vectors have been used as research tools for generating vaccines and have functioned as delivery vehicles for siRNAs, antiviral agents, and other drug candidates. In this review, vectors based on poxvirus, adeno-associated virus, lentivirus and plant viruses are discussed and examples of their applications are provided. Recent innovations with respect to the use of virus expression vectors for the delivery of vaccines or for passive immunization against infectious diseases are outlined. The review concludes with a summary of the current successes and the future challenges that must be addressed for virus vaccine vectors to be utilized for research and medical treatment purposes in the years to come.

Keywords: Adeno-associated virus, HIV-1, immune response, infectious disease, lentivirus, plant virus, poxvirus, vaccine, virus expression vector.

INTRODUCTION

Over the past decade, virus expression vectors have been developed from their wild type counterparts and are playing a role in gene therapy and vaccine development. More recently, these viral vectors have been optimized further to maximize the host immune response, resulting in an effective approach to target cancer cells and a variety of difficulties to treat infectious diseases, including HIV-1/AIDS. At the same time, virus vaccine vectors must be safe enough to use in humans and animals without adverse effects, such as illegitimate recombination events, high toxicity and unwanted virus vector backbone- induced immune

---

*Corresponding Author Kathleen L. Hefferon: Cornell University, Ithaca, NY 14886, USA;
Tel: (607) 387-6304; Fax: (607) 387-6304; E-mail: klh22@cornell.edu

Atta-ur-Rahman / M. Iqbal Choudhary (Eds.)

responses due to pre-existing immunity to the virus in the human population [1]. It is how this vector introduces antigens to specific points of the immune system which determines its efficacy and potency as a vaccine.

Adenovirus expression vectors have been crucial for the development of virus expression vectors for gene therapy as well as for vaccine development. The recent literature relating to adenovirus and other vector strategies is vast and will not be included in this review [2-6]. This review sets out instead to describe some of the most recent studies that have been performed with poxvirus, adeno-associated virus and lentivirus vectors, as well as a plant virus vector derived from Tobacco mosaic virus. The review describes the advantages and hurdles to be addressed by each vaccine vector and concludes with a discussion of the intricacies of virus vaccine vectors and the host immune response as the basis for the next generation of future vaccines to fight infectious diseases.

POXVIRUS VACCINE VECTORS

Poxviruses are double stranded DNA viruses with large, linear genomes that encode many genes and are restricted to the cytoplasm of infected cells. Poxviruses were among the earliest animal viruses to be engineered as gene transfer vectors, and the first heterologous proteins were expressed in vaccinia virus in the early 1980s [7, 8] (Fig. **1**). A number of features make poxviruses excellent vaccine vectors. Among these are the fact that gene expression takes place in the cytoplasm rather than in the nucleus, and the flexibility of the genome to both incorporate large inserts as well as function with substantial amounts of deleted viral DNA without a loss of infectivity. Since smallpox has been eradicated and the vaccine is no longer in use, the general populace should not be affected by pre-existing anti-vector immunity from previous vaccinations. It should be noted that individuals who are immunocompromised are at risk for severe side effects as a result of smallpox vaccination, and thus are an exception to this rule. In addition to this, vaccine proteins expressed in poxviruses appear to induce a strong cytotoxic T cell response [9]. Two different attenuated vaccinia virus strains have been developed as expression vectors; MVA and NYVAC. MVA is derived from a smallpox strain from Turkey known as chorioallantoid vaccinia virus Ankara (CVA). This attenuated strain is missing about 30 kb of its wild type genome. The other attenuated strain, NYVAC, was developed from the Copenhagen vaccine strain (VACV-COP) by the exact removal of eighteen open reading frames that are believed to be involved in pathogenicity and virulence [10]. Other zoonotic viruses such as the closely related canarypox and recombinant fowl pox virus have been shown to be safe in humans and are now used to generate vaccines against other infectious diseases such as tuberculosis [11-13]. Recombinant fowl pox virus is also known to be an excellent mucosal delivery vector [14, 15]. Similarly, aerosol delivery of NYVAC, MVA have also been tested [16]. Some of these have been further modified to extend their host range to include Vero cells, for example, which are most often used for vaccine manufacture. Other studies include the application of an mRNA-Seq transcriptome profiling to further understand the mechanisms behind the immune response to poxvirus produced vaccines [17, 18]. Lauterbach *et al.* (2013) attempted to improve upon the CD8 T cell inducing capacity of the MVA strain of vaccinia virus by adjuvanting the viral genome with a coding sequence of murine CD40L, derived from the tumour necrosis factor superfamily [18]. This improved vector was demonstrated in mice to improve the CD8 T cell response, and more strongly activate dendritic cells, cytotoxic T cells and cytokines, suggesting that this vector could be superior in protecting against specific infectious diseases.

Vaccinia vectors have also been modified to assist in vaccine delivery. Replication competent vectors have been designed by adding an inducible expressed IFN-γ [19]. This SMART (safety mechanism assisted by the repressor of tetracycline) vector system operates under a tetracycline inducible vaccinia promoter and acts as a safety mechanism for controlling vaccinia replication when the vector is used for vaccine or oncolytic cancer therapy. Similarly, genes essential for viral growth can be placed under transcriptional repression by placing the vaccinia early transcription factor, (VETF) under the control of the tet operon. Virus replication, then, becomes dependent upon addition of the antibiotic tetracycline or its derivatives and any adverse reactions could be dealt with easily simply by removal of the antibiotic [20].

Vaccinia has also been used as an antibody discovery platform to express a library of human antibodies on its surface, with one specific type of antibody per virion.

Specific antibodies can then be selected in a manner analogous to phage display, as a rapid and high-throughput selection technique for antibody selection [21].

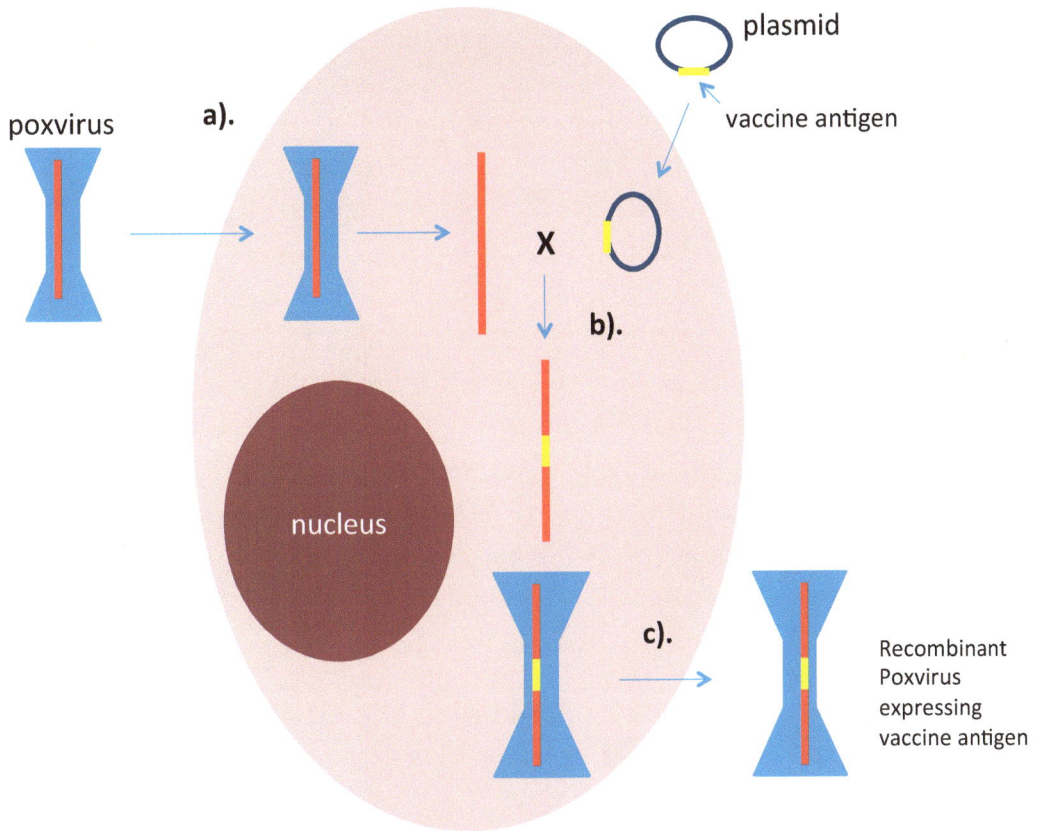

Fig. (1). Vaccine based on poxvirus vector. **a**). Poxvirus and plasmid construct containing both poxvirus sequences and vaccine antigen are transduced into host cell. **b**). A recombination event takes place between the two and results in a recombinant poxvirus harboring the vaccine antigen. **c**) Recombinant poxvirus assembly and exit from cell.

Poxvirus Vectors as Vaccines against HIV

Avipoxviruses (APVs) are found around the world and infect many species of birds by transmission *via* aerosols or insects [11]. The fact that APVs do not produce progeny viruses in mammalian cells and can accommodate large inserts makes them attractive alternatives for vaccine expression vector development [17]. A number of these, including Fowlpox virus (FWPV) and Canarypox virus (ALVAC) have been used in viral vaccine vector development. The most well known use for avipoxvirus as an expression vector has been in vaccine development for prevention against HIV/AIDS [22]. The phase III clinical trial known as RV144 advanced the possibility that a vaccine to HIV could in fact be realized. The trial was conducted in Thailand in 2009 and included 16,402 healthy volunteers [23, 24]. Four doses of ALVAC expressing gag, pol, env and a modified form of gp120 were evaluated in the form of a prime boost. The results of this study demonstrated that 31.2% fewer volunteers from the vaccine group were infected by HIV-1 than volunteers derived from the placebo group. This modest but encouraging protection provided the first glimpse of the potential dream of a vaccine for HIV/AIDS [25]. A modified Ankara poxvirus vector derived from HIV-1 clade B (MVA-B) and expressing Env, Gag, Pol and Nef antigens is also being tested in clinical trials [26]. Not only was MVA-B safe and well tolerated, it induced strong T cell responses in 75% and antibody responses in 95% of uninfected volunteers [27]. Further research is now underway to identify better vaccine candidates using poxviruses as vectors. Improvements include the selective removal of additional poxvirus genes and the addition of genes which broaden host range. A few of the more recent studies in this regard are described here.

More recently, poxviruses have been modified to be more effective at enhancing the cellular immune response. For example, Gomez *et al.*, (2012) analyzed the Ankara strain of poxvirus expressing the HIV-1 antigens Env/Gag-Pol-Nef of HIV-1 clade C, the world's most prevalent subtype [28]. These researchers examined the antiviral response, B and T cell response, cytokine release and antigen presentation in dendritic cells, CD4(+) and CD8(+) cells, as well as the immune memory response [26]. Similarly, Garcia-Arriaza *et al.*, (2013) investigated the immune response to a strain of poxvirus known as MVA-B expressing HIV-1 Env, Gag, Pol and Nef antigens from clade B. A phase I clinical trial in human healthy volunteers has demonstrated MVA-B to be safe and highly immunogenic, capable of sustaining long-lasting CD4(+) and CD8(+) T cell responses to HIV-1 antigens, with preference for memory T cells [29-34]. This trial triggered a predominance of antibodies highly specific to *Env* in most human subjects. The data collected from these clinical trials enabled research groups to create an immunogenicity profile of these candidate vaccine vectors and then to work towards improving upon them further. An example of this is illustrated by Garcia-Arriaza *et al.*, (2013) [35]. This research group constructed a vaccinia virus with deletions in genes coding for inhibitors of interferon signaling pathways. Poxvirus expression vectors containing these deletion mutants upregulated IFN-β and IFNα/β gene expression, in addition to the expression of other cytokines and chemokines. The authors further showed that these deletions blocked the intracellular signal pathway of IFN, thus improving many aspects of the immune response. In the case of MVA vaccines designed against clade B, deletion mutant MVA-B dN2L triggered an increased immune response to HIV antigens without affecting virus replication. The results found by these authors further demonstrated the immunomodulatory role of N2L in poxvirus infection [35].

In another study by Sato *et al.*, (2013), different promoters were used to test a vaccinia vector harboring the gag gene of SIV in a prime/ boost vaccination regimen. The authors determined that they could generate an expression vector that could produce more protein but replicate poorly and elicit long lasting Gag-specific T cells, thus providing a new vaccination strategy against infection [36].

Garcia-Arriza *et al.*, (2012), examined the effect of antiretroviral inhibitors on MVA-B. The most common antiretroviral inhibitors did not effect in any way the kinetics of MVA-B replication or vaccine protein expression [37].

Other Uses of Poxviruses as Expression Vectors

Poxviruses have been used as expression vectors for other purposes as well. For example, the oncolytic vaccina virus GLV-1h109 has been investigated as a novel approach for cancer therapy. Expression of a single-chain antibody to GLAF-1, specific for canine soft tissue sarcomas and prostate carcinomas in xenograft models, resulted in destroying the cancer cell lines [38]. Administration of this virus expression vector was determined to be safe and led to a significant reduction of tumor growth in comparison to mice used as controls.

Other recent examples for the use of poxvirus expression vectors include the generation of Foot-and-mouth disease virus (FMDV) virus- like particles as vaccines *via* a transient vaccinia expression system [39]. This poxvirus system enables viral proteins which are often toxic to the host cell when produced in other viral vectors to be expressed at high levels. Poxvirus has other uses in providing vaccination strategies as well. Different poxvirus vectors, when used in various prime or booster vaccine combinations, can cause different immune outcomes. For example, vectors such as adenovirus frequently cause a vector backbone-based immune response and thus can be limited in its use as a vaccine strategy. Mendes *et al.*, (2013), found that using the vaccinia virus Ankara expressing the parasite *Toxiplasma gondii* antigens as a heterologous prime boost with the adenovirus vector expressing the same antigen reduced this anti-vector immune response while at the same time controlled toxoplasmosis infection in an animal model [40]. Another example of a heterologous prime-boost vaccination strategy is that of the chimpanzee adenovirus ChAd63 along with the poxvirus MVA to combat malaria [41, 42]. Phase II trials using volunteers demonstrated the efficacy of this vaccination strategy [43-45]. Poxvirus vectors can also be improved to induce better immunity by other methods, including the co-expression of immune modulators in conjunction with the vaccine antigen. For example, an Ankara vaccinia virus vector co-expressing granulocyte-macrophage colony stimulating factor (GM-CSF) and SIV glycoprotein enhanced the avidity of SIV specific IgG, neutralizing antibody titres and antibody-dependent cellular cytotoxicity [46]. Furthermore, this co-expressed GM-CSF increased vaccine-induced prevention of infection from 25% for the vaccine group which lacked GM-CSF to 71% for the vaccine group co-expressing GM-CSF [46].

ADENO- ASSOCIATED VIRUS (AAV) VACCINE VECTORS

Adeno-associated virus has been utilized as a vaccine vector as well as for gene therapy. One of the first studies was conducted by Manning *et al.*, (1979), and involved using an AAV vector to induce a strong humoral and cellular response against glycoprotein B of Herpes simplex virus (HSV) type 1 [47]. Since then, many other researchers have explored the use of AAV vectors for genetic vaccination.

AAV offers a number of select advantages for use as vaccine vectors and related applications. AAV is inherently unable to replicate on its own, which provides an attractive safety profile for its use in gene therapy (Fig. **2a**). Since no viral genes are actually encoded by the AAV vector backbone, there is an overall absence of toxicity to the cell. AAV vaccine vectors are able to provide strong and long lasting immune responses, including CD8 (+) T cell responses, and this has been achieved in certain cases upon administration of only a single dosage [48-50]. Furthermore, AAV serotype 2 (AAV2) based transgenes can be packaged into capsids from other AAV serotypes, thus generating rAAV vectors with wide variations in tropism [51, 52]. However, AAV expression vectors have a number of drawbacks for vaccine development, including wide pre-existing immunity in human populations, virus stock preparations that are too low for easy administration, and limitations with respect to transgene capacity. The following section details some of the recent use of AAV vaccine vectors and some of the contributions that have been made to further understand their immunogenic properties.

a).

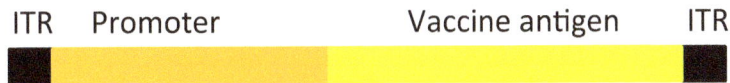

b).

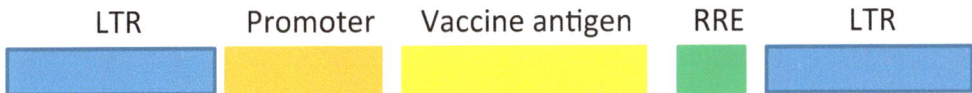

c).

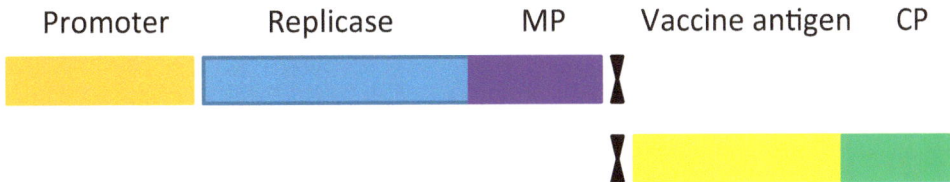

Fig. (2). Schematic diagram of virus vector backbones described in text. **a**) AAV vector backbone. ITR; inverted terminal repeat. **b**) LV vector backbones. LTR; Long Terminal Repeat, RRE, Rev Response Element. **c**) TMV vector backbone; MP; movement protein, CP, coat protein; hourglass represents site of recombination.

Ussher and Taylor, (2010) examined the ability of AAV to transduce dendritic cells, one of the antigen-presenting cells that plays a role in the immune response and thus stimulates T cell immunity [53]. The authors were able to engineer a recombinant AAV vector that was encapsidated with coat protein from AAV type 6. This pseudotyped vector was better able to target and infect human monocyte-derived dendritic cells (MoDCs) [54]. The capsid was genetically engineered through a mutation of Tyr-731, which further enhanced MoDC transduction of AAV6. These pseudotyped rAAV2/6 vectors could elicit a CD8(+) T cell clone specific for the antigen, indicating that modifications such as these could be useful for AAV vaccine vector development [53, 54].

AAV vectors have been utilized to express neutralizing antibodies *in vivo*. To ensure equimolar amounts of antibody components, these antibodies are produced as heavy and light chains that are linked by a self-processing peptide 2A of Foot and mouth disease virus [29]. This circumvents the need for multiple administrations of high doses of antibody that is often required for clinical efficacy. AAV vectors allow for the sustained and continuous expression of the neutralizing antibody at high levels after a single administration [55]. An example of how this strategy has been used is the AAV expression of a murine antibody against respiratory syncytial virus (RSV). Intrapleural administration of this vector resulted in the long-term production of anti-RSV neutralizing antibody in serum and lungs. The vaccine was able to partially protect the animals against virus challenge [56].

AAV has been used as a vector for a number of infectious diseases, a few selected examples are described here.

AAV Vectors to Combat HIV-1

Early studies using AAV vectors to express the HIV-1 antigens *env, tat* and *rev* in BALB/c mice resulted in high levels of serum IgG and fecal IgA production, in addition to a cytotoxic T cell response [57]. Similarly, Johnson *et al.* (2005), expressed several SIV genes (*rev-gag, rev-env,* and RT-IN) in an AAV vector that was injected intramuscularly [58]. Strong T cell and antibody responses were observed upon a single vaccination, and the animals were protected completely against intravenous challenge with low doses of SIV. Higher doses of SIV resulted in only partial protection.

Lin *et al.*, (2009), designed a chimeric AAV vector (AAVrh32.33) based on two rhesus macaque AAV strains [59, 60]. The AAVrh32.33 vector expressing Gag of HIV was injected into mice and elicited a strong CD8(+) T-cell response and high levels of Gag-specific antibodies. Macaques were administered with different vectors expressing gp140 and elicited an antibody and CD8 T cell response similar to the mice, suggesting that AAV may be a feasible HIV-1 vaccination platform [59, 60].

Further research studies have been conducted using recombinant AAV vaccines against HIV-1, and have been taken to the clinical trial stage [60, 61]. The vaccine vector tgAAC09, which encodes a number of HIV-1 gene products, was demonstrated to induce a strong immune response in monkeys [62]. Based on these results, a preliminary clinical trial consisting of 80 healthy adults showed that the vaccine is safe and presented no adverse effects. A second phase II study was also conducted involving 91 healthy Africans provided with one of three possible doses of tgAAC09. HIV-specific T cell responses were identified in 25% of the vaccine recipients with 38% of the responders originating from the highest dosage group [63].

Passive immunotherapy has also been used to provide an AAV vector based protection against HIV and SIV. Johnson and colleagues expressed imunoadhesins (IA) (antibody-like molecules) against SIV in macaques in a double-stranded AAV1 vector [64]. This research group demonstrated that intra-muscular injection of the AAV vector resulted in a high level of secretion of IA and provided long lasting neutralizing activity in serum; most animals were protected against infection with SIV and all animals in the study were protected against the disease. These initial efforts have been supported by Balazs *et al.*, (2012), who were able to protect humanized mice against very high doses of HIV with a single intra-muscular injection of an AAV8 vector expressing a monoclonal antibody against HIV [55].

AAV Vectors and other Infectious Diseases

AAV vectors have been generated which express HA, nucleoprotein and matrix proteins of a Mexican strain of pandemic influenza virus H1N1. A single injection of an AAV vector expressing these proteins resulted in full protection against challenge with homologous virus and partial protection against challenge with a heterologous and highly virulent strain of influenza [65]. Broadly neutralizing antibodies (bnAb) and immunoadhesins (IA), which bind to the conserved stem region of HA have been produced in AAV vectors for passive immunotherapy [66, 67]. One research group injected an AAV8 vector expressing bnAb to influenza virus HA intramuscularly in mice and ferrets and observed a long-term production of this antibody in serum which offered complete protection against five different influenza strains [37]. IA expressed from an AAV9 vector that was intranasally administered was observed to be localized to only the nose and lungs [67]. Since the nasal epithelia undergoes a natural turnover, the vector would not be present permanently in the body, an attractive feature for immunization. Animals expressing this vaccine vector were protected against challenge with different strains of influenza strains, and the time taken between AAV injection and challenge was determined to be as short as three days and yet remain effective [67].

Another example of the use of AAV vaccine vectors to treat infectious diseases is that of the henipaviruses, including nipahvirus (NiV) and hendravirus (HeV). These paramyxoviruses can be responsible for causing considerable morbidity and mortality in both humans and other mammals [68]. Currently, there is no adequate vaccine against henipavirus, thus they are considered to be potential biowarfare agents that could be utilized in acts of terrorism (48). AAV vectors have been engineered to express the G protein of nipahvirus, and mouse studies have demonstrated that a potent and sustained IgG response could be elicited using this approach. Furthermore, studies using hamsters showed that a single administration of the AAV vector expressing NiV G could protect all animals against lethal challenge with NiV and half of the animals against a challenge with HeV [69].

Li *et al.*, (2012) developed an AAV vector vaccine that expressed the Dengue fever virus carboxy-terminal truncated envelope protein known as 79E. Mice intramuscularly injected with the vaccine vector generated a sustained antibody response against Dengue virus that remained present 20 weeks post-immunization and was capable of neutralizing homogeneous viruses, indicating that AAV vectors could be considered for the future development of a Dengue vaccine [70].

Immunogenicity and Vaccine Vector Development

AAV vectors have the obvious advantage of providing safe and long lasting expression of vaccine proteins and antibodies at high levels *via* a single injection, while at the same time providing a low profile of vector immunogenicity [71]. This latter characteristic can be explained at least in part by the lack of functional CD8(+) T-cell based immunity found in natural AAV infections [71, 72]. However, this fact itself poses a problem for any form of vaccination which would require the induction of a strong cytotoxic T-cell response. The next step, therefore, would be to alter AAV in such a way that these immunogenic properties are enhanced. Since the immune response can vary so significantly between different serotypes of AAV, and since there are over 100 variants that have been identified so far, the manipulation of the capsid protein to produce new artificial variants with the necessary immunogenic profile seems to be one worthwhile approach to improving AAV vaccine vector immunogenicity [73]. For example, the new variant described earlier as AAVrh32.33, designed as a hybrid between two natural AAV rhesus macaque isolates, could induce a robust CD8C T-cell response directed against a selected antigen [59]. Further structural analysis was used to determine that this response was derived from a location within the viral capsid protein. This knowledge will be helpful for the design of future vaccine vectors which can selectively elicit a particular immune response.

Alternatively, AAV capsid proteins can be modified to express specific epitopes of infectious diseases, so that upon virus assembly, they can act as epitope presentation systems. An example of this vaccine vector strategy was demonstrated by the insertion of two neutralizing epitopes from the L2 protein of HPV16 and HPV31 into two different locations of one of the capsid proteins (VP3) [74, 75]. Virus-like particles assembled from these chimeric capsid proteins were then used to vaccinate mice and rabbits, and were shown to induce high levels of antibodies that had the capacity to cross neutralize several HPV serotypes. Nieto *et al.*, (2012) immunized rhesus macaques *via* intranasal administration with a recombinant AAV vector that expresses L1 of HPV16 and elicited L1-specific antibodies which were not only able to neutralize HPV16 pseudovirions, but also remained viable over 7 months post-inoculation, further implicating that AAV shows promise as a noninvasive nasal vaccination strategy [76]. Artificially designed AAV variants can also exhibit a much lower seroprevalence than natural serotypes, which are present in the vast majority of the world's population [77-80].

As another example, Rybniker *et al.*, (2012) demonstrated that genetic modification of AAV capsids for the display of the antigen Ag85A, a well-known target antigen used for *Mycobacterium tuberculosis* vaccines, resulted in an increase in antigen-specific immunogenicity. The authors combined peptide display with vector-based production of the same antigen and found that they could achieve a significantly faster immune response in a single inoculation [73].

LENTIVIRUS VACCINE VECTORS

Lentiviruses, a genus of the retroviruses including HIV-1 and SIV, are RNA viruses which contain a reverse transcriptase and have the ability to integrate a cDNA copy of their genome into the host chromosome. Lentiviruses have also been successfully used to activate cellular immunity and humoral responses against vaccine antigens. Lentiviruses can infect dendritic cells and other antigen presenting cells, thus making them effective vectors to target a broad range of different cancers and infectious diseases [81-83]. Their capacity to encode fairly large transgenes that can be transduced into both dividing and nondividing cells, and then become integrated into the host genome makes lentiviruses attractive as delivery vehicles for vaccines and therapeutic proteins [84, 85].

Lentivirus vectors (LVs) today are commonly derived from HIV-1 and have been genetically modified to increase efficacy and safety [86] (Fig. **2b**). For example, viral genes which are nonessential for vector function such as *vif, vpr, nef,* and *vpu* are often removed. Hybrid constructs utilizing CMV/LTR and codon optimization have also resulted in an increase in efficacy of vector production. As a further safety measure, LVs have been developed which are self-inactivating, through the generation of deletions in the transcriptional activation unit of the 3' LTR's U3 region. Today's LVs also contain a rev-responsive element (RRE) which binds to the rev protein and enables the viral genome to be exported from the nucleus. A polypurine tract has been included in the polymerase open reading frame to improve nuclear import of the proviral DNA [87]. microRNAs have also been included to assist in suppressing unwanted immune responses [88, 89]. The risk of insertional mutagenesis has been addressed through the creation of integration-deficient LVs, or IDLVs (these vectors have a defective integrase function or disabled attachment site within the LTR) [90-92]. Finally, LVs have been pseudotyped with surface glycoproteins derived from viruses such as vesicular stomatitis virus (VSV-G) to broaden LV host range. LVs alternatively can be provided with tissue-specific promoters to drive transgene expression in target cells only, in a process known as transcriptional targeting [93, 94]. Stable packaging cell lines have been developed to assist in LV production. LVs have also been engineered with ligands or antibodies bound to the vector envelope to assist in targeting specific cell types.

The fact that LVs can transduce pluripotent stem cells have made them a powerful tool for gene therapy [82, 85, 95]. Similarly, since LVs are easily transduced into dendritic cells, presentation of antigens such as lymphocyic choriomeningitis virus glycoprotein, influenza HA or tumour-associated antigens is greatly sustained and a more potent T cell response can be induced [96, 97]. This characteristic enables LVs to become highly effective vaccine vectors for infectious diseases. A number of *ex vivo* vaccination studies using dendritic cells which have been transduced by LVs and then directly immunized into the host subcutaneously have demonstrated strong and highly specialized immune responses *via* the migration of these antigen presenting cells into the skin-draining lymph nodes where they can prime the immune system [98-101]. Other routes of LV injection, including intramuscular and intraperitoneal, are also effective at inducing a robust immune response and at maintaining vector expression for extended periods of time. This long term antigen presentation is directly correlated with a more efficacious immune response and T cell memory [102, 103].

Lentiviruses as Vaccine Vectors against Infectious Diseases

One of the earliest examples of the utilization of LVs to combat infectious diseases was conducted against Hepatitis B virus. LVs expressing HBV surface antigen could generate a fast and robust immune response that offered protection against the virus in both rabbits and chimps [104]. LVs have also been effectively used in animal models to protect against challenge by West Nile virus, SIV and HIV [105, 106]. For example, mice immunized singly with LV expressing a secreted form of the WDV envelope protein were protected against a lethal dose of the virus for up to three months post-inoculation [107, 108]. Similarly, an LV expressing gag, pol and rev of HIV elicited antigen specific T cells and an IgG response [109, 110]. Further homozygous and heterozygous prime boost vaccination strategies using solely LV or LV and other virus vectors such as adenovirus (Ad) also enhanced the anti-HIV immune response [103, 111]. Based on these studies, more efforts were made to characterize the LV vaccine vector immune response to HIV using non-human primates [108]. LVs that were pseudotyped with G proteins from VSV and expressed a codon-optimized *gag* gene for SIV could generate both T and B cell responses and protect cynomolgous macaques against challenge with SIV [108]. Macaques who were vaccinated using this vector exhibited reduced viremia and preserved memory CD4(+) T cells at the most severe phase of infection, indicating that protection using this viral vaccine vector was significant [108].

In other studies, mouse dendritic cells expressing the glycoprotein of lymphocytic choriomeningitis virus (LCMV) and monkey cells expressing gag of SIV were able to produce highly specific cytotoxic T cell responses, as could human derived dendritic cells transduced with LVs expressing epitopes derived from influenza virus and hepatitis C virus [115, 116]. Other researchers found that immunizing mice with LVs that expressed the LCMV glycoprotein were protected against challenge with LCMV [117].

Non primate lentiviruses have a number of advantages over their primate counterparts such as HIV and SIV. There are substantial records of human exposure to nonprimate lentiviruses that are uneventful. Nonprimate lentiviruses lack cross reactivity to HIV in humans, and it is more likely that patients would be comfortable using a non-HIV system for their medical treatment. Nonprimate lentiviruses including those derived from Feline Immunodeficiency Virus (FIV), EIAV and Visna virus have also been used as expression vectors [112, 116- 118]. For example, Sinn *et al.*, 2007, 2008, were able to show stable gene expression for over eleven months post infection, following a single application of GP64-FIV into the nasal epithelia of mice [113, 114]. The authors found that repeated administration of this lentivirus vector resulted in an increase in gene expression as well as an increase in the number of epithelial cells that were infected. From the ungulate group, EIAV is also being developed as an HIV-1 vaccine and has been pseudotyped with HA to enable it to be effectively transferred to the nose, trachea and lungs [119- 122].

The results of these studies support the further use of lentiviruses as vaccine vectors, however, several hurdles still need to be addressed. For example, unexpected recombination events and vector mobilization and escape are worries that remain under consideration [123].

PLANT VIRUS VACCINE VECTORS

Recently, plant viruses have been engineered for pharmaceutical protein production and also as research tools for plant functional genomics studies. Incorporation of virus induced gene silencing (VIGS) technology into the plant virus vector enables specific host transcripts to become down-regulated, thus enabling their function to be identified, a key step toward the development of crops with improved characteristics. Plant viruses have also been developed as expression vectors for the production of vaccines against infectious diseases [124, 125]. Plant-derived vaccines are safe, efficacious and easy to produce en mass. The fact that they can provide inexpensive medicines that lack cold chain requirements make them attractive candidates for the world's rural poor. Their ease of production and storage enable plant-made vaccines to be stockpiled in preparation of global pandemics as well as against the threat of biowarfare agents [126, 127].

As is the case with the animal virus expression vectors discussed in this review, plant viruses have been extensively modified to remove some of their unwanted attributes. For example, the removal of the genes encoding virus movement and/or coat proteins reduces concerns about unintended vector transmission to other plants. Today, many plant virus expression vectors are introduced to the host plant *via* agroinfiltration, which involves the use of a syringe or vacuum. This enables virus infection to be synchronous and robust, and infected plants can be rapidly harvested for the pharmaceutical protein of interest under greenhouse conditions [128].

One of the most well characterized plant viruses used for vaccine production is Tobacco mosaic virus (TMV) (Fig. **2c**). TMV has been used to produce in large quantities the broadly neutralizing antibody VRCO1 against HIV-1 [91]. VRC01 is planned to be used as part of a topical microbicide to block HIV-1 transmission, and while conventionally produced monoclonal antibodies are expensive to manufacture, a plant-derived version is both inexpensive and efficacious, being produced at approximately 150 mg/kg fresh leaf material within days 5-7 post agroinoculation. Plant-produced VCR01 exhibited identical gp120 binding and neutralization activities as its human cell-produced counterpart. The glycosylation profile of the plant produced *versus* the conventional VCR01 were also similar [129].

TMV has also been used to generate on a large scale a vaccine for pandemic influenza virus. The demand for flu vaccines worldwide is enormous and is out of reach for many in developing countries. TMV capsid protein has been used as an epitope presentation system to express three different versions of the epitope M2e of influenza virus on the surface of the virus particle [130]. Mice immunized with this TMV chimera were found to resist challenge by lethal doses of influenza H1N1 virus [130]. Another research group has generated a subunit vaccine to the haemmaglutinin (HA) of H1N1 pandemic flu virus using TMV as the expression vector [131]. Clinical trials revealed that this plant-derived vaccine is as efficacious and free of adverse effects as the currently used approved vaccine for

H1N1 [132, 133]. Similarly, human clinical trials demonstrated that this plant virus produced vaccine was capable of re-activating an influenza-specific T cell response [28].

A number of other plant virus vectors have now been developed for vaccine production, including Cowpea mosaic virus (CPMV) expressing Bluetongue virus-like particles, Potato virus X (PVX) expressing human papillomavirus-like particles and the geminivirus Bean yellow dwarf virus (BeYDV) expressing a monoclonal antibody to Ebola virus [124, 134]. In addition to this, transgenic plants have been used to generate a variety of pharmaceuticals, such as monoclonal antibodies for rabies [124]. Advancements in vaccine vector technology has raised the possibility that vaccines could be produced inexpensively for developing countries or even produced by the countries themselves, as the manufacturing requirements are relatively unsophisticated. Vaccines produced in plants need only be partially purified, in the form of cornmeal, for example, or soymilk, and administered orally in order to be effective. This attribute offers promise to those who have little access to the same pharmaceuticals as are taken for granted in industrialized countries.

CONCLUSION

Virus vectors have been engineered to act as novel delivery platforms for gene therapy as well as for infectious disease research [135]. This review has served to provide recent developments in the use of virus vectors to combat infectious diseases (Table **1**). Of great current interest in all of the examples presented here is the relationship between the virus vector itself and the immune response, either through the vector's capacity to generate a robust and sustainable response against a select antigen, or through its action as a production platform by which to deliver antibodies in the form of passive immunotherapy [136, 137].

This review has explored the use of virus expression vectors to combat HIV/SIV infection as a point of focus. Improvements in vaccine vector development have led to success from previous failures [138]. It is noteworthy to mention that other vaccine vectors have also been successful in HIV/SIV vaccine development. For

Table 1. **Selected Examples of Current Vectors undergoing Clinical Trials to Combat Infectious Disease**

Virus Vector	Immunization Strategy	Results of Clinical Trial	References
FWPV	Prime: 2 x DNA-HIV-B consisting of Gag, Pol, Env, Vpu, Tat and Rev (clade B) Boost: 1 x FPV-HIV-B Gag and Pol (clade B)	No T cell responses.	[142]
	Prime: 3 x DNA-HIV-AE Gag, Pol, Rev, Tat, Env and Nef (clade A/E) Boost: 1 x FPV-HIV-AE Gag/Pol, Env, Tat/Rev (clade A/E)	ICS : No vaccine-induced CD4(+) or CD8(+) T cell responses.	[143]
	5 x FPV- HIV Env/Gag, Tat/Rev/Nef-RT (clade B	ICS: Poorly immunogenic, short-lived	[144]
ALVAC	Prime: 2 x ALVAC-HIV (vCP125) Boost: 2 x rgp160	Env-specific CD8(+) CTL activity in 39% of volunteers and still present 2 y after initial immunization in 2/3 of subjects tested.	[145, 146]
	Prime: 2, 4 xx ALVAC-HIV (gp160) (effect of dose) Boost: (x gp120	For high-dose regimen, vCP125 + rgp120 regimen elicited CD8(+) CTL activity more often (37%) than immunization with vCP125 (22%) or rgp120 (10%) alone. Memory CD8(+) T cell response against HIV-1$_{MN}$ rgp160 in 22% of vCP125 + rgp120 recipients. Reported cross-clade CTL reactivities.	[147-149]
	Prime: 4 x ALVAC-HIV (gp120 (HIV-1$_{MN}$) linked to TM domain of gp41 (HIV-1$_{LAI}$); Gag and protease (HIV-1$_{LAI}$)) Boost: 2 x SF-2 rgp120	Env/Gag-specific CD8(+) CTLs induced at least once in 64% of volunteers	[150]
NYVAC	2 x NYVAC-C Env, Gag-Pol-Nef (HIV-1 clade C)	ELISPOT: Vaccine-induced T cell responses in 50% of vaccines. Not durable and mainly against Env.	[151]
	2 x NYVAC-C Env, Gag-Pol-Nef (HIV-1 clade C)	ELISPOT: Vaccine-induced T cell responses in 33% of vaccines. Not durable.	[152, 153]
	NYVAC, expressing Gag, Pol, Nef, and Env from an HIV clade B isolate	Expansion of preexisting T-cell responses, and the appearance of newly detected HIV-specific CD4(+) and CD8(+) T-cell responses were observed. NYVAC-B immunization induces broad, vigorous, and polyfunctional HIV-specific T-cell responses.	[154]
	vaccinia-vectored vaccine for hemorrhagic fever with renal syndrome, Two subcutaneous vaccinations were administered at 4-week intervals.	Neutralizing antibodies to Hantaan virus or to vaccinia virus were detected in 72% or 98% of vaccinia virus-naive volunteers	[155]

Table 1 contd…..

Virus Vector	Immunization Strategy	Results of Clinical Trial	References
NYVAC	Modified Vaccinia virus Ankara (MVA) vector encoding nucleoprotein and matrix protein 1	Higher T cell responses than those induced by any other influenza vaccination approach	[156]
	Prime is ChAd63 Boost (eight weeks later) with an attenuated modified vaccinia virus Ankara (MVA) vector of malarial antigens MSP1 and AMA1	Both antibody and CD8(+) and CD4(+) T cell responses	[43-45]
Lentivirus	VRX496-T (Lexgenleucel-T)	Long antisense RNA to HIV-1	[157]

example, the research of Louis Picker and coworkers have demonstrated the ability of a cytomegalovirus (CMV) based vaccine vector to completely clear SIV infection in monkeys [139]. The authors found that half of the monkeys who were vaccinated and then administered a highly pathogenic form of SIV became infected, but eliminated all trace of the virus over time. This vector is currently being used in phase I clinical trials and also as a vaccine vector against tuberculosis (TB) which is fatal to monkeys. The authors found that at 14 weeks, five out of seven monkeys were protected from TB, while nearly all of the uninoculated control group that were infected with TB had died. A CMV-based vaccine may also soon be examined as a means to combat malaria [139, 140].

While the examples presented in this review have focused on difficult to treat infectious diseases such as HIV-1/AIDS, virus vectors have also been successful for targeting the host immune system against other pathologies such as a variety of cancer cells and tumors. The ability to induce a prolonged immune response, including the generation of memory T cells after a single injection of several of the virus vectors described here has been one of the achievements that has been highlighted in this review. Challenges that remain include the further optimization of the virus vector to enhance immunogenicity of the vaccine antigen in question, while at the same time reduce pre-existing immunity to the vector itself. Further insight into the relationship between recombinant virus vectors, including chimeric and artificial vectors, with respect to the immune response will greatly improve the potential of poxviruses, adeno-associated viruses and lentiviruses as vaccine vectors. In the same way, plant viruses have also been used as immunogens and several have been demonstrated to elicit improved immune responses [141]. Further elucidation of the mechanisms behind these immune responses will result in the design of superior and highly optimized vaccine vectors.

Another challenge that is currently being addressed is the precise nature of the heterogeneous prime/boost vaccine vector strategy to improve the immune response. Although several of the studies provided in this review indicate that this issue is currently under close scrutiny, much more information is needed to fully comprehend the effects of virus vectors in prime/boost vaccination to improve the host response to a given pathogen. It is time consuming and costly to determine the best route of administration for each vector. Furthermore, non-primate and even primate models do not always successfully represent a human model. Often, virus expression vectors are difficult and expensive to produce at yields sufficient for medical application. In addition to this, issues such as genetic stability of the vector, ease of scalability, purification and storage can be serious hurdles in virus vector development. Also, dose escalation, managing toxicity problems and improvements in vector safety are timely but important steps in moving vaccine vector technology forward past the research and development stage. The consequence of these efforts will be safe and efficacious virus vectors that generate broad based and robust responses, which in turn could be utilized for novel vaccine regimens as well as for a myriad of other applications.

ACKNOWLEDGEMENTS

None declared.

CONFLICT OF INTEREST

The author confirms that this chapter contents have no conflict of interest.

REFERENCES

[1]   Rollier CS, Reyes-Sandoval A, Cottingham MG, Ewer K, Hill AV. Viral vectors as vaccine platforms: deployment in sight. Curr Opin Immunol 2011; 23(3): 377-82.
[2]   Wong CM, McFall ER, Burns JK, Parkes RJ. The Role of Chromatin in Adenoviral Vector Function Viruses 2013; 5(6): 1500-15.

[3]   Deal, C, Pekosz, A., Ketner, G. Prospects for oral replicating adenovirus-vectored vaccines. Vaccine 2013; 31(32): 3236-43

[4]   Deisseroth A, Tang Y, Zhang L, Akbulut H, Habib N. TAA/ecdCD40L adenoviral prime-protein boost vaccine for cancer and infectious diseases. Cancer Gene Ther 2013; 20(2): 65-9.

[5]   Zhang, J, Tarbet EB, Toro, H, Tang, DC. Adenovirus-vectored drug-vaccine duo as a potential driver for conferring mass protection against infectious diseases. Expert Review of Vaccines 2011; 10(11): 1539-52

[6]   Bassett, JD, Swift, SL, Bramson, JL. Optimizing vaccine-induced CD8+ T-cell immunity: focus on recombinant adenovirus vectors. Expert Rev Vaccines 2011; 10(9): 1307-19.

[7]   Smith GL, Mackett M, Moss B. Infectious vaccinia virus recombinants that express hepatitis B virus surface antigen. Nature 1983; 302: 490-95.

[8]   Moss B, Smith GL, Gerin JL, Purcell RH. Live recombinant vaccinia virus protects chimpanzees against hepatitis B. Nature 1984; 311: 67-9.

[9]   Draper, SJ, Cottingham, MG, Gilbert, SC. Utilizing poxviral vectored vaccines for antibody induction - Progress and prospects. Vaccine 2013; 31(39): 4223-30.

[10]   Melamed S, Wyatt LS, Kastenmayer RJ, Moss B. Attenuation and immunogenicity of host-range extended modified vaccinia virus Ankara recombinants. Vaccine 2013; 31(41): 4569-77.

[11]   Weli SC, Tryland M. Avipoxviruses: infection biology and their use as vaccine vectors. Virol J 2011; 8: 49.

[12]   Pacchioni SM, Bissa M, Zanotto C, Morghen Cde G, Illiano E, Radaelli A. L1R, A27L, A33R and B5R vaccinia virus genes expressed by fowlpox recombinants as putative novel orthopoxvirus vaccines. J Transl Med 2013; 11: 95.

[13]   Barbara EH, Coupar, BEH, Damian FJ. Purcell, DFJ, Scott A. Thomson, SA, Ian A. Ramshaw, IA, Stephen J. Kent, SJ, David B. Boyle, DB. Fowlpox virus vaccines for HIV and SHIV clinical and pre-clinical trials. Vaccine 2006; 24(9): 1378-88.

[14]   Ranasinghe, C, Medveczky, JC, Woltring, D, Gao, K, Thomson, S, Coupar, BEH, Boyle, DB, Ramsay, AJ, Ramshaw, IA. Evaluation of fowlpox-vaccinia virus prime-boost vaccine strategies for high-level mucosal and systemic immunity against HIV-1. Vaccine 2006; 24(31-32): 5881-95.

[15]   Ranasinghe, C, Trivedi, S, Stambas, J Jackson, RJ. Unique IL-13Rα2-based HIV-1 vaccine strategy to enhance mucosal immunity, CD8+ T-cell avidity and protective immunity. Mucosal Immunol 2013; 6(6):1068-80.

[16]   Corbett, M, Bogers, WM, Heeney, JL, Gerber, S, Genin, C, Didierlaurent, A, *et al.* Aerosol immunization with NYVAC and MVA vectored vaccines is safe, simple, and immunogenic. Proc Natl Acad Sci U S A 2008; 105(6): 2046-51.

[17]   Kennedy RB, Oberg AL, Ovsyannikova IG, Haralambieva IH, Grill D, Poland GA. Transcriptomic profiles of high and low antibody responders to smallpox vaccine. Genes Immun 2013; 14(5): 277-85.

[18]   Lauterbach H, Pätzold J, Kassub R, Bathke B, Brinkmann K, Chaplin P, *et al.* Genetic Adjuvantation of Recombinant MVA with CD40L Potentiates CD8 T Cell Mediated Immunity. Front Immunol 2013; 4: 251.

[19]   Grigg P, Titong A, Jones LA, Yilma TD, Verardi PH. Safety mechanism assisted by the repressor of tetracycline (SMART) vaccinia virus vectors for vaccines and therapeutics. Proc Natl Acad Sci U S A 2013; 110(38): 15407-12.

[20] Hagen CJ, Titong A, Sarnoski EA, Verardi PH. Antibiotic-dependent expression of early transcription factor subunits leads to stringent control of vaccinia virus replication. Virus Res 2014; 181: 43-52.

[21] Smith ES, Zauderer M. Antibody library display on a Mammalian virus vector: combining the advantages of both phage and yeast display into one technology. Curr Drug Discov Technol 2014; 11(1): 48-55.

[22] Montefiori DC, Karnasuta C, Huang Y, Ahmed H, Gilbert P, de Souza MS, *et al.* Magnitude and breadth of the neutralizing antibody response in the RV144 and Vax003 HIV-1 vaccine efficacy trials. J Infect Dis 2012; 206(3): 431-41.

[23] McElrath MJ, Haynes BF. Induction of immunity to human immunodeficiency virus type-1 by vaccination. Immunity 2010; 33(4): 542-54.

[24] Gómez CE, Perdiguero B, Garcia-Arriaza J, Esteban M. Poxvirus vectors as HIV/AIDS vaccines in humans. Hum Vaccin Immunother 2012; 8(9): 1192-207.

[25] Vaccari M, Poonam P, Franchini G. Phase III HIV vaccine trial in Thailand: a step toward a protective vaccine for HIV. Expert Rev Vaccines 2010; 9(9): 997-1005.

[26] Pantaleo G, Esteban M, Jacobs B, Tartaglia J. Poxvirus vector-based HIV vaccines. Curr Opin HIV AIDS 2010; 5(5): 391-6.

[27] García, F, López, JC, de Quirós, B, Gómez, CE, Perdiguero, B, Nájera, JL, *et al.* Safety and immunogenicity of a modified pox vector-based HIV/AIDS vaccine candidate expressing Env, Gag, Pol and Nef proteins of HIV-1 subtype B (MVA-B) in healthy HIV-1-uninfected volunteers: A phase I clinical trial (RISVAC02). Vaccine 2011; 29(46): 8309-16.

[28] Gómez CE, Perdiguero B, Jiménez V, Filali-Mouhim A, Ghneim K, Haddad EK, *et al.* Systems analysis of MVA-C induced immune response reveals its significance as a vaccine candidate against HIV/AIDS of clade C. PLoS One 2012; 7(4): e35485.

[29] García-Arriaza J, Arnáez P, Gómez CE, Sorzano CO, Esteban M. Improving Adaptive and Memory Immune Responses of an HIV/AIDS Vaccine Candidate MVA-B by Deletion of Vaccinia Virus Genes (C6L and K7R) Blocking Interferon Signaling Pathways. PLoS One 2013; 8(6): e66894.

[30] O'Connell RJ, Kim JH, Corey L, Michael NL. Human immunodeficiency virus vaccine trials. Cold Spring Harb Perspect Med 2012; 2(12): a007351.

[31] Walsh SR, Seaman MS, Grandpre LE, Charbonneau C, Yanosick KE, Metch B, *et al.* Impact of anti-orthopoxvirus neutralizing antibodies induced by a heterologous prime-boost HIV-1 vaccine on insert-specific immune responses. Vaccine 2012; 31(1): 114-9.

[32] Cebere, I, Dorrell, L, McShane, H, Simmons, A, McCormack, S, Schmidt, C *et al.* Phase I clinical trial safety of DNA- and modified virus Ankara-vectored human immunodeficiency virus type 1 (HIV-1) vaccines administered alone and in a prime-boost regime to healthy HIV-1-uninfected volunteers. Vaccine 2006; 24(4): 417-25.

[33] Gilbert SC. Clinical development of Modified Vaccinia virus Ankara vaccines. Vaccine 2013; 31(39): 4241-6.

[34] Johnson JA, Barouch DH, Baden LR. Nonreplicating vectors in HIV vaccines. Curr Opin HIV AIDS 2013; 8(5): 412-20.

[35] García-Arriaza J, Gómez CE, Sorzano CO, Esteban M. Deletion of the vaccinia virus N2L gene encoding an inhibitor of IRF3 improves the immunogenicity of MVA expressing HIV-1 antigens. J. Virol 2014; 88(6): 3392-410.

[36] Sato H, Jing C, Isshiki M, Matsuo K, Kidokoro M, Takamura S, *et al.* Immunogenicity and safety of the vaccinia virus LC16m8Δ vector expressing SIV Gag under a strong or moderate promoter in a recombinant BCG prime-recombinant vaccinia virus boost protocol. Vaccine 2013; 31(35): 3549-57.

[37] García-Arriaza J, Arnáez P, Jiménez JL, Gómez CE, Muñoz-Fernández MÁ, Esteban M. Vector replication and expression of HIV-1 antigens by the HIV/AIDS vaccine candidate MVA-B is not affected by HIV-1 protease inhibitors. Virus Res 2012; 167(2): 391-6.

[38] Patil SS, Gentschev I, Adelfinger M, Donat U, Hess M, Weibel S, *et al.* Virotherapy of canine tumors with oncolytic vaccinia virus GLV-1h109 expressing an anti-VEGF single-chain antibody. PLoS One 2012; 7(10): e47472.

[39] Gullberg M, Muszynski B, Organtini LJ, Ashley RE, Hafenstein SL, Belsham GJ, *et al.* Assembly and characterization of foot-and-mouth disease virus empty capsid particles expressed within mammalian cells. J Gen Virol 2013; 94(Pt 8): 1769-79.

[40] Mendes ÉA, Fonseca FG, Casério BM, Colina JP, Gazzinelli RT, Caetano BC. Recombinant vaccines against T. gondii: comparison between homologous and heterologous vaccination protocols using two viral vectors expressing SAG1. PLoS One 2013; 8(5): e63201.

[41] Elias, SC, Choudhary, P, de Cassan, SC, Biswas, S, Collins, KA, Halstead, FD, *et al.* Analysis of human B-cell responses following ChAd63-MVA MSP1 and AMA1 immunization and controlled malaria infection. Immunology 2014; 141(4): 628-44.

[42] Bauza, K, Malinauskas, T, Pfander, C, Anar, B, E Jones, EY, Oliver Billker, O, *et al.* Efficacy of a Plasmodium vivax Malaria Vaccine Using ChAd63 and Modified Vaccinia Ankara Expressing Thrombospondin-Related Anonymous Protein as Assessed with Transgenic Plasmodium berghei Parasites Infect. Immun 2014; 82(3): 1277-86.

[43] Elias SC, Collins KA, Halstead FD, Choudhary P, Bliss CM, Ewer KJ, *et al.* Assessment of immune interference, antagonism, and diversion following human immunization with biallelic blood-stage malaria viral-vectored vaccines and controlled malaria infection. J Immunol 2013; 190(3): 1135-47.

[44] Betts, G, Poyntz, H, Stylianou, E, Reyes-Sandoval, A, Cottingham, M, Hill, A. *et al.* Optimising Immunogenicity with Viral Vectors: Mixing MVA and HAdV-5 Expressing the Mycobacterial Antigen Ag85A in a Single Injection. PLoS One 2012; 7(12): e50447.

[45] Ogwang, C, Afolabi, M, Kimani, D, Jagne, YJ, Sheehy, SH, Bliss, CM, *et al.* Safety and Immunogenicity of Heterologous Prime-Boost Immunisation with *Plasmodium falciparum* Malaria Candidate Vaccines, ChAd63 ME-TRAP and MVA ME-TRAP, in Healthy Gambian and Kenyan Adults. PLoS One 2013; 8(3): e57726.

[46] Lai, L, Kwa, SF, Kozlowski, PA, Montefiori, DC, Ferrari, G, Johnson, WE, *et al.* Prevention of Infection by a Granulocyte-Macrophage Colony-Stimulating Factor Co-Expressing DNA/Modified Vaccinia Ankara Simian Immunodeficiency Virus Vaccine. J Infect Dis Jul 1, 2011; 204(1): 164-73.

[47] Manning WC, Paliard X, Zhou S, Bland MP, Lee AY, Hong K, *et al.* Genetic immunization with adeno-associated virus vectors expressing herpes simplex virus type 2 glycoprotein B and D. J Virol 1997; 71(10): 7960-2.

[48] Nieto K, Salvetti A. AAV Vectors Vaccines Against Infectious Diseases. Front Immunol 2014; 5: 5.

[49] Flotte, TR, Berns, KI. Adeno-associated virus:a ubiquitous commensal of mammals. Hum Gene Ther 2005; 16: 401-7.

[50]   Dismuke DJ, Tenenbaum L, Samulski RJ. Biosafety of recombinante adeno- associated vírus vectors. Curr Gene Ther 2013; 13: 434-52.

[51]   Rabinowitz, JE, Rolling, F, Li C, Conrath, H, Xiao, W, Xiao, X, *et al.* Cross-packaging of a single adeno-associated virus (AAV) type 2 vector genome into multiple AAV serotypes enables transduction with broad specificity. J Virol 2002; 76: 791-801.

[52]   Mitchell, AM, Nicolson, SC, Warischalk, JK, Samulski, RJ. AAV's Anatomy: Roadmap for Optimizing Vectors for Translational Success. Curr Gene Ther 2010; 10(5): 319-40

[53]   Ussher, JE, Taylor, JA. Optimized transduction of human monocyte-derived dendritic cells by recombinant adeno-associated virus serotype 6. Hum Gene Ther 2010; 21(12): 1675-86.

[54]   Sheppard, HM, Ussher, JE, Verdon, D, Chen, J, Taylor, JA, Dunbar, PR. Recombinant Adeno-Associated Virus Serotype 6 Efficiently Transduces Primary Human Melanocytes PLoS One 2013; 8(4): e62753.

[55]   Balazs AB, Chen J, Hong CM, Rao DS, Yang L, Baltimore D. Antibody-based protection against HIV infection by vectored immunoprophylaxis. Nature 2012; 481: 81-4.

[56]   Skaricic D, Traube C, De B, Joh J, Boyer J, Crystal RG, *et al.* Genetic delivery of an anti-RSV antibody to protect against pulmonary infection with RSV. Virology 2008; 378: 79-85.

[57]   Xin KQ, Urabe M, Yang J, Nomiyama K, Mizukami H, Hamajima H, *et al.* A novel recombinant adeno-associated virus vaccine induces a long-term humoral immune response to human immunodeficiency virus. Hum Gene Ther 2001; 12: 1047-61.

[58]   Johnson PR, Schnepp BC, Connell MJ, Rohne D, Robinson S, Krivulka GR, *et al.* Novel adeno-associated virus vector vaccine restricts replication of simian immunodeficiency virus in macaques. J Virol 2005; 79: 955-65.

[59]   Lin J, Calcedo R, Vandenberghe LH, Bell P, Somanathan S, Wilson JM. A new genetic vaccine platform based on an adeno-associated virus isolated from a rhesus macaque. J Virol 2009; 83(24): 12738-50.

[60]   Mays, LE, Vandenberghe, LH, Xiao, R, Bell, P, Nam, H-J, *et al.* Adeno-Associated Virus Capsid Structure Drives CD4-Dependent CD8$^+$ T Cell Response to Vector Encoded Proteins. The Journal of Immunology 2009; 182 (10): 6051-60.

[61]   Xin KQ, Mizukami H, Urabe M, Toda Y, Shinoda K, Yoshida A, *et al.* Induction of robust immune responses against human immunodeficiency virus is supported by the in her enttropismofadeno-associatedvirustype5fordendriticcells. J Virol 2006; 80: 11899-910.

[62]   Tatalick, LM, Gerard, CJ, Takeya, R, Price, DN, Thorne, BA, Wyatt, LM, *et al.* Safety characterization of HeLa-based cell substrates used in the manufacture of a recombinant adeno-associated virus-HIV vaccine. Vaccine 2005; 23(20): 2628-38.

[63]   Vardas E, Kaleebu P, Bekker LG, Hoosen A, Chomba E, Johnson PR, *et al.* A phase 2 study to evaluate the safety and immunogenicity of a recombinant HIV type 1 vaccine based on adeno-associated virus. AIDS Res Hum Retroviruses 2010; 26(8): 933-42.

[64]   Johnson PR, Schnepp BC, Zhang J, Connell MJ, Greene SM, Yuste E, *et al.* Vector-mediated gene transfer engenders long-lived neutralizing activity and protection against SIV infection in monkeys. Nat Med 2009; 15: 901-6.

[65]   Sipo I, Knauf M, Fechner H, PollerW, Planz O, Kurth R, *et al.* Vaccine protection against lethal homologous and heterologous challenge using recombinant AAV vectors expressing codon-optimized genes from pandemic swine origin influenza virus(SOIV). Vaccine 2011; 29: 1690-9.

[66]   Balazs AB, Bloom JD, Hong CM, Rao DS, Baltimore D. Broad protection against influenza infection by vectored immunoprophylaxis in mice. Nat Biotechnol 2013; 31: 647-52.

[67]   Limberis MP, Adam VS, Wong G, Gren J, Kobasa D, Ross TM, *et al.* Intranasal antibody gene transfer in mice and ferrets elicits broad protection against pandemic influenza. Sci Transl Med 2013; 5: 187.

[68]   Eaton BT, Broder CC, Middleton D, Wang LF. Hendra and Nipah viruses: different and dangerous. Nat Rev Microbiol 2006; 4: 23-35.

[69]   Ploquin A, Szecsi J, Mathieu C, Guillaume V, Barateau V, Ong KC, *et al.* Protection against henipavirus infection by use of recombinant adeno-associated virus-vector vaccines. J Infect Dis 2013; 207: 469-78.

[70]   Li X, Cao H, Wang Q, Di B, Wang M, Lu J, Pan L, Yang L, Mei M, Pan X, Li G, Wang L. Novel AAV-based genetic vaccines encoding truncated dengue virus envelope proteins elicit humoral immune responses in mice. Microbes Infect 2012; 14(11): 1000-7.

[71]   Rogers GL, Martino AT, Aslanidi GV, Jayandharan GR, Srivastava A, Herzog RW. Innate immune responses to AAV vectors. Front Microbiol 2011; 2: 194.

[72]   Calcedo R, Vandenberghe LH, Gao G, Lin J, Wilson JM. Worldwide epidemiology of neutralizing antibodies to adeno-associated viruses. J Infect Dis 2009; 199: 381-90.

[73]   Rybniker J, Nowag A, Janicki H, Demant K, Hartmann P, Büning H. Incorporation of antigens into viral capsids augments immunogenicity of adeno-associated virus vector-based vaccines. J Virol 2012; 86(24): 13800-4.

[74]   Nieto K, Kern A, Leuchs B, Gissmann L, Muller M, Klein Schmidt JA. Combined prophylactic and therapeutic intranasal vaccination against human papillomavirus type-16 using different adeno-associated virus serotype vectors. Antivir Ther 2009; 14: 1125-37.

[75]   Nieto K, Weghofer M, Sehr P, Ritter M, Sedlmeier S, Karanam B, *et al.* Development of AAVLP(HPV16/31L2) particles as broadly protective HPV vaccine candidate. PLoS One 2012; 7: e39741.

[76]   Nieto K, Stahl-Hennig C, Leuchs B, Müller M, Gissmann L, Kleinschmidt JA. Intranasal vaccination with AAV5 and 9 vectors against human papillomavirus type 16 in rhesus macaques. Hum Gene Ther 2012; 23(7): 733-41.

[77]   Liu DW, Chang JL, TsaoYP, Huang CW, Kuo SW, Chen SL. Co-vaccination with adeno-associated virus vectors encoding human papillomavirus 16 L1 proteins and adenovirus encoding murine GM-CSF can elicit strong and prolonged neutralizing antibody. Int J Cancer 2005; 113: 93-100.

[78]   Liu Q, Huang W, Zhao C, Zhang L, Meng S, Gao D, Wang Y. The prevalence of neutralizing antibodies against AAV serotype 1 in healthy subjects in China: implications for gene therapy and vaccines using AAV1 vector. J Med Virol 2013; 85(9): 1550-6.

[79]   Mingozzi F, Maus MV, Hui DJ, Sabatino DE, Murphy SL, Rasko JE, *et al.* CD8(+) T-cell responses to adeno-associated virus capsid in humans. Nat Med 2007; 13: 419-22.

[80]   Murphy SL, Li H, Mingozzi F, Sabatino DE, Hui DJ, Edmonson SA, *et al.* Diverse IgG subclass responses to adeno-associated virus infection and vector administration. J Med Virol 2009; 81: 65-74.

[81]   Emeagi PU, Goyvaerts C, Maenhout S, Pen J, Thielemans K, Breckpot K. Lentiviral vectors: a versatile tool to fight cancer. Curr Mol Med 2013; 13(4): 602-25.

[82]   Picanco-Castro V, de Sousa Russo-Carbolante EM, Tadeu Covas D. Advances in lentiviral vectors: a patent review. Recent Pat DNA Gene Seq 2012; 6(2): 82-90.

[83]   Sakuma T, Barry MA, Ikeda Y. Lentiviral vectors: basic to translational. Biochem J 2012; 443(3): 603-18.

[84]   Negri DR, Michelini Z, Bona R, Blasi M, Filati P, Leone P, Rossi A, Franco M, Cara A. Integrase-defective lentiviral-vector-based vaccine: a new vector for induction of T cell immunity. Expert Opin Biol Ther 2011; 11(6): 739-50.

[85]   Kumar P, Woon-Khiong C. Optimization of lentiviral vectors generation for biomedical and clinical research purposes: contemporary trends in technology development and applications. Curr Gene Ther 2011; 11(2): 144-53.

[86]   Hu B, Tai A, Wang P. Immunization delivered by lentiviral vectors for cancer and infectious diseases. Immunol Rev 2011; 239(1): 45-61.

[87]   Follenzi A, Ailles LE, Bakovic S, Geuna M, Naldini L. Gene transfer by lentiviral vectors is limited by nuclear translocation and rescued by HIV-1 pol sequences. Nat Genet 2000; 25(2): 217-22.

[88]   Brown BD, Venneri MA, Zingale A, Sergi L, Naldini L. Endogenous microRNA regulation suppresses transgene expression in hematopoietic lineages and enables stable gene transfer. Nat Med 2006; 12: 585-91.

[89]   Brown BD, Cantore A, Annoni A, Sergi LS, Lombardo A, Della Valle P, *et al.* A microRNA-regulated lentiviral vector mediates stable correction of hemophilia B mice. Blood 2007; 110: 4144-52.

[90]   Banasik MB, McCray PB., Jr Integrase-defective lentiviral vectors: progress and applications. Gene Ther 2010; 17: 150-57.

[91]   Negri DR, Michelini Z, Cara A. Toward integrase defective lentiviral vectors for genetic immunization. Curr HIV Res 2010; 8: 274-81.

[92]   Sarkis C, Philippe S, Mallet J, Serguera C. Non-integrating lentiviral vectors. Curr Gene Ther 2008; 8: 430-37.

[93]   Froelich S, Tai A, Wang P. Lentiviral vectors for immune cells targeting. Immunopharmacol Immunotoxicol 2010; 32(2): 208-18.

[94]   D'Costa J, Mansfield SG, Humeau LM. Lentiviral vectors in clinical trials: Current status. Curr Opin Mol Ther 2009; 11(5): 554-64.

[95]   Matrai J, Chuah MK, VandenDriessche T. Recent advances in lentiviral vector development and applications. Mol Ther 2010; 18: 477-90.

[96]   He Y, Falo LD., Jr Lentivirus as a potent and mechanistically distinct vector for genetic immunization. Curr Opin Mol Ther 2007; 9: 439-46.

[97]   Pincha M, Sundarasetty BS, Stripecke R. Lentiviral vectors for immunization: an inflammatory field. Expert Rev Vaccines 2010; 9: 309-21.

[98]   He Y, Zhang J, Donahue C, Falo LD., Jr Skin-derived dendritic cells induce potent CD8(+) T cell immunity in recombinant lentivector-mediated genetic immunization. Immunity 2006; 24: 643-56.

[99]   Arce F, Rowe HM, Chain B, Lopes L, Collins MK. Lentiviral vectors transduce proliferating dendritic cell precursors leading to persistent antigen presentation and immunization. Mol Ther 2009; 17: 1643-50.

[100] Barouch DH. The quest for an HIV-1 vaccine--moving forward. N Engl J Med 2013; 369(22): 2073-6.

[101] Negri DR, Michelini Z, Baroncelli S, Spada M, Vendetti S, Bona R, *et al.* Nonintegrating lentiviral vector-based vaccine efficiently induces functional and persistent CD8+ T cell responses in mice. J Biomed Biotechnol 2010; 534501.

[102] Negri DR, Michelini Z, Baroncelli S, Spada M, Vendetti S, Buffa V, *et al*. Successful immunization with a single injection of non-integrating lentiviral vector. Mol Ther 2007; 15: 1716-23.

[103] Buffa V, Negri DR, Leone P, Bona R, Borghi M, Bacigalupo I, *et al*. A single administration of lentiviral vectors expressing either full-length human immunodeficiency virus 1 (HIV-1)(HXB2) Rev/Env or codon-optimized HIV-1(JR-FL) gp120 generates durable immune responses in mice. J Gen Virol 2006; 87: 1625-34.

[104] Hong, Y., Peng, Y., Mi, M., Xiao, H., Munn, DH., Wang, GQ, *et al*. Lentivirus expressing HBsAg and immunoglobulin Fc fusion antigen induces potent immune responses and results in seroconversion in HBsAg transgenic mice. Vaccine 2011; 29(22): 3909-16.

[105] Iglesias MC, Frenkiel MP, Mollier K, Souque P, Despres P, Charneau P. A single immunization with a minute dose of a lentiviral vector-based vaccine is highly effective at eliciting protective humoral immunity against West Nile virus. J Gene Med 2006; 8: 265-74.

[106] Iglesias MC, Mollier K, Beignon AS, Souque P, Adotevi O, Lemonnier F, Charneau P. Lentiviral vectors encoding HIV-1 polyepitopes induce broad CTL responses *in vivo*. Mol Ther 2007; 15(6): 1203-10.

[107] Coutant F, Frenkiel MP, Despres P, Charneau P. Protective antiviral immunity conferred by a nonintegrative lentiviral vector-based vaccine. PLoS One 2008; 3: e3973.

[108] Beignon AS, Mollier K, Liard C, Coutant F, Munier S, Rivière J, *et al*. Lentiviral vector-based prime/boost vaccination against AIDS: pilot study shows protection against Simian immunodeficiency virus SIVmac251 challenge in macaques. J Virol 2009; 83: 10963-74.

[109] Asefa B, Korokhov N, Lemiale F. Heterologous HIV-based lentiviral/adenoviral vectors immunizations result in enhanced HIV-specific immunity. Vaccine 2010; 28: 3617-24.

[110] Dai B, Yang L, Yang H, Hu B, Baltimore D, Wang P. HIV-1 Gag-specific immunity induced by a lentivector-based vaccine directed to dendritic cells. Proc Natl Acad Sci U S A 2009; 106: 20382-87.

[111] Appay V, Iglesias MC. Antigen sensitivity and T-cell receptor avidity as critical determinants of HIV control. Curr Opin HIV AIDS 2011; 6(3): 157-62.

[112] Dai B, Yang L, Yang H, Hu B, Baltimore D, Wang P. HIV-1 Gag-specific immunity induced by a lentivector-based vaccine directed to dendritic cells. Proc Natl Acad Sci U S A 2009; 106: 20382-7.

[113] Uchida N, Hsieh MM, Washington KN, Tisdale JF. Efficient transduction of human hematopoietic repopulating cells with a chimeric HIV1-based vector including SIV capsid. Exp Hematol 2013; 41(9): 779-88.

[114] Coutant F, Frenkiel MP, Despres P, Charneau P. Protective antiviral immunity conferred by a nonintegrative lentiviral vector-based vaccine. PLoS One 2008; 3: e3973.

[115] Negri DR, Bona R, Michelini Z, Leone P, Macchia I, Klotman ME, *et al*. Transduction of human antigen-presenting cells with integrase-defective lentiviral vector enables functional expansion of primed antigen-specific CD8(+) T cells. Hum Gene Ther 2010; 21(8): 1029-35.

[116] Walker BD, Burton DR. Toward an AIDS vaccine. Science 2008; 320: 760-64.

[117] Woolard SN, Kumaraguru U. Viral vaccines and CTL response. J Biomed Biotechnol 2010; 2010: 141657.

[118] Sinn PL, Arias AC, Brogden KA, McCray PB Jr. Lentivirus vector can be readministered to nasal epithelia without blocking immune responses. J Virol 2008 82(21): 10684-92.

[119] Sinn PL, Goreham-Voss JD, Arias AC, Hickey MA, Maury W, *et al.* Enhanced gene expression conferred by stepwise modification of a nonprimate lentiviral vector. Hum Gene Ther 2007; 18(12): 1244-52.

[120] Barraza RA, Poeschla EM. Human gene therapy vectors derived from feline lentiviruses. Vet Immunol Immunopathol 2008; 123(1-2): 23-31.

[121] Farley DC, Bannister R, Leroux-Carlucci MA, Evans NE, Miskin JE, Mitrophanous KA. Development of an equine-tropic replication-competent lentivirus assay for equine infectious anemia virus-based lentiviral vectors. Hum Gene Ther Methods 2012; 23(5): 309-23.

[122] Patel M, Giddings AM, Sechelski J, Olsen JC. High efficiency gene transfer to airways of mice using influenza hemagglutinin pseudotyped lentiviral vectors. J Gene Med 2013; 15(1): 51-62.

[123] Hacein-Bey-Abina S, von Kalle C, Schmidt M, Le Deist F, Wulffraat N, McIntyre E, *et al.* A serious adverse event after successful gene therapy for X-linked severe combined immunodeficiency. N Engl J Med 2003; 348: 255-56.

[124] Hefferon KL. (2012). Plant virus expression vectors set the stage as production platforms for biopharmaceutical proteins. Virology Nov 10; 433(1): 1-6.

[125] Ko, K, Koprowski, H. Plant biopharming of monoclonal antibodies Virus Research 2005; 111: 93-100

[126] Yusibov V, Shivprasad S, Turpen TH, Dawson W, Koprowski H. Plant viral vectors based on tobamoviruses. Curr Top Microbiol Immunol 1999; 240: 81-94.

[127] Rybicki EP. Plant-produced vaccines: promise and reality. Drug Discov Today 2009; 14(1-2): 16-24.

[128] Leuzinger K, Dent M, Hurtado J, Stahnke J, Lai H, Zhou X, *et al.* Efficient agroinfiltration of plants for h igh-level transient expression of recombinant proteins. Journal of Visual Experimentation 2013; (77).

[129] Hamorsky KT, Grooms-Williams TW, Husk AS, Bennett LJ, Palmer KE, Nobuyuki Matoba N. Efficient Single Tobamoviral Vector-Based Bioproduction of Broadly Neutralizing Anti-HIV-1 Monoclonal Antibody VRC01 in *Nicotiana benthamiana* Plants and Utility of VRC01 in Combination Microbicides Antimicrobial Agents and Chemotherapy 2013; 57(5): 2076-86.

[130] Petukhova NV, Gasanova TV, Stepanova LA, Rusova OA, Potapchuk MV, Korotkov AV, *et al.* Immunogenicity and protective efficacy of candidate universal influenza A nanovaccines produced in plants by Tobacco mosaic virus-based vectors. Current Pharmaceutical Design 2013; 19(31): 5587-600.

[131] Yusibov V, Streatfield SJ, Kushnir N, Roy G, Padmanaban A. Hybrid viral vectors for vaccine and antibody production in plants. Current Pharmaceutical Design 2013; 19(31): 5574-86.

[132] Shoji Y, Jones RM, Mett V, Chichester JA, Musiychuk K, Sun X, *et al.* A plant-produced H1N1 trimeric hemagglutinin protects mice from a lethal influenza virus challenge. Human Vaccine Immunotherapy 2013; 9(3): 23234.

[133] Cummings JF, Guerrero ML, Moon JE, Waterman P, Nielsen RK, Jefferson SF, *et al.* Safety and immunogenicity of a plant-produced recombinant monomer hemagglutinin-based influenza vaccine derived from influenza A (H1N1)pdm09 virus: A Phase 1 dose-escalation study in healthy adults. Vaccine Journal 2013; 32(19): 2251-9.

[134]   Vezina L-P, D'Aoust MA, Landry N, Couture MJ, Charland N. Plants As an Innovative and Accelerated Vaccine-Manufacturing Solution. BioPharmaceutical International 2011; Supplementary 24: s27-30.

[135]   Draper SJ, Heeney JL. Viruses as vaccine vectors for infectious diseases and cancer. Nat Rev Microbiol 2010; 8: 62-73.

[136]   Krause A, Worgall S. Delivery of antigens by viral vectors for vaccination. Ther Deliv 2011; 2(1): 51-70.

[137]   Liu MA. Immunologic basis of vaccine vectors. Immunity 2010; 33: 504-15.

[138]   Rafick-Pierre Sekaly The failed HIV Merck vaccine study: a step back or a launching point for future vaccine development? J Exp Med Jan 21, 2008; 205(1): 7-12.

[139]   Hansen, SG, Sacha, JB, Hughes, CM, Ford, JC, Burwitz, BJ, Scholz, I, *et al.* Cytomegalovirus vectors violate CD8+ T cell epitope recognition paradigms. Science 2013; 340 (6135): 1237874.

[140]   Hansen, SG, Ford, JC, Lewis, MS, Ventura, Ab, Hughes, CM, Coyne-Johnson, L, *et al.* Profound early control of highly pathogenic SIV by an effector-memory T cell vaccine. Nature 2011; 473(7348): 523-27.

[141]   McCormick AA, Corbo TA, Wykoff-Clary S, Nguyen LV, Smith ML, *et al.* TMV-peptide fusion vaccines induce cell-mediated immune responses and tumor protection in two murine models. Vaccine 2006; 24(40-41): 6414-23.

[142]   Kelleher AD, Puls RL, Bebbington M, Boyle D, Ffrench R, Kent SJ, *et al.* A randomized, placebo-controlled phase I trial of DNA prime, recombinant fowlpox virus boost prophylactic vaccine for HIV-1. AIDS 2006; 20: 294-7.

[143]   Hemachandra A, Puls RL, Sirivichayakul S, Kerr S, Thantiworasit P, Ubolyam S, *et al.* An HIV-1 clade A/E DNA prime, recombinant fowlpox virus boost vaccine is safe, but non-immunogenic in a randomized phase I/IIa trial in Thai volunteers at low risk of HIV infection. Hum Vaccin 2010; 6: 835-40.

[144]   Keefer MC, Frey SE, Elizaga M, Metch B, De Rosa SC, Barroso PF, *et al.* NIAID HIV Vaccine Trials Network A phase I trial of preventive HIV vaccination with heterologous poxviral-vectors containing matching HIV-1 inserts in healthy HIV-uninfected subjects. Vaccine 2011; 29: 1948-58.

[145]   Pialoux G, Excler JL, Rivière Y, Gonzalez-Canali G, Feuillie V, Coulaud P, *et al.* A prime-boost approach to HIV preventive vaccine using a recombinant canarypox virus expressing glycoprotein 160 (MN) followed by a recombinant glycoprotein 160 (MN/LAI). The AGIS Group, and l'Agence Nationale de Recherche sur le SIDA. AIDS Res Hum Retroviruses 1995; 11: 373-81.

[146]   Fleury B, Janvier G, Pialoux G, Buseyne F, Robertson MN, Tartaglia J, *et al.* Memory cytotoxic T lymphocyte responses in human immunodeficiency virus type 1 (HIV-1)-negative volunteers immunized with a recombinant canarypox expressing gp 160 of HIV-1 and boosted with a recombinant gp160. J Infect Dis 1996; 174: 734-8.

[147]   Egan MA, Pavlat WA, Tartaglia J, Paoletti E, Weinhold KJ, Clements ML, *et al.* Induction of human immunodeficiency virus type 1 (HIV-1)-specific cytolytic T lymphocyte responses in seronegative adults by a nonreplicating, host-range-restricted canarypox vector (ALVAC) carrying the HIV-1MN env gene. J Infect Dis 1995; 171: 1623-7.

[148]   Clements-Mann ML, Weinhold K, Matthews TJ, Graham BS, Gorse GJ, Keefer MC, *et al.* NIAID AIDS Vaccine Evaluation Group Immune responses to human immunodeficiency virus (HIV) type 1 induced by canarypox expressing HIV-1MN gp120, HIV-1SF2

recombinant gp120, or both vaccines in seronegative adults. J Infect Dis 1998; 177: 1230-46.

[149] Ferrari G, Humphrey W, McElrath MJ, Excler JL, Duliege AM, Clements ML, *et al.* Clade B-based HIV-1 vaccines elicit cross-clade cytotoxic T lymphocyte reactivities in uninfected volunteers. Proc Natl Acad Sci U S A 1997; 94: 1396-401.

[150] Belshe RB, Gorse GJ, Mulligan MJ, Evans TG, Keefer MC, Excler JL, *et al.* NIAID AIDS Vaccine Evaluation Group Induction of immune responses to HIV-1 by canarypox virus (ALVAC) HIV-1 and gp120 SF-2 recombinant vaccines in uninfected volunteers. AIDS 1998; 12: 2407-15

[151] Bart PA, Goodall R, Barber T, Harari A, Guimaraes-Walker A, Khonkarly M, *et al.* EuroVacc Consortium EV01: a phase I trial in healthy HIV negative volunteers to evaluate a clade C HIV vaccine, NYVAC-C undertaken by the EuroVacc Consortium. Vaccine 2008; 26: 3153-61.

[152] Harari A, Bart PA, Stöhr W, Tapia G, Garcia M, Medjitna-Rais E, *et al.* An HIV-1 clade C DNA prime, NYVAC boost vaccine regimen induces reliable, polyfunctional, and long-lasting T cell responses. J Exp Med 2008; 205: 63-77.

[153] McCormack S, Stöhr W, Barber T, Bart PA, Harari A, Moog C, *et al.* EV02: a Phase I trial to compare the safety and immunogenicity of HIV DNA-C prime-NYVAC-C boost to NYVAC-C alone. Vaccine 2008; 26: 3162-74.

[154] Harari A, Rozot V, Cavassini M, Enders FB, Vigano S, Tapia G, *et al.* NYVAC immunization induces polyfunctional HIV-specific T-cell responses in chronically-infected, ART-treated HIV patients. Eur J Immunol 2012; 42(11): 3038-48.

[155] McClain DJ, Summers PL, Harrison SA, Schmaljohn AL, Schmaljohn CS. Clinical evaluation of a vaccinia-vectored Hantaan virus vaccine. J Med Virol 2000; 60(1): 77-85.

[156] Berthoud TK, Hamill M, Lillie PJ, Hwenda L, Collins KA, Ewer KJ, *et al.* Potent CD8+ T-cell immunogenicity in humans of a novel heterosubtypic influenza A vaccine, MVA-NP+M1. Clin Infect Dis 2011; 52(1): 1-7.

[157] Tebas P, Stein D, Binder-Scholl G, Mukherjee R, Brady T, Rebello T, *et al.* Antiviral effects of autologous CD4 T cells genetically modified with a conditionally replicating lentiviral vector expressing long antisense to HIV. Blood 2013; 121(9): 1524-33.

CHAPTER 4

Newcastle Disease Virus as a Promising Vector against Infectious Diseases and as a Potential Agent against Cancers

Xiaodong Zhang[*,1], Mingming Han[1], Chao Gao[1], Renfu Yin[1], Donald L. Reynolds[2], Dylan Frabutt[3], Liangxue Lai[1], Minhua Sun[4], Ying Chen[5], Xiang Li[1] and Zhuang Ding[*,1]

[1]*Key Laboratory of Zoonosis Research, Ministry of Education, Institute of Zoonosis, College of Veterinary Medicine, Jilin University, Changchun 130062, China;* [2]*Atlantic Veterinary College, University of Prince Edward Island, Prince Edward Island, Canada;* [3]*Michigan State University, East Lansing, MI 48824, USA;* [4]*Institute of Animal Health, Guangdong Academy of Agriculture Sciences, Guangzhou, China; and* [5]*College of Animal Science and Technology, Guangxi University, Nanning, China*

Abstract: The continual emergence of viral pathogens highlights the need for effective vaccine systems that can rapidly adapt to changing or novel pathogens. The use of Newcastle disease virus (NDV)-based vector vaccines may be one of the most feasible approaches for achieving protection against such pathogens. ND is one of the most important infectious diseases of poultry. However, the use of this poultry pathogen as a vaccine vector to offer protection against other pathogens has become of interest to researchers worldwide. For example, a study has demonstrated that an NDV-based influenza A virus (H5N1) vaccine could provide complete protection of chickens and mice from lethal challenge of homologous and heterologous H5N1 avian influenza viruses. Furthermore, naturally occurring strains of NDV have demonstrated oncolytic therapeutic potency in preclinical and clinical studies. With the development of reverse genetics technology, modifications of oncolytic NDVs resulting in increased targeting and oncolytic potency become feasible. Such strategies may become a promising novel therapeutic approach against cancers. Therefore, NDV can be used as a vaccine vector to immunize against emerging or reemerging pathogens and may have great potential to be used for cancer treatment in the future.

Keywords: Newcastle disease virus, vaccine vector, reverse genetics, infectious disease, cancer treatment.

---

*Corresponding Author Xiaodong Zhang: College of Veterinary Medicine, Jilin University, No.5333 Xi'an Street, Changchun, 130062, China; Tel: 86-431-84533422 & 86-0431-87836160; Fax: 86-431-84533431 & 86-0431-87836160; E-mails: zhang_xd@jlu.edu.cn & Zhuang_Ding@yahoo.com.cn, respectively.

The continual emergence of viral pathogens, such as novel avian influenza A (H7N9) virus, newly emerged Middle East respiratory syndrome coronavirus, highly pathogenic avian influenza A (H5N1) virus, severe acute respiratory syndrome coronavirus, Ebola virus, novel phlebovirus and other viral pathogens highlights the need for effective vaccine systems that can be rapidly adapted to changing or novel pathogens. Viral vectored vaccines are one of the most promising approaches for achieving protection against such pathogens [1, 2]. Newcastle disease virus (NDV) is an ideal candidate for such viral vectors.

NDV is an important avian pathogen that can cause severe economic losses to the poultry industry [3]. NDV, an avian paramyxovirus, has a negative-sense, single-stranded RNA genome (15~16 kb in length). The genome of NDV mainly contains six genes encoding six major structural proteins: nucleoprotein (NP), phosphoprotein (P), matrix protein (M), fusion protein (F), hemagglutinin-neuraminidase (HN), and RNA-dependent RNA polymerase (L), as shown in Fig. (1). The RNA together with NP, P, and L proteins forms the ribonucleoprotein complex (RNP), which serves as the template for RNA synthesis [4, 5]. Protruding on the virion surface, the HN protein mediates receptor attachment, while the F protein directs the fusion of the virus membrane with the cell membrane. The M protein inside the envelope stabilizes virus structure. Different strains of NDV share the six common genes, each with its own transcription start and stop signals. These genes appear in the following order from the 3' end to the 5' end in the genome: NP, P, M, F, HN, and L [6], and are separated by junction sequences that consist of three elements, known as gene-end (GE), intergenic (IG) and gene-start (GS) sequences [7]. The viral RNA polymerase complex is supposed to enter the genomic RNA at a single 3' entry site and to transcribe the genome by a sequential start–stop mechanism. The aforementioned characteristics are fundamental for the genetic manipulation of NDV *in vitro*.

The modular nature of gene transcription and the lack of a DNA phase in the replication cycle make NDV a suitable candidate for the rational design of a safe and stable vaccine and gene therapy vector [8]. Reverse genetics has made it possible to clone the NDV genome and to introduce new foreign genes to cells or tumors. In this review, it will be demonstrated that recombinant NDV is suitable as a live attenuated vaccine against infections in multiple animals and may also have potential use in some human populations. Furthermore, naturally occurring strains of NDV have shown oncolytic therapeutic potency in preclinical and clinical studies. With the development of reverse genetics technology, recombinant NDVs with increased targeting and oncolytic potency become possible. In this review, we will focus first on the recent progress in NDV research as a promising vaccine vector for combating infectious diseases and then on the development of NDV as a potential anticancer agent.

NEWCASTLE DISEASE VIRUS AS A VECTOR

Properties of NDV Suitable as a Vector

NDV is considered to be a suitable viral vector candidate because of its viral characteristics and desirable properties for a vector. First, much is known about attenuating NDV [6, 9]. Live attenuated vaccines are still considered to be highly efficient and the ideal approach for immunization. Second, NDV is efficient in inducing local IgA, systemic IgG, and cell-mediated protective immune responses when administered by the intranasal route [6]. Third, NDV replicates in the cytoplasm of the host cell and does not integrate into the host genome, obviating concerns about cellular transformation or viral persistence [6]. Fourth, NDV has a relatively simple genome and the genes of NDV are nonoverlapping, making them easy to manipulate [6]. Fifth, previous studies have shown that various foreign proteins expressed from recombinant NDVs can be maintained stably during serial passages [9, 10]. Sixth, controversial low rate of recombination. As pointed out in the article of Song *et al.* [11], more and more recombination events have been reported in recent years for NDVs, with the recombination occurring throughout the whole genome, but the authors' investigation indicates that the recombination of NDV is not as common as has been reported. Moreover, Miller *et al.* [12] pointed out that previous studies reporting recombination in NDV sequences failed to demonstrate recombination as an evolutionary force, as viable recombinant progenies in nature had not been identified. So they evaluated a comprehensive dataset of NDV genome sequences using bioinformatics to characterize the evolutionary forces affecting NDV genomes, and found out that despite evidence of recombination in most genes, only one event in the fusion gene of genotype V viruses produced evolutionarily viable progenies. Therefore, we agree with the need for caution in the use of live NDV-based vector vaccines, but caution in the analyses of the data is also needed [11, 13]. We believe that all these reasons make NDV a suitable candidate as a vector.

Reverse Genetics and Its Application in Negative-strand RNA Viruses

In classical genetics, the specific genes in an organism are deduced from observations of the phenotype of the organism. However, reverse genetics is a term coined to describe the processes where information flows in the opposite direction, that is, the gene is determined or altered directly and the resultant phenotype is observed [14]. In other words, reverse genetics tries to find what phenotypes appear as a result of particular genetic sequences.

Reverse genetics in molecular virology provides for the generation of viruses possessing a genome derived from cloned complementary DNA (cDNA) [15]. In fact, the technology has already revolutionized research on RNA viruses. As summarized by Michele and Ramon [16]: "Reverse genetics technology makes it possible to manipulate viral RNA molecules using cDNA copies so one can study the effects of genetic changes on the biology of the virus. This technology was applied to the modification of plus-stranded RNA virus genomes and to the recovery (rescue) of infectious virus from cDNA because plus-stranded RNA viruses are able to utilize the host cell DNA replication machinery to initiate their life cycles. Thus, plasmid-encoded or *in vitro* synthesized genomic RNA of these viruses is infectious when introduced into permissive cells. However, recovery of negative-strand RNA viruses from either cDNA or synthetic RNA was a substantial challenge because, unlike the plus-stranded RNA viruses, replication initiation requires *de novo* protein synthesis mediated by viral RNA-dependent RNA polymerase, and the input genomic or antigenomic RNA needs to be encapsidated with the viral nucleoprotein before it can serve as a functional template to initiate transcription/replication. After the successful application of reverse genetics technology for the manipulation of negative-strand RNA virus genomes, much has been elucidated about the molecular characteristics and pathogenesis of these viruses, and the insights obtained from such studies have provided new impetus for the development of rationally designed vaccines." By reverse genetics, researchers can engineer changes introduced directly into the cDNA used to generate infectious RNA virus, in order to study the function of specific gene sequences and proteins. It is a powerful tool both for the generation of modified viruses, which can act as vaccines or vectors, and for the analysis of viral genes and non-coding sequences [14].

In 1989, influenza virus became the first negative-strand RNA virus to yield to genetic manipulation. Initial strategies were designed to reconstitute a biologically active RNP complex, consisting of a synthetic RNA and purified nucleoproteins. Then the complex was transfected into cells that had previously been infected with a helper virus which provided those proteins *in trans* that are necessary for the replication and encapsidation of the synthetic RNA [17, 18]. Afterwards, 12-plasmid DNA transfection system [19] and eight-plasmid DNA transfection system [20] for the recovery of infectious influenza virus from cloned cDNA were developed. In contrast to the earlier helper virus-based recovery methods, the plasmid-based system can be easily used for the generation of infectious influenza viruses containing multiple mutations in different genes at the same time.

However, the manipulation of the genomes of nonsegmented negative-strand (NSNS) RNA viruses occurred later, being first achieved for rabies virus in 1994 [21]. The manipulation requires the reconstruction of full-length RNP complexes. The recovery of rabies virus was achieved by transfecting cells with four plasmids (one plasmid encoding the full-length antigenomic viral RNA and three expression plasmids respectively encoding N, L, and P proteins), under the control of the T7 polymerase provided by a further expression system [18]. Afterwards, similar strategies have been adopted for other NSNS RNA viruses, such as vesicular stomatitis virus [22], human respiratory syncytial virus [23], and Sendai virus [24].

The Application of Reverse Genetics in NDV

In 1999, Peeters *et al.* first reported the generation of infectious NDV entirely from cloned full-length cDNA [25]. The naked RNA alone is not infectious, and the RNP, namely NP, P, and L proteins, are essential to initiate the first round of RNA synthesis and establish infection [9]. So, the recovery was finally accomplished by using an approach in which cDNA-encoded antigenomic RNA is synthesized by means of the T7 RNA polymerase in cells that simultaneously express the viral replication proteins NP, P, and L from cotransfected plasmids [25]. Afterwards, using similar approaches of recovery, other researchers have achieved the generation of multiple strains of NDV from cloned full-length cDNA, such as Clone 30 [26], Beaudette C [9], Hitchner B1 [27], Herts/33 [28], ZJ1 [29], and 9a5b-D5C1 [30].

NDV as a Vector to Express Foreign Genes

The successful recovery of NDV from cDNA clones allows genetic manipulation of the entire genome of NDV, and the established reverse genetics system permits the generation of a genetically altered NDV. Therefore, over the past decade, researchers from around the world have been expending much effort in exploring NDV as a vaccine vector. The foreign proteins are inserted into the genome of NDV and are under control of NDV transcriptional start and stop signals. Surprisingly, as pointed out by Krishnamurthy *et al.* [9], it had been demonstrated in previous studies that the expression levels of foreign proteins are quite high and foreign genes are very stable after many passages both *in vitro* and *in vivo*. For example, Huang *et al.* [31] constructed a recombinant NDV expressing a foreign gene—CAT. The CAT gene was inserted into NDV antigenomic cDNA in the upstream region of the 3'-proximal NP gene open reading frame (ORF). The experimental results showed that the recombinant virus expressed a high level of the CAT protein and the expression of the CAT protein was stable over 12 low-dilution passages. Additionally, the replication and pathogenesis of the CAT-expressing recombinant virus were not significantly modified. Moreover, Engel-Herbert *et al.* [10] generated a recombinant NDV possessing the green fluorescent protein (GFP) gene between F and HN genes. Their experimental results showed that the expression of the heterologous gene was maintained stably for at least five passages in embryonated eggs. The replication kinetics in embryonated eggs and pathogenicity in chickens of the recombinant virus did not differ significantly from those of the parent virus.

Besides, reverse genetics enables NDV to be used as a vector to generate recombinant viruses for the expression of foreign protective antigens. For example, Khattar *et al.* [32] generated a recombinant NDV possessing human immunodeficiency virus type 1 envelope glycoprotein (gp160) gene between the

P and M genes. Experimental results showed that the recombinant virus grew efficiently in cell culture and in embryonated eggs. The expressed gp160 protein was incorporated into the NDV virion, with no effect on vector virus replication and pathogenicity. Immunization with the recombinant NDV elicited the Th1-type response. In this study, it is demonstrated that it is feasible to use NDV as a vaccine vector to induce strong mucosal and systemic neutralizing antibody responses to the HIV-1 envelope protein in guinea pigs. All above-mentioned studies illustrate that recombinant NDVs are able to express exogenetic genes and NDV may have great potential to be used as a broad-spectrum vaccine vector to provide protection against NDV as well as other pathogens. Fig. (**1**) is a schematic diagram, showing the use of NDV as a vaccine vector to generate recombinant viruses expressing a foreign protective antigen of a pathogen.

Locations for the Insertion of Foreign Genes in the NDV Genome

If NDV is used as a vector, the relationship between the insertion of foreign genes in the NDV genome and the expression level of the foreign genes needs to be addressed. This knowledge would lead to a finer insertion strategy for the foreign gene.

The expression level of the foreign gene in NDV was originally thought to be high when placed near the 3' end of the genome [9, 33]. Moreover, according to the tentatively deduction by Huang *et al.* [31], the expression level of the foreign gene in NDV was highest when placed near the 3' end of the genome (namely, inserted before the ORF of the 3'-proximal NP gene).

Later studies make us gradually closer to the truth. Zhao and Peeters [7] inserted a reporter gene encoding secreted alkaline phosphatase (SEAP) at four different positions distributed along the NDV genome between NP and P, M and F, HN and L genes, and behind the L gene. Their results demonstrated that NDV could be used as a vector to deliver foreign genes by insertion at different positions without severely affecting virus replication efficiency or virus yield. Quantification of the SEAP gene

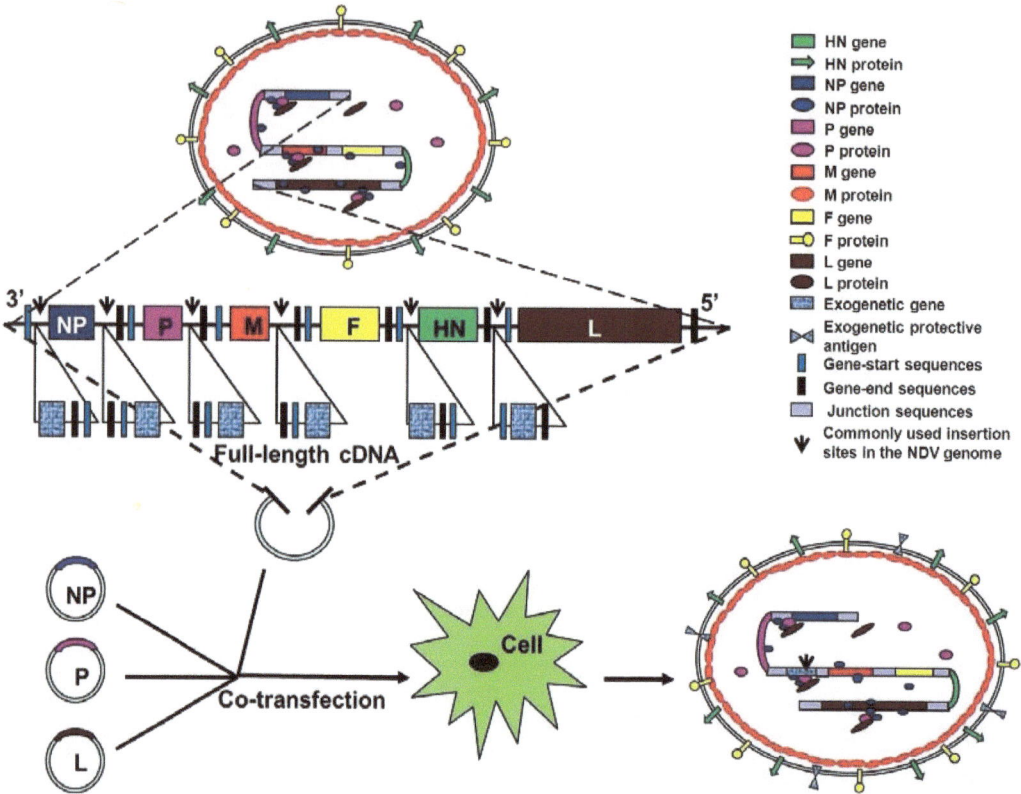

Fig. (1). Schematic representation of the utilization of NDV as a vector to generate a recombinant virus expressing an exogenetic protective antigen of a pathogen. An exogenetic gene can be inserted in different positions in the NDV genome, but the nucleotides should be added in the untranslated region to follow the rule of six. Here, the exogenetic gene is inserted between the P and M genes. Finally, recombinant virus expressing an exogenetic protective antigen is rescued and the exogenetic protective protein is incorporated into the NDV envelope.

expression by different recombinants in CEF cells showed high expression levels when the SEAP gene was located between the NP and P, M and F, and HN and L genes. In contrast, very low levels were expressed when the SEAP gene was inserted behind the L gene. However, in embryonated eggs, SEAP expression levels at 4 days after inoculation were 2–3 times lower when the SEAP gene was inserted between the NP and P genes than when it was inserted between the M and F genes. In another study, Carnero [34] determined the optimal insertion site into the NDV genome. They generated recombinant NDV-HIVGag viruses in which HIV *gag* was inserted at different transcriptional positions throughout the NDV genome. It was expected that higher levels of expression of Gag could be observed when the insertion was closer to the 3' end. This gradient of expression was the case when Gag was located between the P and M genes and positions located after the M gene (in the order of greatest to least expression). However, the Gag expression level was considerably lower when the gene was located between the NP and P genes. Unfortunately, they were not able to rescue a recombinant virus expressing HIV Gag in front of the NP gene of NDV. Furthermore, their *in vivo* experiments revealed that higher HIV Gag protein expression positively correlates with an enhanced CD8+ T-cell-mediated immune response and protective immunity against challenge with vaccinia virus expressing HIV Gag. This study illustrated that the location of *gag* between the P and M genes elicited the highest expression of this foreign protein and this location would be a finer insertion site for the foreign gene into the NDV genome.

Currently, the upper size limit of foreign genes that can be inserted into the NDV genome is unknown. Some aspects of the NDV vectors regarding expression levels, size of the foreign gene, and attenuation level of the recombinant virus need to be further investigated and elucidated.

Chimeric NDV-Based Vector as a Novel Solution to Eliminate Interference with Maternally Derived NDV Antibodies

NDV is a promising viral vector for the expression of foreign proteins from a variety of unrelated viruses. However, in reality, commercial chickens often have maternally derived NDV antibodies because of natural infection or vaccination, and the preexisting antibodies may impair vector replication, leading to a low immune response against the foreign antigen. A chimeric NDV-based vector with functional surface glycoproteins unrelated to NDV may well solve this problem. Steglich *et al.* (2013) constructed an NDV vector that carries the F and HN proteins of avian paramyxovirus type 8 instead of the corresponding NDV proteins in an NDV backbone (derived from Clone 30 strain of NDV) and that contains a foreign gene expressing HPAIV H5 inserted between the F and HN genes. After successful virus rescue, the expression and virion incorporation of the foreign proteins were confirmed respectively by western blot and electron microscopy. Replication of the rescued recombinant virus was comparable to parental NDV in embryonated chicken eggs. Immunization with the recombinant virus induced full protection against lethal HPAIV infection in chickens with NDV specific-maternally derived antibodies, which illustrates the substantial benefit of the chimeric NDV-based vector in protecting chickens with maternally derived NDV antibodies [35].

NDV-BASED VECTOR VACCINES AGAINST ANIMAL INFECTIOUS DISEASES

Infectious Bursal Disease Virus

Infectious bursal disease (IBD) is a highly contagious disease affecting major poultry production areas throughout the world [36]. Available live IBDV vaccines may lead to the generation of variant viruses [37], so alternative vaccines that would not create variant IBDV strains are needed. Therefore, Huang *et al.* designed a recombinant virus derived from LaSota strain of NDV to express the host-protective immunogen VP2 of a variant IBDV strain GLS-5 (rLaSota/VP2). Vaccination with rLaSota/VP2 provided 90% protection against NDV and IBDV, and booster immunization even provided complete protections against both viruses. Their results demonstrated that NDV could be a suitable vaccine vector candidate for other avian pathogens [37]. Furthermore, in another study, Ge *et al.* devised a recombinant NDV (rLaSota-VP2) expressing VP2 protein of the very virulent IBDV (vvIBDV) Gx strain. The foreign gene was inserted between the P and M of full-length genomic cDNA of NDV LaSota strain. Vaccination with rLaSota-VP2 in 7-day old specific-pathogen-free chickens conferred complete protection against a highly virulent NDV F48E9 strain and provided over 90% protection against vvIBDV Gx strain three weeks after vaccination. This study demonstrated that the recombinant NDV (rLaSota-VP2) could be used as a bivalent vaccine against NDV and IBDV [38]. A patent application on the method to produce the recombinant NDV (rLaSota-VP2) and on its use for the prevention of ND and IBD has been filed by Bu *et al.* [39].

Bovine Herpesvirus-1

Bovine herpesvirus-1 (BHV-1) is a pathogen of great economic importance in the global cattle industry [40, 41]. As described by Khattar *et al.* [41], currently used vaccines against BHV-1, formulated with either inactivated or modified live virus, have many disadvantages. Hence, they devised two recombinant NDVs respectively expressing the glycoprotein D of BHV-1 from a foreign gene. One-time intranasal and intratracheal inoculation of calves with either recombinant NDV could induce mucosal and systemic antibodies specific to BHV-1. After challenge with BHV-1, calves immunized with the recombinant NDVs had lower titers and earlier clearance of challenge virus in contrast to the empty vector control. Therefore, it was suggested that NDV is suitable as a vaccine vector to be used in bovines.

Herpesviruses are a large family of DNA viruses that can cause diseases in animals and humans. It has been difficult to develop effective vaccines against these viruses, because many of them have complex life cycles and lie dormant in the body for long periods of time. So scientists have never stopped exploring for effective vaccines against such notorious viruses. A patent application filed by Bublot *et al.* [42] encompasses recombinant NDV-Herpesvirus vaccines. The invention encompasses recombinant NDVs that can express herpesvirus pathogen, antigens, proteins, epitopes or immunogens. Such vaccines may be used to protect animals against the disease.

NDV-BASED VECTOR VACCINES AGAINST ZOONOSES

Highly Pathogenic Avian Influenza A (H5N1) Virus

The highly pathogenic avian influenza H5N1 virus (HPAIV) has strong zoonotic characteristics and can be transmitted from birds to different mammalian species including humans [43]. The HPAIV H5N1 was first detected in human infections in 1997 in HongKong [44]. It appears that H5N1 influenza viruses pose a serious threat to both domestic poultry and public health. Because the relatively high cost of production and the laborsome administration of traditional vaccines had limited their widespread application in the field in animals, Ge *et al.* [45] devised a novel NDV-based vector vaccine targeted against AIV for the use in the field in the control of infection and spread of AIV. They constructed a recombinant NDV expressing an H5 subtype AIV hemagglutinin (HA). BALB/c mice and chickens immunized with the recombinant NDV-based vector vaccine were completely protected from challenge with a lethal dose of homologous and heterologous H5N1 HPAIV. Their results demonstrated that the recombinant NDV can be used as a live attenuated vaccine against NDV and AIV infections in poultry and suggested that recombinant NDV may also have potential use in high-risk human individuals to control the pandemic spread of lethal avian influenza. Two patents on the recombinant NDV-based vector vaccines expressing wild or mutant AIV H5 subtype HA protein have been applied for by Bu and Chen [46, 47].

Rabies Virus

Rabies virus (RV) can cause a fatal neurologic disease in humans and animals. Rabies occurs in more than 150 countries and territories around the world. More than 55,000 people (another estimation is 60,000) die each year of rabies, mostly in Asia and Africa [48, 49]. So, there is still a need for the effective, safe and affordable rabies vaccines. Ge *et al.* [50] had generated a recombinant LaSota strain of NDV expressing the RV glycoprotein (rL-RVG). Intramuscular vaccination with the recombinant virus stimulated a substantial RV neutralizing antibody response and could offer complete protection from challenge with circulating rabies virus strains. Furthermore, the recombinant virus could stimulate strong and long-lasting protective neutralizing antibody responses to RV in dogs and cats. The vaccinated dogs were completely protected from RV street virus challenge after a year, displaying no signs of disease or death. This study demonstrated that immunization with an NDV-based vector vaccine could induce long-lasting protective immunity against rabies in dogs and cats, and suggested that the vaccine may also have potential use in high-risk human individuals to control rabies infections.

Rift Valley Fever Virus

Rift Valley fever (RVF) is a mosquito-borne zoonosis that primarily affects ruminants but also has the capacity to infect humans. Infections can cause severe disease in both animals and humans. RVF is generally found in Africa and the Arabian Peninsula, but the worldwide distribution of potential RVFV mosquito vectors raises the concerns that it could extend to other parts of the world [51-53]. Currently, there is still a need for a safe and effective vaccine against the disease. Thus, Kortekaas *et al.* [53] tried to use recombinant NDV as a vector vaccine for the prevention of RVF. They constructed a recombinant NDV (NDFL-Gn) expressing the RVF virus Gn glycoprotein. Intramuscular vaccination with the recombinant virus induced antibodies against both NDV and Gn protein. The RVFV-neutralizing activity of the antisera from the intramuscularly vaccinated calves was demonstrated in the study. The study suggested that NDV is a promising vaccine vector for the prevention of RVF in calves.

Indeed, live-attenuated NDV-based vector vaccines have some advantages. First, the NDV-based vector vaccines can potentially be administered by aerosol sprays or drinking water for poultry, thus reducing the cost of mass administration. Second, the ability to differentiate infected from vaccinated animals (DIVA) is another major advantage for NDV-based vector vaccines. A vaccine that can be distinguished serologically from a field strain is called a DIVA or marker vaccine. Peeters *et al.* first chose to modify the HN protein of NDV to generate a genetically modified marker vaccine, which can be differentiated from wild-type NDV on the basis of different antibodies induced by their HN proteins [54]. Furthermore, a NDV-based vector vaccine inserted with an exogenetic gene of a pathogen which can only induce an immune response against the exogenetic protein in animals makes serological surveillance against the pathogen possible, since vaccinated animals lack immune responses against antigens present in the whole pathogen [35, 55-57].

NDV-BASED VECTOR VACCINE AGAINST HUMAN INFECTIOUS DISEASE

Human Immunodeficiency Virus

Human Immunodeficiency Virus (HIV) remains one of the most serious global public health challenges, particularly in low- and middle-income countries. It has been over 30 years since the identification of HIV as the causative agent of the acquired immunodeficiency syndrome [58]. However, there is still an urgent need for the development of an effective vaccine to halt the HIV pandemic [32]. Maamary *et al.* [59] devised an rNDV vector vaccine expressing a dendritic cell-targeted HIV Gag protein. The mice immunized with the recombinant virus vaccine were better protected from challenge with a recombinant vaccinia virus expressing the HIV Gag protein than those immunized with rNDV expressing a non-targeted HIV Gag antigen. This study supported the use of NDV as a vaccine vector for further studies aiming at the development of an effective HIV vaccine. Additionally, two authors of this article, Garcia-Sastre and Palese have applied for a patent regarding genetically engineered NDVs expressing heterologous gene products including a peptide or protein derived from the genome of a human immunodeficiency virus [60].

It is worth mentioning here that since the majority of human infectious diseases have animal origins, the prevention and control of disease in animals should be considered as one of the primary lines of defense for protecting human populations as well as animals and their associated economic importance [61].

Finally, all these studies warrant further study on the use of NDV as a promising vaccine vector for combating infectious animal diseases, zoonotic diseases and human infectious diseases.

ONCOLYTIC NEWCASTLE DISEASE VIRUS FOR CANCER TREATMENT

Cancer remains a major cause of death in humans. In the past, virotherapy using oncolytic viruses (OVs) was proposed as a potent cancer therapy [62]. Increasing problems with tumor resistance to chemotherapeutic agents resulting in cancer relapses have been noted. Because of this trend, there has been a renewed interest from clinicians in using OVs as tumor cell killers [63, 64]. Naturally occurring strains of NDV have been demonstrated to possess significant oncolytic activity against cancers in preclinical and clinical studies.

Clinical Trials with Oncolytic NDVs

The first utilization of NDV for human tumor therapy was documented in 1964 by Dr. Wheelock and Dr. Dingle. A patient with acute myelogenous leukemia, after receiving intravenous inoculation with NDV Hickman strain, showed rapid reduction in leukemic blast count and improvement in symptoms. However, these improvements were short-lived and only lasted for approximately two weeks [65, 66]. Afterwards, multiple oncolytic NDV strains, such as MTH-68 [67], PV-701 [68] or HUJ [69], were used in succession in treating cancer patients, mainly *via* inhalation and intravenous administration. From these clinical studies, the effect of NDV as an anticancer agent has been observed, warranting further study on the virus as a novel therapeutic agent for cancer patients. Additionally, encouraging results of using NDV as an anticancer agent were also noted in some preclinical studies, such as breast carcinoma [70], melanoma [71], gastric carcinoma [72], leukemia [73], lymphoma [74, 75]. As a result, the focus on the use of oncolytic strains of NDV as an anticancer agent has generated some patent applications [76-78].

The use of NDV as an oncolytic agent exhibits several advantages: (1) the virus is an economically important pathogen in multiple avian species but nonpathogenic to humans and other domestic animals; (2) the viral genome can allow for the introduction and stable expression of foreign genes; (3) the virus has a wide variety of anticancer properties, which were detailed and summarized by Lam *et al.* [62]. Additionally, the mechanisms of NDV-mediated oncolysis (direct mechanism *via* NDV-induced apoptosis and indirect mechanism *via* NDV-activated innate and adaptive anti-tumor immune responses) and the mechanisms of NDV specificity for tumor cells were summarized for further reading by Zamarin and Palese [66]. However, there are limitations of using NDV as an oncolytic agent in clinical oncology. Systemically delivered NDV may fail to reach solid tumors in therapeutic concentrations and may also spread poorly within the tumors due to barriers including complement, innate immunity, and the extracellular matrix [79]. So improving the tumor-specific targeting of oncolytic NDV and the delivery efficiency (*e.g.*, avoiding the neutralizing immune response to oncolytic NDV which may limit its therapeutic efficacy) are truly big challenges. Therefore, overcoming these obstacles seems more important than realizing the oncolytic potency of NDV. Reverse genetics technology may be instrumental in overcoming these obstacles.

Enhancing Oncolytic Activity of NDV through Reverse Genetics

As previously described by Zamarin and Palese [66], reverse genetics has been explored as an approach to enhance the oncolytic potency of NDV mainly by following strategies: (1) engineering fusogenic NDV to increase viral spread from cell to cell so as to enhance the oncolytic potency; (2) engineering NDV armed with immunostimulatory cytokines results in activation and recruitment of lymphocytes and dendritic cells; (3) engineering NDV to modulate innate immune responses to enhance viral replication and thus to improve the oncolytic efficacy;

(4) engineering NDV to express immunoglobulins, apoptin, or tumor-associated antigens for the enhancement of oncolytic potency.

Besides, a recent report is noteworthy. Shobana *et al.* [79] constructed a recombinant NDV (rNDV) whose F protein could only be cleaved by prostate-specific antigen (PSA). The recombinant virus showed efficient and specific replication in prostate cancer cells and 3-dimensional prostaspheres but failed to replicate in the absence of PSA. Moreover, PSA-retargeted NDV also showed its potential efficacy *in vivo* by efficiently lysing prostasphere tumor mimics. Hence, prostate-specific antigen targeting is likely to improve the oncolytic efficacy of rNDV because of tumor-restricted replication and enhanced fusogenicity.

Additionally, patent applications have been generated for genetically engineered NDVs to be used as oncolytic agents (such as comprising a binding protein gene when expressed by the virus-infected tumor cell that has a therapeutic activity, incorporating therapeutic transgenes, or expressing a heterologous interferon antagonist) [80-82].

The observations made during the past decades have demonstrated the feasibility of NDV as a therapeutic agent against cancers. Furthermore, by reverse genetics, modifications of oncolytic NDVs lead to increased targeting and oncolytic potency, potentially resulting in strengthening the feasibility of the use of NDV as a cancer therapy.

CURRENT AND FUTURE DEVELOPMENTS

We have reviewed some (but not all) excellent examples of advances using reverse genetics to generate recombinant NDV strains to combat infectious diseases and to treat cancers. NDV has become one of the most promising vaccine vectors against pathogens. Furthermore, the ongoing studies using reverse genetics to develop enhanced recombinant NDVs as cancer therapeutic agents, may allow for crucial improvements for oncolytic NDV to be used in the clinical treatment of malignant tumors. Besides, new insights into the virus life cycle and the continued development of reverse genetics technology may make an enormous contribution to the use of NDV as a vaccine vector or as an anticancer agent in the future.

ACKNOWLEDGEMENTS

Grant support: the Research Fund for the Doctoral Program of Higher Education by the Ministry of Education of China (20100061120038) (to X. Zhang).

CONFLICT OF INTEREST

The authors confirm that this chapter contents have no conflict of interest.

REFERENCES

[1]   Bukreyev A, Skiadopoulos MH, Murphy BR, Collins PL. Nonsegmented negative-strand viruses as vaccine vectors. J Virol 2006; 80: 10293-306.
[2]   DiNapoli JM, Ward JM, Cheng L, Yang L, Elankumaran S, Murphy BR, Samal SK, Collins PL, Bukreyev A. Delivery to the lower respiratory tract is required for effective immunization with Newcastle disease virus-vectored vaccines intended for humans. Vaccine 2009; 27: 1530-9.
[3]   Alexander DJ. & Senne DA. Newcastle disease, other avian paramyxoviruses, and pneumovirus infections. In Diseases of poultry (Saif YM, ed.), 12th ed. Blackwell Publishing, Ames, Iowa, 2008; 75-115.
[4]   Lamb RA, Kolakofsky D. Paramyxoviridae: the viruses and their replication. In Fields BN, Eds. Fields virology, 3rd ed. LippincottRaven Press, Philadelphia, Pa. 1996.
[5]   Mebatsion T, Koolen MJ, de Vaan LT, de Haas N, Braber M, Römer-Oberdörfer A, van den Elzen P, van der Marel P. Newcastle disease virus (NDV) marker vaccine: an immunodominant epitope on the nucleoprotein gene of NDV can be deleted or replaced by a foreign epitope. J Virol 2002; 76: 10138-46.
[6]   Sato H, Yoneda M, Honda T, Kai C. Recombinant vaccines against the mononegaviruses-- what we have learned from animal disease controls. Virus Res 2011; 162: 63-71.
[7]   Zhao H, Peeters BPH. Recombinant Newcastle Disease virus as a viral vector: effect of genomic location of foreign gene on gene expression and virus replication. J Gen Virol 2003; 84: 781-8.
[8]   Schirrmacher V, Fournier P. Newcastle disease virus: a promising vector for viral therapy, immune therapy, and gene therapy of cancer. Methods Mol Biol 2009; 542: 565-605.
[9]   Krishnamurthy S, Huang Z, Samal SK. Recovery of a virulent strain of newcastle disease virus from cloned cDNA: expression of a foreign gene results in growth retardation and attenuation. Virology 2000; 278: 168-82.
[10]   Engel-Herbert I, Werner O, Teifke JP, Mebatsion T, Mettenleiter TC, Römer-Oberdörfer A. Characterization of a recombinant Newcastle Disease virus expressing the green fluorescent protein. J Virol Methods 2003; 108: 19-28.

[11]   Song Q, Cao Y, Li Q, Gu M, Zhong L, Hu S, Wan H, Liu X. Artificial recombination may influence the evolutionary analysis of Newcastle disease virus. J Virol 2011; 85: 10409-14.

[12]   Miller PJ, Kim LM, Ip HS, Afonso CL. Evolutionary dynamics of Newcastle disease virus. Virology 2009; 391: 64-72.

[13]   Afonso CL. Not so fast on recombination analysis of Newcastle disease virus. J Virol 2008; 82: 9303.

[14]   Bridgen A. Reverse genetics of RNA viruses : applications and perspectives. Chichester, West Sussex: Wiley-Blackwell, 2013.

[15]   Neumann G, Whitt MA, Kawaoka Y. A decade after the generation of a negative-sense RNA virus from cloned cDNA -- what have we learned? J Gen Virol 2002; 83: 2635-62.

[16]   Bouloy M, Flick R. Reverse genetics technology for Rift Valley fever virus: Current and future applications of the development of therapeutics and vaccines. Antiviral Research 2009; 84: 101-18.

[17]   Luytjes W, Krystal M, Enami M, Parvin JD, Palese P. Amplification, expression and packaging of a foreign gene by influenza virus. Cell 1989; 59: 1107-13.

[18]   Hewson R. RNA viruses: emerging vectors for vaccination and gene therapy. Mol Med Today 2000; 6: 28-35.

[19]   Fodor E, Devenish L, Engelhardt OG, Palese P, Brownlee GG, García-Sastre A. Rescue of influenza A virus from recombinant DNA. J Vriol 1999; 11: 9679-82.

[20]   Hoffmann E, Neumann G, Kawaoka Y, Hobom G, Webster RG. A DNA transfection system for generation of influenza A virus from eight plasmids. Proc Natl Acad Sci U S A 2000; 97: 6108-13.

[21]   Schnell MJ, Mebatsion T, Conzelmann KK. Infectious rabies viruses from cloned cDNA. EMBO Journal 1994; 13: 4195-203.

[22]   Whelan SP, Ball LA, Barr JN, Wertz GT. Efficient recovery of infectious vesicular stomatitis virus entirely from cDNA clones. Proc Natl Acad Sci U S A 1995; 92: 8388-92.

[23]   Collins PL, Hill MG, Camargo E, Grosfeld H, Chanock RM, Murphy BR. Production of infectious human respiratory syncytial virus from cloned cDNA confirms an essential role for the transcription elongation factor from the 5' proximal open reading frame of the M2 mRNA in gene expression and provides a capability for vaccine development. Proc Natl Acad Sci U S A 1995; 92: 11563-7.

[24]   Kato A, Sakai Y, Shioda T, Kondo T, Nakanishi M, Nagai Y. Initiation of Sendai virus multiplication from transfected cDNA or RNA with negative or positive sense. Genes Cells 1996; 1: 569-79.

[25]   Peeters BP, de Leeuw OS, Koch G, Gielkens AL. Rescue of Newcastle disease virus from cloned cDNA: Evidence that cleavability of the fusion protein is a major determinant for virulence. J Virol 1999; 73: 5001-9.

[26]   Römer-Oberdörfer A, Mundt E, Mebatsion T, Buchholz UJ, Mettenleiter TC. Generation of recombinant lentogenic Newcastle disease virus from cDNA. J Gen Virol 1999; 80: 2987-95.

[27]   Nakaya T, Cros J, Park MS, Nakaya Y, Zheng H, Sagrera A, Villar E, García-Sastre A, Palese P. Recombinant Newcastle disease virus as a vaccine vector. J Virol 2001; 75: 11868-73.

[28]   de Leeuw OS, Koch G, Hartog L, Ravenshorst N, Peeters BP. Virulence of Newcastle disease virus is determined by the cleavage site of the fusion protein and by both the stem

region and globular head of the haemagglutinin-neuraminidase protein. J Gen Virol 2005; 86: 1759-69.

[29]   Liu YL, Hu SL, Zhang YM, Sun SJ, Romer-Oberdorfer A, Veits J, Wu YT, Wan HQ, Liu XF. Generation of a velogenic Newcastle disease virus from Cdna and expression of the green fluorescent protein. Arch Virol 2007; 153: 1241-9.

[30]   Yu Y, Qiu X, Xu D, Zhan Y, Meng C, Wei N, Chen H, Tan L, Yu S, Liu X, Qin A, Ding C. Rescue of virulent class I Newcastle disease virus variant 9a5b-D5C1. Virol J 2012; 9: 120-8.

[31]   Huang Z, Krishnamurthy S, Panda A, Samal SK. High-level expression of a foreign gene from the most 3'-proximal locus of a recombinant Newcastle disease virus. J Gen Virol 2001; 82: 1729-36.

[32]   Khattar SK, Samal S, Devico AL, Collins PL, Samal SK. Newcastle disease virus expressing Human immunodeficiency virus type 1 envelope glycoprotein induces strong mucosal and serum antibody responses in Guinea pigs. J. Virol 2011; 85: 10529-41.

[33]   Wertz GW, Perepelitsa VP, Ball LA. Gene rearrangement attenuates expression and lethality of a nonsegmented negative strand RNA virus. Proc Natl Acad Sci U S A 1998; 95: 3501-6.

[34]   Carnero E, Li W, Borderia AV, Moltedo B, Moran T, García-Sastre A. Optimization of human immunodeficiency virus gag expression by newcastle disease virus vectors for the induction of potent immune responses. J Virol 2009; 83: 584-97.

[35]   Steglich C, Grund C, Ramp K, Breithaupt A, Höper D, Keil G, Veits J, Ziller M, Granzow H, Mettenleiter TC, Römer-Oberdörfer A. Chimeric newcastle disease virus protects chickens against avian influenza in the presence of maternally derived NDV immunity. PLoS One 2013; 8: e72530.

[36]   Alfonso-Morales A, Martínez-Pérez O, Dolz R, Valle R, Perera CL, Bertran K, Frías MT, Majó N, Ganges L, Pérez LJ. Spatiotemporal Phylogenetic Analysis and Molecular Characterisation of Infectious Bursal Disease Viruses Based on the VP2 Hyper-Variable Region. PLoS One 2013; 8: e65999.

[37]   Huang Z, Elankumaran S, Yunus AS, Samal SK. A recombinant Newcastle Disease Virus (NDV) expressing VP2 protein of Infectious Bursal Disease Virus (IBDV) protects against NDV and IBDV. J Virol 2004; 78: 10054-63.

[38]   Ge J, Wen Z, Gao H, Wang Y, Hu S, Bao E, Wang X, Bu Z. Generation of recombinant Newcastle Disease Virus LaSota vaccine strain expressing VP2 gene of very virulent infectious bursal disease virus isolated from cDNA clone by reverse genetic. Scientia Agricultura Sinica 2008; 41: 243-51.

[39]   Bu, Z., Wang, X., Chen, H.: WO2007/025431A1 (**2007**).

[40]   van Drunen Littel-van den Hurk S, Parker MD, Massie B, van den Hurk JV, Harland R, Babiuk LA, Zamb TJ. Protection of cattle from BHV-1 infection by immunization with recombinant glycoprotein gIV. Vaccine 1993; 11: 25-35.

[41]   Khattar SK, Collins PL, Samal SK. Immunization of cattle with recombinant Newcastle disease virus expressing bovine herpesvirus-1 (BHV-1) glycoprotein D induces mucosal and serum antibody responses and provides partial protection against BHV-1. Vaccine 2010; 28: 3159-70.

[42]   Bublot, M., Reynard, F., Poulet, H., David, F.R.: WO2012/030720A1 (**2012**).

[43]   Kalthoff D, Globig A, Beer M. (Highly pathogenic) avian influenza as a zoonotic agent. Vet Microbiol 2010; 140: 237-45.

[44]   Chen H, Deng G, Li Z, Tian G, Li Y, Jiao P, Zhang L, Liu Z, Webster RG., Yu K. The evolution of H5N1 influenza viruses in ducks in southern China. Proc Natl Acad Sci U S A 2004; 101: 10452-7.

[45]   Ge J, Deng G, Wen Z, Tian G, Wang Y, Shi J, Wang X, Li Y, Hu S, Jiang Y, Yang C, Yu K, Bu Z, Chen H. Newcastle Disease Virus-based live attenuated vaccine completely protects chickens and mice from lethal challenge of homologous and heterologous H5N1 Avian Influenza Viruses. J Virol 2007; 81: 150-8.

[46]   Bu, Z., Chen, H.: WO2007/128169A1 (**2007**).

[47]   Bu, Z., Chen, H.: WO2007/025420A1 (**2007**).

[48]   Dietzschold B, Schnell M, Koprowski H. Pathogenesis of rabies. Current Topics in Microbiology and Immunology 2005; 292: 45-56.

[49]   World Health Organization. Rabies. Updated July 2013, http://www.who.int/mediacentre/factsheets/fs099/en/

[50]   Ge J, Wang X, Tao L, Wen Z, Feng N, Yang S, Xia X, Yang C, Chen H, Bu Z. Newcastle Disease Virus-Vectored Rabies Vaccine Is Safe, Highly Immunogenic, and Provides Long-Lasting Protection in Dogs and Cats. J Virol 2011; 85: 8241-52.

[51]   Flick R, Bouloy M. Rift Valley fever virus. Curr Mol Med 2005; 5: 827-34.

[52]   Bird BH, Ksiazek TG, Nichol ST, Maclachlan NJ. Rift Valley fever virus. J Am Vet Med Assoc 2009; 234: 883-93.

[53]   Kortekaas J, Dekker A, de Boer SM, Weerdmeester K, Vloet RP, de Wit AA, Peeters BP, Moormann RJ. Intramuscular inoculation of calves with an experimental Newcastle disease virus-based vector vaccine elicits neutralizing antibodies against Rift Valley fever virus. Vaccine 2010; 28: 2271-6.

[54]   Peeters BP, de Leeuw OS, Verstegen I, Koch G, Gielkens AL. Generation of a recombinant chimeric Newcastle disease virus vaccine that allows serological differentiation between vaccinated and infected animals. Vaccine 2001; 19: 1616-27.

[55]   Veits J, Wiesner D, Fuchs W, Hoffmann B, Granzow H, Starick E, Mundt E, Schirrmeier H, Mebatsion T, Mettenleiter TC, Römer-Oberdörfer A. Newcastle disease virus expressing H5 hemagglutinin gene protects chickens against Newcastle disease and avian influenza. Proc Natl Acad Sci U S A 2006; 103: 8197-202.

[56]   Park MS, Steel J, García-Sastre A, Swayne D, Palese P. Engineered viral vaccine constructs with dual specificity: avian influenza and Newcastle disease. Proc Natl Acad Sci U S A 2006; 103: 8203-8.

[57]   Nayak B, Rout SN, Kumar S, Khalil MS, Fouda MM, Ahmed LE, Earhart KC, Perez DR, Collins PL, Samal SK. Immunization of chickens with Newcastle disease virus expressing H5 hemagglutinin protects against highly pathogenic H5N1 avian influenza viruses. PLoS One 2009; 4: e6509.

[58]   Gallo RC, Montagnier L. The discovery of HIV as the cause of AIDS. N Engl J Med 2003; 349: 2283-5.

[59]   Maamary J, Array F, Gao Q, García-Sastre A, Steinman RM, Palese P, Nchinda G. Newcastle disease virus expressing a dendritic cell-targeted HIV gag protein induces a potent gag-specific immune response in mice. J Virol 2011; 85: 2235-46.

[60]   Garcia-Sastre, A., Palese, P.: US2009/0280144A1 (**2009**).

[61]   Zhang X. Deeper system reforms are urgently needed to ensure functional anti-animal disease epidemic personnel in China. Int J Infect Dis 2012; 16: e640.

[62]   Lam HY, Yeap SK, Rasoli M, Omar AR, Yusoff K, Suraini AA, Alitheen NB. Safety and clinical usage of newcastle disease virus in cancer therapy. J Biomed Biotechnol 2011; 2011: 718710.

[63]   Nelson NJ. Scientific interest in Newcastle disease virus is reviving. J Natl Cancer Inst. 1999; 91: 1708-10.

[64]   Fournier P, Schirrmacher V. Oncolytic Newcastle disease virus as cutting edge between tumor and host. Biology 2013; 2: 936-75.

[65]   Wheelock EF, Dingle JH. Observations on the repeated administration of viruses to a patient with acute leukemia — a preliminary report. N Engl J Med 1964; 271: 645-51.

[66]   Zamarin D, Palese P. Oncolytic Newcastle disease virus for cancer therapy: old challenges and new directions. Future Microbiol 2012; 7: 347-67.

[67]   Csatary LK, Eckhardt S, Bukosza I, Czegledi F, Fenyvesi C, Gergely P, Bodey B, Csatary CM. Attenuated veterinary virus vaccine for the treatment of cancer. Cancer Detect Prev 1993; 17: 619-27.

[68]   Pecora AL, Rizvi N, Cohen GI, Meropol NJ, Sterman D, Marshall JL, Goldberg S, Gross P, O'Neil JD, Groene WS, Roberts MS, Rabin H, Bamat MK, Lorence RM. Phase I trial of intravenous administration of PV701, an oncolytic virus, in patients with advanced solid cancers. J Clin Oncol 2002; 20: 2251-66.

[69]   Freeman AI, Zakay-Rones Z, Gomori JM, Linetsky E, Rasooly L, Greenbaum E, Rozenman-Yair S, Panet A, Libson E, Irving CS, Galun E, Siegal T. Phase I/II trial of intravenous NDV-HUJ oncolytic virus in recurrent glioblastoma multiforme. Mol Ther 2006; 13: 221-8.

[70]   Ghrici M, El Zowalaty M, Omar AR, Ideris A. Newcastle disease virus Malaysian strain AF2240 induces apoptosis in MCF-7 human breast carcinoma cells at an early stage of the virus life cycle. Int J Mol Med 2013; 31: 525-32.

[71]   Termeer CC, Schirrmacher V, Brocker EB, Becker JC. Newcastle disease virus infection induces B7–1/B7–2-independent T-cell costimulatory activity in human melanoma cells. Cancer Gene Ther 2000; 7: 316-23.

[72]   Song KY, Wong J, Gonzalez L, Sheng G, Zamarin D, Fong Y. Antitumor efficacy of viral therapy using genetically engineered Newcastle disease virus [NDV(F3aa)-GFP] for peritoneally disseminated gastric cancer. J Mol Med (Berl) 2010; 88: 589-96.

[73]   Alabsi AM, Ali R, Ideris A, Omar AR, Bejo MH, Yusoff K, Ali AM. Anti-leukemic activity of Newcastle disease virus strains AF2240 and V4-UPM in murine myelomonocytic leukemia *in vivo*. Leuk Res. 2012; 36: 634-45.

[74]   Bar-Eli N, Giloh H, Schlesinger M, Zakay-Rones Z. Preferential cytotoxic effect of Newcastle disease virus on lymphoma cells. J Cancer Res Clin Oncol 1996; 122: 409-15.

[75]   Eaton MD, Levinthal JD, Scala AR. Contribution of antiviral immunity to oncolysis by Newcastle disease virus in a murine lymphoma. J Natl Cancer Inst 1967; 39: 1089-97.

[76]   Csatary, L.K., Szeberenyi, J., Fabian, Z.: US2006/0018836A1 (**2006**).

[77]   Csatary, L.K., Szeberenyi, J., Fabian, Z.: US2006/0018884A1 (**2006**).

[78]   Csatary, C.M., Csatary, L.K.: WO2011/064630A1 (**2011**).

[79]   Shobana R, Samal SK, Elankumaran S. Prostate-specific antigen-retargeted recombinant newcastle disease virus for prostate cancer virotherapy. J Virol 2013; 87: 3792-800.

[80]   Beier, R., Puhler, F.: WO2006/050984A2 (**2006**).

[81]   Subbiah, E., Samal, S.K.: US2009/0175826A1 (**2009**)

[82]   Zamarin, D., García-Sastre, A., Palese, P., Fong, Y.: WO2010/091262A1 (**2010**).

CHAPTER 5

Basis of Anti-Infective Therapy against *Leishmaniasis* and Future Perspectives

Adil M. Allahverdiyev[*,1], Tanil Kocagoz[*,2], Melahat Bagirova[1], Emrah Sefik Abamor[1], Sinem Oktem Okullu[2], Nihan Aytekin Unubol[2], Rabia Cakir Koc[1], Sezen Canim Ates[1], Meral Miraloglu[3] and Serhat Elcicek[4]

[1]*Yildiz Technical University, Department of Bioengineering, Istanbul, Turkey;* [2]*Acibadem University, School of Medicine, Department of Microbiology, Istanbul, Turkey;* [3]*Cukurova University, Vocational School of Health, Adana, Turkey; and* [4]*Firat University, Department of Bioengineering, Elazig, Turkey*

Abstract: *Leishmaniasis* is a group of diseases caused by protozoa of the genus *Leishmania*. The disease is transmitted to humans *via* bites of female phlebotomies sand flies that are infected with *Leishmania* parasites. *Leishmaniasis* affects 12 million people in the world, and it is known that nearly 350 million people are under risk of infection. *Leishmania* parasites are responsible for cutaneous, mucocutaneous, and visceral forms of *Leishmaniasis*. Every year, approximately 1.5 million *Cutaneous Leishmaniasis* (CL) and 500,000 *Visceral Leishmaniasis* cases are reported in the world. Due to several factors such as cross-country travel, co-infections between human immunodeficiency virus (HIV) and *Leishmaniasis*, resistance to antileishmanial drugs in parasites, resistance to insecticides in vectors, and global warming, all types of *Leishmaniasis* are rapidly spreading all around the world. In order to combat *Leishmaniasis*, various approaches such as vaccine development, chemotherapy, physical treatment methods, immunotherapy, applications of natural plant products, phototherapy, and nanotechnologic approaches are used in the treatment. In this review, we will mention these approaches, which compose the basis of anti-infective therapy against *Leishmaniasis* and suggest new future perspectives for treatment of this serious disease.

Keywords: Anti-*Leishmanial*, cutaneous, diagnosis, drugs, essential oils, immune therapy, *Leishmania*, *Leishmaniasis*, photo dynamic therapy, plant extracts, therapy, vaccine, visceral.

*Corresponding Author Adil M. Allahverdiyev: Yildiz Technical University, Department of Bioengineering, Istanbul, Turkey; Tel: +90 212 383 46 39; Fax: +90 212 383 46 25; E-mail: adilmoglu@gmail.com

INTRODUCTION

Leishmaniasis is one of the major tropical diseases in the world caused by intracellular protozoan parasites, which belong to the genus *Leishmania* [1]. According to the World Health Organization (WHO), *Leishmaniasis* threatens about 350 million people in 98 countries around the world [2]. There are an estimated 12 million people infected by *Leishmania*, and approximately 2 million new cases occur every year [2, 3]. It is known that approximately 21 of 30 species of *Leishmania* parasites are pathogenic for human [4, 5]. The species are found in two morphologic forms during their life cycle. In humans and other mammalian hosts, they exist within macrophages and monocytes as round to oval nonflagellate. These forms are called amastigotes. The other parasite form is called promastigotes, which has flagella and exists in the gastrointestinal system of vectors (sand flies) [6, 7]. The promastigote form resides in the midgut of infected sand flies [8]. The disease is transmitted generally by the bite of female sand flies, which belong to the *Phlebotomus* and *Lutzomyia* genus of *phlebotomine* [4]. However, other means of transmission are possible. Healthy people are infected in a variety of ways by *Leishmania* parasites [9, 10]. Transmission of *Leishmania* by blood transfusion has been reported [10-16]. Other means of transmission, such as needle sharing among intravenous drug users, have also been reported and experimentally confirmed [2]. Occasionally, infection also occurs congenitally from mother to infant [17], sexual transmission [10, 18], laboratory accidents [6, 19, 20], and through organ [10, 21] and stem-cell transplantation [22, 23]. Additionally, in recent years there have been studies regarding spread of the disease among donor blood [10, 24-29]. These findings are important for the asymptomatic *Leishmaniasis*, which are characterized in individuals who are infected by the *Leishmania* parasite but are apparently healthy. *Leishmaniasis* is a serious public health problem all over the world; it is known that it shows differences in epidemiological and clinical aspects [30].

Epidemiological Aspects of *Leishmaniasis*

Leishmaniasis has a worldwide distribution, and the disease occurs on all continents except Antarctica [3, 31]. The geographical distribution of *Leishmaniasis* changes due to the natural habitats of the sand fly. The characteristics of the parasite species, the local ecological feature of the transmission types, and the current and past exposure to the human population affect the epidemiology of *Leishmaniasis* [2]. In spite of fighting against *Leishmaniasis* for many years, the spread of the disease increasingly continues [2]. *Leishmaniasis*, which is endemic in many countries, indicates that country-specific regional character. As with many other tropical diseases, this depends on factors such as heat, humidity, altitude of the region, and vegetation. In addition, factors such as economic development of the region and man-made environmental changes, which increase exposure to the sand fly species as vectors, all play a role. Trade in forest products, mining, dam construction, agricultural extension, destruction of forest areas, and the concentration of people in these regions, rural-urban migration, and rapid urbanization are causes of increasing the spread of *Leishmaniasis* in the world [32-34]

As a result of economic development, widespread urbanization, deforestation, and migration to urban areas, new settlements have been established, which can cause the spread of sand flies (the reservoirs of *Leishmania*). In addition, the number of new host populations [for example, the patient population infected with human immunodeficiency virus (HIV) and VL] at the same time has increased, especially in southern Europe and Africa [6].

The major cause of the spread of *Leishmaniasis* is mainly through dogs, but it is also spread through mice, foxes, and cats [35]. The reservoirs for the disease are everywhere, including rural areas and particularly in vectors that can obtain the parasites from this source before infecting humans. In addition, the insecticides against the disease vectors and the used drugs against disease factors are important in the development of resistance [36]. There are many factors for spreading of the disease: untreated patients, facilitation of travel between cities and migrations to endemic regions, war, AIDS and other immune deficiencies, the increase of agricultural land and irrigation, forest destruction, dam construction, and ineffective implementation of insecticide, which cause the vector-gaining resistance against insecticide [2, 6, 37, 38].

Clinical Aspects of *Leishmaniasis*

There are three most common clinical forms of the disease: *Visceral Leishmaniasis* (VL), *Cutaneous Leishmaniasis* (CL), *Muco-cutaneous Leishmaniasis* (MCL) [2, 39]. There are also other clinical variants of *Leishmaniasis* called *Diffuse Cutaneous Leishmaniasis* (DCL) and *Post-Kala-azar Dermal Leishmaniasis* (PKDL) [2]. Additionally, relatively uncommon clinical variants of *Leishmaniasis* are *Leishmaniasis* recidivans (LR) [40] and disseminated Cutaneous *Leishmaniasis* [2]. *Leishmania* species lead to different clinical forms (the main distribution countries are shown at Table **1**). In recent years, endemic studies have shown that asymptomatic *Leishmaniasis* (AL) is also quite common as a subclinical form [41].

The symptoms produced by *Leishmania* parasites can vary from mild (in cases of chronic *Leishmaniasis*, CL) to more severe forms such as VL [42]. The severity of the clinical disease is also dependent on several confounding factors, including the genetic nature of the host organism, the type or strains/species of the parasite, and the environment. CL is by far the most common clinical form of the disease and experimentally the most studied among all other forms. In contrast, VL is a common and clinically relevant disease owing to its high morbidity and mortality in untreated cases. A great number of reported treatments for CL indicate that no single and ideal therapy has to date been identified [43].

Visceral Leishmaniasis (VL)

VL, which is also known by the Hindi name "kala-azar," means "black fever" or "deadly fever" and affects the organs of the reticuloendothelial system [2]. If left untreated, it can result in death [6]. The parasites colonize in the internal organs, *e.g.*, spleen, bone marrow, liver, and lymph nodes [2, 50]. VL can easily occur with malnutrition and immune deficiency as a result of organ transplants. Especially in endemic areas, VL has become a common disease of HIV-positive individuals who have suppressed immune systems [51]. However, it can be seen in the lungs and intestines where the mononuclear phagocytic system cells exist [52]. In recent years, it is remarkable that increased cases of immune deficiency patients parallel cases of VL.

Table 1.   *Leishmaniasis* Species Based on Clinical Forms

Clinical Forms	Species	Country or Territory	References
Visceral *Leishmaniasis*	*L. donovani*	Africa, Bangladesh, India, Sudan	[31, 41, 44, 45]
	L. infantum	Afghanistan, African Republic, Albania, Brazil, Central Asia, Central Iraq, France, Mediterranean basin, Tunisia and Turkey New World	[6, 41, 45]
	L. chagasi		[6, 41]
Cutanoeus *Leishmaniasis*	*L. tropica*	Afghanistan, Azerbaijan, Egypt, Ethiopia, Turkey	[2, 31, 39]
	L. major	Afghanistan, Azerbaijan, Egypt, Ethiopia India, Iran, Iraq, Kenya, Morocco, Nigeria, Pakistan, Tunisia, and Yemen	[2, 31, 39]
	L. infantum		[2, 31]
	L. aethiopica	Albania, Bulgaria, China	[2, 31, 39]
	L. donovani	Ethiopia, Kenya	[2]
	L. mexicana	Cyprus, Israel	[31, 39]
	L. braziliensis	Belize, Colombia, Mexico	[2]
	L. guyanensis	Argentina, Brazil, Bolivia, Colombia, Mexico, Panama, Paraguay and Peru	[2, 46]
	L. panamensis	Argentina, Brazil, Guyana, Peru and Venezuela	[2]
	L. peruviana	Colombia, Costa Rica, Ecuador, Honduras and Panama	[2]
		Peru	
Muco-cutaneous *Leishmaniasis*	*L. braziliensis*	Argentina, Bolivia, Brazil, Colombia, Mexico, Paraguay, Peru	[2]
	L. major	America, Mexico	[2]
	L. panamensis	Colombia, Costa Rica, Honduras, Panama	[2, 31, 47]
	L. braziliensis guyanensis	Peru	[31, 48]
Diffuse cutaneous *Leishmaniasis*	*L. aethiopica*	Ethiopia, Kenya	[2, 31]
	L. Mexicana	America, Costa Rica, Ecuador, Mexico Guatemala	[2]
	L. amazonensis	Bolivia, Colombia, Ecuador, Venezuela	[2, 31]
Post-kala-azar dermal *Leishmaniasis*	*L. donovani*	Bangladesh, Ethiopia, India, Nepal, Sudan	[31, 49]

Cutaneous Leishmaniasis (CL)

CL has local names such as "Delhi ulcer," "Aleppo boil," "one-year boil," "Baghdad boil," "Biskra button," and "Chiclero ulcer" [53]. These *Leishmaniasis* forms cause chronic skin ulcers [54]. Lesions start generally with a papule or nodule at the site of inoculation and grow slowly [2]; CL can be seen at any age and usually occurs on the uncovered body parts such as face, neck, and arms. However, it also has been reported that it can be seen on the scalp and even also on the penis [55].

Muco-Cutaneous Leishmaniasis (MCL)

MCL is also called "Espundia" in South America. This form is characterized with skin erosions in mucosal membranes such as the nose, mouth, pharynx, and larynx. MCL begins with erythema and ulcerations at the nares and can be distinguished from the CL due to occurring in mucosal membranes. Insufficient treatment of *Leishmaniasis* can cause MCL, and, if not treated, it can cause painful injuries, even death [39, 56, 57].

Diffuse Cutaneous Leishmaniasis (DCL)

Characteristics of DCL have been described as diffusion of lesions, great abundance of parasites, anergy to skin tests, and also resistance to treatment [58]. Patients with DCL have multiple widespread cutaneous papules and nodules without ulceration, involving almost the entire body [59].

Post Kala Azar Dermal Leishmaniasis (PKDL)

This form of *Leishmaniasis* develops within months to years after the patient's improvement from VL. Macular, maculopapular, and nodular rashes can be seen in patients [60]. Depigmented eruption is typically found on the face, arms, and upper part of the body. PKDL requires prolonged and expensive treatment [61]. Patients with PKDL also play an important role in the transmission of VL [6, 62].

Leishmaniasis Recidivans or Recurrent (LR)

LR presents as a recurrence of lesions at the site of apparently healed disease years after the original infection [40]. Typically, LR lesions occur on the face with an enlarging papule, plaque, or coalescence of papules that heals with central scarring. Expansion at the periphery may cause significant facial destruction similar to the lupus vulgaris variant of cutaneous tuberculosis [63].

Asymptomatic Leishmaniasis (AL)

It is shown that the *Leishmania* parasites could still remain in the body after clinical recovery [64-66]. The cause of asymptomatic infection may depend on the patient's immune system [41]. According to WHO, the number of symptomatic patients is 5-20% of the asymptomatic individuals [10, 66]. The existence of mild and hidden *Leishmania* infections has been reported at the beginning of the twentieth century with very few signs of VL and spontaneously diagnosed VL [67]. Epidemiological reports published in Brazil show that, in contrast to previous opinions infectious, disease factors due to mild or asymptomatic *L. chagas* or *L. infantum* are seen more frequently than the diseases showing few signs [68, 69]. Also in the Mediterranean region, long-lasting subclinical *Leishmaniasis* has been reported in healthy and HIV-infected cases [24, 25, 70-72]. Individuals may be asymptomatic carriers of the disease for many years [38]. It has been reported that the incubation period of asymptomatic *Leishmania* can be up to 30 years [10]. In recent studies, it has been demonstrated that donor blood plays an important role in the epidemiology of asymptomatic *Leishmaniasis* [10, 26, 65, 68]. Also in our recent study, we have shown that there are *Leishmania* parasites in blood bank donors in Turkey [73].

Diagnosis of *Leishmaniasis*

It is possible to use different clinical and laboratory methods for the diagnosis of *Leishmaniasis*. Clinical diagnosis is the first and most important one. Diagnosis of VL cannot be done with only clinical symptoms and signs. Because the VL may be confused with diseases such as malaria, diseases that cause hepatomegaly and splenomegaly or cirrhosis develop secondary to portal hypertension [1]. On the other hand, in CL the diagnosis can be confused with other skin diseases (impetigo, leprosy, lupus vulgaris, syphilis, skin lesions, Blastomycosis, skin cancer) instead of CL [1, 74]. Laboratory diagnosis methods of *Leishmaniasis* are mainly microscopic, cultural, serological, and molecular techniques. Moreover, there are also some applications on experimental animals [1, 75, 76].

Microscopic Methods

Microscopic methods are the most commonly used in laboratory diagnosis. Obtaining samples from spleen, bone marrow, liver, skin lesions, and lymph nodes are accepted as invasive methods, while obtaining samples from peripheral blood is used as a noninvasive method. After staining of the sample with Giemsa stain, the microscopic diagnosis based on the presence of amastigote form of *Leishmania* parasites can be performed [1, 6, 74].

The material for skin lesions obtained from the lower edge of ulcers can be used for microscopic examination, but today biopsy is preferred instead of this method. Smears from biopsy samples stained with Giemsa and hematoxylin and eosin indicate the existence of parasites by histology [20]. Microscopic methods are based on accurate detection of parasites, but the high rate of undiagnosed cases associated with this method shows its deficiency [77].

Culture Methods

The culture methods are based on the transformation of amastigote forms of parasites to promastigote forms following inoculating patient samples into a relevant medium [78]. In 1994, McNeal and Novy prepared the biphasic medium to obtain a culture of *Trypanosoma*. Later this medium had been modified for the cultivation of *Leishmania* promastigotes by Nicole, and the medium was named the Nicole Novy-MacNeal (NNN) medium due to successful diagnosis of *Leishmania* parasites. Afterward, this method became the classical cultivation method all over the world and is still being performed in various endemic regions [78, 79].

Nowadays for *Leishmania* cultivation, monophase (Schineder's medium, M199, or Grace's medium), or di-phase (NNN medium and Tobies medium), mediums are used [6]. In biochemical studies, the liquid medium is recommended, but for isolation the modified NNN medium is recommended [78]. For diagnosis of *Leishmaniasis*, the sensitivity of the culture methods is excessively high, since the main mechanism of the method depends on directly detection of the presence of parasites in the obtained sample [77, 80, 81].

Microculture Method

In recent years, Allahverdiyev *et al*. [77] developed the microculture method, which has rapid and sensitive results in diagnosis of VL and CL cases, and it is easy to apply [82-87]. The main mechanism of MCM relies on transformation of intracellular amastigotes into extracellular promastigotes in a microaerophylic environment. Therefore, these motile promastigotes can be easily detected in a liquid media by using an inverted microscope [77, 82, 83, 85-87]. This method, unlike the conventional culture method, can diagnose the disease within one to three days [65, 77, 83]. In our recent studies, it has been shown that the MCM is also sensitive in asymptomatic animal models (unpublished) and in blood donors [73]. Nowadays, this method is being used in several regions of the world [85-88].

Leishmania species also can be produced in experimental animals with inoculation [78, 89]. The continuous culture of *Leishmania* species can be achieved with long-term storage in liquid nitrogen by freezing the promastigote and amastigote cultures [78, 89].

Molecular Methods

The value of molecular biology is rapidly rising in terms of diagnosis and control of infectious diseases. Information on DNA sequences has been extensively exploited for the development of polymerase chain reaction (PCR)-based techniques for a variety of applications in the understanding of the parasite and the diseases [90-92]. A diversity of nucleic-acid-sensing procedures targeting DNA and RNA genes has been developed. However, amongst all the molecular advances, gene amplification techniques have been most satisfying as far as diagnosis and disease manipulation [91]. Identification of the *Leishmania* species is significant for the appropriate treatment since different species cause different clinical manifestations of the disease [93]. A number of molecular markers and PCR assays for the detection or identification of *Leishmania* on different taxonomical levels (genus, complex, and species) has been showed [94, 95]. Molecular methods for identifying *Leishmania* [50, 96-98] are, at times, overwhelming and expensive for diagnostic resolves.

On the other side, a specific PCR-based method is appealing as it is rapid, sensitive, and specific, avoiding culturing of parasites, thus being suitable for *Leishmaniasis* surveillance programs that command efficient laboratorial response for rapid and useful actions. Several molecular techniques, remarkably those based on the PCR, have been developed for the diagnosis and identification of *Leishmania* species [99-102]. The PCR is now a basic molecular tool that has been proven to be more specific and emotional than conventional diagnostic methods [103] and can be performed on any biological sample. However, PCR is far from being standardized for the routine diagnosis of the disease [104].

Serological Methods

Serological methods are based on the determination of the antibody response against the parasite by serological tests in patient serum or urine. The specificity of the antibody used in the tests depend on the antigen or epitope [6]. Antigen can be detected in early stages of the infection [6]. Several serological tests show high sensitivity and specificity independent from the region where the specimen is obtained [105]. To determine nonspecific immunoglobulins, there are tests such as Napier's formalin gel, aldehyde, and Chopra antimony. Several serological methods, which are more sensitive and more specific, have been developed in recent years.

There are also feasible serological methods, such as the *Leishmanin* skin test, immunofluorescence antibody test [20, 73, 106-111], enzyme-linked immunoassay [112], direct agglutination test (DAT), indirect hemagglutination test (IHA), gel diffusion, complement fixation, latex agglutination, rk39 immunochromatographic dipstick rapid test (ICT), and western blotting (WB), which are mostly used in diagnosis of *Leishmaniasis* in various endemic regions of the world [112].

However, serological methods are not preferred as much in diagnosis because of a very low titer of antibodies to be detected or not detected by serological testing. In addition, serologic tests cannot distinguish between old and new infections [113]. Further, it is not safe in individuals with compromised immune systems and can give cross-reactions [114].

As can be seen, a variety of methods are used in the diagnosis of *Leishmaniasis*. Sensitivity and specification of these used methods are high in symptomatic *Leishmaniasis* but lower in the asymptomatic *Leishmaniasis*. The MCM, which has been developed in recent years, could lead to new hopes in this respect.

IMMUNOLOGY OF *LEISHMANIASIS*

The following points are in regards to the activation and modulation of innate immunity by *Leishmania*:

First: Leishmania promastigotes enter macrophages by a quiescent mechanism that fails to induce innate immune responses; this may result in a delayed induction of an adaptive immune response. This delay in the development of adaptive immunity may provide opportunity for the parasite to replicate within macrophages.

Second: Parasite replication disrupts the ability of macrophages to respond to the eventually generated immune signals.

Third: Amastigote entry into macrophages also may be the harbinger for successful parasitism. Amastigotes coat themselves in host IgG, which binds macrophage FcγR, resulting in the hyperproduction of IL-10 from infected macrophages. IL-10 can prevent macrophages responses to IFN γ, allowing the parasites to survive even in the immunologically intact host [115].

The immune response that occurs in host cells against *Leishmania* is comprehensive and can be altered by various factors such as the species and strain of the parasite and the genetics of the host. Both the innate and adaptive components of the immune system play crucial roles for determination of *Leishmania* infection progress. A small pool of blood is formed when a female sand fly takes a blood meal. Infectious promastigotes (metacyclics) are regurgitated into this pool of blood, where they enter the human host. Phagocytic cells recruited to the site of infection rapidly internalize the promastigotes. The parasites not only survive but replicate within the acidic phagolysosome. Studies show that the first phase of the infection involves the initial uptake of the *Leishmania* parasites by cells of immune defense system such as neutrophils, macrophages, and dendritic cells [116].

Among other immune system components, dendritic cells play essential roles in the adaptive immunity raised against *Leishmania*. Uptake of promastigotes is usually followed by the inhibition of cellular apoptotic signaling, which can lead to an increase in their lifespan [117]. It also has been shown that spontaneous production of IFN-γ can activate infected macrophages, thereby leading to the upregulation of inducible nitric oxide (NO) synthesis. NO has been recently shown to be the key molecule for killing *Leishmania* organisms.

In *Leishmaniasis*, cellular immune responses are involved in healing from the disease. In general, spontaneous *Leishmania*-specific T cell response initially develops after infection. At first, the parasites multiply as amastigotes into the phagolysosome within the macrophage. Then either intact parasites or *Leishmanial* antigens are picked up by antigen-presenting cells, which transfer them to CD4+ and CD8+ T cells. These cells activate specific T cells in the production of different cytokines (IL-22, interferon-gamma and granulocyte macrophage colony-stimulating factor) and induce the macrophage to kill the intracellular parasite [118]. CD8+ T cells are involved in cytolytic antileishmanial activity by inducing the production of IFN- γ and transforming growth factor beta. Activation in the presence of IL-2 or TGF β 4 leads to the development of cytolytic cells producing IFN- γ . Beside this, activation in the presence of IL-4, noncytolytic CD8-CD4-T cells are developed and lead to IL-4, IL-5, and IL-10 production and inflammation of the disease. IL-12 is an additional essential cytokine involved in inducing cell-mediated immunity, cell proliferation, and secretion of IFN- γ by T and natural killer cells. It supports the development of CD4 Th1 cells, which are important in the protective immunity against the disease.

Healing and protection against *Leishmaniasis* results from a strong and specific cellular immune response, followed by the development of long-term protection. CL generally causes self-healing disease with life-long immunity against reinfections. Healing is characterized by induction of specific IFN-γ responses from *Leishmania*-specific CD4$^+$ T cells [119]. Increased expression of IL-10 in *L. major* lesions was found to be associated with progressive disease [120]. Studies have also highlighted a dichotomy between Th1 *versus* Th2 responses in simple *versus* diffuse CL in humans [121].

Acute VL patients generally demonstrate anergy with a negative skin test to *Leishmania* antigens. Peripheral blood mononuclear cells from such individuals fail to proliferate or to produce IFN-γ when exposed to the specific antigen *in vitro* [122]. In addition to anti-IL-10R antibody to T cells produced from disease, further studies show that, for IL-10, IL-10 mRNA expression is in bone marrow [122, 123], lymph nodes [122], and the spleen [124]. Cure from disease has been associated with a fall in IL-10 mRNA levels [122, 123]. Increased expression of classical Th2 cytokines has been reported in VL with elevated IL-4, which has been especially associated with treatment failure [125]. Elevated levels of IL-13 have been observed in acute disease that returned to normal following successful treatment [126].

Several key cytokines and their possible but intriguing roles have recently been elucidated and confirmed in mice. It was shown that production of IL-12, together with the degree of responsiveness of T cells to IL-12, has been key in affecting the outcome of *L. major* infection [127-129]. DCs isolated from BALB/c mice were shown to produce less IL-12 following *L. major* infection, and T cells from these mice have been found to poorly respond to the IL-12 due to IL-12 receptor (γ)-chain downregulation [130]. On the contrary, C57BL/6 mice produced more IL-12 and maintained their IL-12 levels during the entire course of infection. It is greatly accepted that the outcome of *Leishmania* infection in mice depends on the relative ability of host T cells to produce IFN-γ [131, 132]. In contrast to IL-12 action, early production of IL-4 by a unique population of CD4+ T cells (which support the development and expansion of Th2 cells) increases the susceptibility [133-136]. IL-10 also plays an important role in the regulation of *Leishmaniasis*. It was demonstrated that lack of the IL-10 gene made infected mice resistant to *L. major* infection [137]. On the other hand, mice that synthetized a large amount of IL-10 were susceptible to infection [138]. Other cytokines, which were demonstrated to contribute to resistance or susceptibility against *L. major* infection, are the tumor necrosis factor (TNF) [139], TGF [140, 141], membrane lymphotoxin (LT) [142], and LT-like cytokines [139].

VL is generally seen in visceral organs; resistance is, however, associated with the type and severity of immune response in the infected organs. Similar to the CL response, local production of IFN-γ is thought to play an important role in defense against infection by activating infected macrophages to mediate NO production and parasite killing in this method [142]. Numerous researchers have shown that

CD8+ and CD4+ T cells act in cooperation for disease progression upon VL infection: CD4+ T cells can function in the control of primary infection, and CD8+ T cells can participate in secondary immune response [143].

L. donovani infection causes decreased production of Th1 cytokines (*i.e.*, IFN-γ) and thereby results in impaired cell-mediated immunity [144]. Upon infection, infected Kupffer cells (KCs) releases chemokines, including chemokine ligand (CCL) 2 and 3 in a T-cell-independent manner. It is because studies have shown that this release also occurs in T-cell-deficient mice, indicating its T-cell independent nature. However, sustained production or these chemokines necessitates the presence of hepatic lymphocytes [145]. Upon chemokine stimuli, T cells can function to develop granulomas, and the number of CD4+ and CD8+ T cells increase within one week of infection [146]. Such responses are thought to be the primary parasite control in the liver. In contrast, although the reason is not clear, unlike in the liver, infection in the spleen and bone marrow becomes chronic [147]. However, it recently has been shown that production of certain chemokines (TGF-γ and IL-10) has been found to be related to local immunosuppression and persistence of *Leishmania* parasites within infected mice spleens [148]. Parasite persistence can then be associated with the absence of splenomegaly, granulomosis, and lymphoid disruptions [149, 150].

Although Th1/Th2dilemma (dichotomy) in T-cell responses can be seen in mice studies, human infections (experimental and natural) have shown that it is not the case in humans [151]. Flow cytometry analysis of CL patients exhibited significant differences in the frequency of cells that secrete cytokines such as IFN-γ, TNF-γ, and IL-10 in one study [152]. It was also demonstrated that IFN-γ response varied in the early and late stages of CL. Levels of IFN-γ were very low in 50% of patients diagnosed with early CL. On the other hand, it is rapidly enhanced in the late stages of the disease [153]. For immunity against *Leishmania*, host factors are also important.

Leishmania's host factors are age, nutritional status, pregnancy, and HIV infection, which [154] contribute to varied disease for intensity. But in many infected people, it can develop subclinical infections. These facts emphasize the importance of host immunity to disease pathogenesis. CL patients who heal from the first infection, either spontaneously or with medical therapy, have lifelong immunity. Besides this, in both CL and VL, after a subclinical infection, many patients in endemic areas develop persistent immunity, as it can be obviously seen by a positive *Leishmanin* skin test. Healing of *Leishmania* infection is associated with presentation of *Leishmania* antigens by macrophages and DCs. These cells can secrete CD4 and CD8 lymphocytes. Recent studies have shown that the contention of sustained immunity may require persistent low-level infection with parasites [155-157].

Leishmania infection can be arranged at many times, including control of the first infection by innate immune cells such as neutrophils, natural killer (NK) cells, mast cells, and macrophages or during development of lasting immunity. B cells are responsible for controlling parasite load, and adaptive immunity components such as antigen presenting cells (APC) have important roles in the progress of the disease [158].

There are many suggested mechanisms for *Leishmania*'s recovering effector mechanisms against immune systems:

1.   Prevention of macrophage phagosomal killing functions (NO and ROS mediated).

2.   Prevention of macrophage phagosomal maturation [155].

3.   Prevention of DC maturation and chemotaxis [159].

4.   Strengthening of inhibitory CD41, CD251, Fox P31 regulatory T cells [156, 160, 161].

5.   The immune program is biasing away from the effective cellular response [coordinated by Th1-type CD41 helper T cells in association with interleukin (IL)-12 and IFN-g] and toward the ineffective humoral/antihelminthic response, which is typified by Th2-type CD41 helper T cells in association with IL-4, IL-5, and IL-13 [156, 160, 162].

Additionally, natural T-regs that express FoxP3 and other regulatory T-cell subsets that secrete IL-10 and/or TGF-β have been implicated in chronic or nonhealing disease states in animal models and human patients.

The role of adaptive immunity is well known in *Leishmania* studies. The innate immune system consists of fungible cells of the hematopoietic family such as macrophages, DCs, NK cells, neutrophils, eosinophils, and mast cells. This system plays a role as phagocytes, pathogen killers, antigen-presenting cells, and producers of biochemical signals. In addition, they do participate in the specificity of the immune response *via* the mechanism of pattern recognition receptors (PRR). Further, it recognizes stereotypical biochemical motifs on foreign organisms and identifies those potentially dangerous. Additionally, the innate immune system includes a kind of soluble antimicrobial substance; for example, antimicrobial peptides, the protein components of the complement system, PRR on adaptive immune cells, and non-hematopoietic cells. The skin participates in innate immunity as if it were a mechanical barrier to infections. However, no specific evidence suggests skin barrier facilitates infections with *Leishmania*.

The innate immune system cells recognize conserved components of microbial pathogens, which are called pathogen-associated molecular patterns (PAMPs) [163] *via* PRR [164-167]. Besides toll-like receptors (TLRs), other examples of PRRs include intracellular NOD-like receptors [166-168], and sweeper receptors [169]. Activation of TLRs by PAMPs leads to inflammatory cytokine production. A characteristic antimicrobial immune response is generated by innate immune cells such as macrophages, DC, NK cells, and granulocytes [164-166, 170].

Despite *in vivo* studies, which suggest a role for innate immunity, *in vitro* infections emphasize basic differences in the innate response of macrophages and DCs to bacteria. Even small numbers of bacteria, which are phagocytosed, are invariably associated with the rapid translocation of NF-KB [171] and with the secretion of a big array of cytokines such as TNF, IL-1, and IL-12. This activation of the innate immune system does not seem to occur following *Leishmania* infections because the phagocytosis of the microorganism results in no detectable NF-KB activation. As a result, promastigote phagocytosis reduces minimal cytokine secretion by infected macrophages, which are specific for *Leishmania* species.

IMMUNOTHERAPY FOR *LEISHMANIA*

The human immune system is unique in its defense mechanisms, which are capable of protecting the body against many diseases. In its simple terms, disease occurs when there is either a lack of suboptimal immune reaction. Excessive immune reaction is also harmful for the system, indicating that there should be limits for the immune reaction to properly serve as a defense. Immunotherapy is therefore widely accepted as a form of treatment modality in which biological agents are utilized in order to modulate and/or modify immune responses and achieve an optimal level of immunity for prophylactic and therapeutic results. Immunotherapeutic agents can be biological or chemical and exert their effects, either directly or indirectly, by increasing the host natural defenses. Research on such compounds and their immune-modulatory effects has been performed for over 30 years. Although positive results could be obtained in animal models, the use of nonspecific immunomodulators, including certain chemicals, bacterial extracts, and viruses, were found to be noneffective in clinical trials [172]. However, highly purified biological compounds, which are produced by genetic engineering techniques, are also being tested in clinical trials [172].

Contemporary medicine used in the treatment for *Leishmaniasis* in general includes sodium stilbogluconate (SSG) [173], amphotericin B [174], paramycin sulphate [175], and meglumine antimoniate [176]. Likewise, topical paromomycin sulphate with methylbenzethonium chloride (MBCL) or urea is used in the treatment of CL, and amphotercin B is used in acute VL and is effective in children and adults in all endemic areas [177-179].

Treatment of *Leishmaniasis* is known to be influenced by the factors related to lesions (size, number, and location); duration of the disease after first treatment; frequency of reinfections; severity; immunosuppression; co-infections; and age of the patient [180]. If patients have multiple large lesion(s) or lesion(s) on the face, over joints, or close to vital organs, *Leishmaniasis* is generally treated by antimonials. However, patients with small lesion(s) that is/are localized at cosmetically nonimportant sites are treated intralesionally or left uncured if patients live in regions endemic for CL. It is important to note that, upon diagnosis, treatment should immediately start due to the high morbidity and mortality rates of the disease.

Unfortunately, in some places in the world (such as Bihar, India, where 45% of worldwide VL cases occurs) resistance to antimonials has made the use of such treatment approach needless. Instead, amphotericin B (lipid formulation) is enormously effective against VL and can demonstrate sufficient efficacy in a short time [181]. Moreover, the use of paromomycin and miltefosine also has improved the success rates in the treatment of VL [182].

The disease is characterized by the development of ulcerative skin lesions lasting for months and, in most cases, is resolved by Th1 T-cell activity. Although, in patients with a defective cellular immune response, a long-lasting chronic disease (recurrent CL or DCL) may develop [183]. Nearly all patients recover from the disease after primary exposure to the parasite, but a small percentage may develop severe secondary life-persisting lesions in the MCL. The disease is well developed in the presence of Th2 T-cell-mediated immunity. The visceral form caused by *L. donovani* and *L. infantum* is characterized by systemic infection of the reticuloendothelial system [188, 189].

As of publication, there is no vaccine or prophylactic available for use in humans. Also, the number of available drugs for treating the disease is limited, and most parasites develop drug resistance. In the last 20 years, immunotherapy has been developed as additional treatment for *Leishmaniasis*. Immunotherapy has been used to accelerate the specific immune response in immunologically responsive patients and to establish an effective reaction in those who are nonresponsive [183].

Even for patients with refractive *Leishmaniasis*, several murine and human studies indicate the presence of promising alternatives to conventional chemotherapy. However, there is considerable need to standardize immunotherapeutic protocols used in treatment of *Leishmaniasis* [184, 185].

VACCINE DEVELOPMENT

The first vaccine studies against *Leishmaniasis* started in 1908 with the discovery of promastigote growth in *in vitro* culture conditions [186, 187]. After that, with developing technology, *Leishmania* vaccine studies have spread to different areas such as genetic engineering or recombinant protein technologies.

Leishmania vaccines generally are grouped in three generations:

- first generation is vaccination with live virulent parasites (termed *Leishmanization*) and vaccination with killed parasites;

- second generation is vaccination with subunits, purified fractions, recombinant vaccines in heterologous microbial vectors, and genetically or otherwise attenuated live parasites (second-generation vaccines);

- third generation is DNA-based vaccines [188].

FIRST-GENERATION VACCINES

Leishmania parasites can be easily grown in cultures with low cost, which provides early vaccine studies with killed organisms, as for many other infection diseases [189]. It was suggested that the whole killed parasites provide prophylactic and therapeutic effects [190]. A cocktail of killed promastigotes, which belongs to five different *Leishmania* species, was found safe, but its therapeutic effect was 50% [191]. Leishvacin (killed *L. amazonensis* promastigotes) is also safe, but the prophylactic effect was found low with clinical tests (Phase III) [192].

First-generation vaccines have been tested on humans and dogs in Phase III trials in Asia and South America since 1930s and 1940s and used for over 60 years in several countries [199]. The vaccine was tested in Phase III trials in Colombia [195] and in several Phase I-III trials against CL in Iran [196] and against VL in Sudan [197]. Some studies showed that vaccination with killed *Leishmania* parasites provides 53.3% efficacy. Whole cell killed parasites provide safety but a poorly defined variable in potency and inefficiency against *Leishmaniasis* [190].

Since their effectiveness in the treatment has been lower than expected levels, some studies argue that the prospects of using first-generation vaccines should be assessed [198]. The first prophylactic vaccine that consisted of killed *Leishmania* promastigotes was investigated in 1992 for its immunotherapeutic efficacy against American cutaneous *Leishmaniasis* (ACL) [199]. Some adjuvants were also administered together with the vaccine in order to improve effectiveness. One of the most usually used adjuvants is bacillus Calmette-Guerin (BCG). Several studies have shown positive contribution of BCG inclusion in the vaccine treatment approach [200, 201].

The use of pasteurized *Leishmania* promastigotes as a vaccine is shown to be an effective immunotherapeutic component [202]. On the other hand, studies also indicate that vaccine-based treatment options are only effective against active lesions, which occurred following infection with parasites that are included in the New World, as no reports yet exist in the literature on the effective utilization of killed parasites for VL treatment. Recently it was reported in Sudan that a combination of killed parasites with BCG as a form of vaccine therapy was effective for controlling post-VL dermatitis [203].

Live attenuated *Leishmania* parasites are also used for vaccination against *Leishmaniasis*. The aim of a live attenuated vaccine provides more and longer protection than does killed parasites. For safety, virulence of parasites were decreased by a long-term culture [204], exposure to gamma irradiation [205], chemical agents, or antibiotics [206, 207].

Inoculation of live virulent *Leishmania* parasites is known as *Leishmanization*. *Leishmaniazation* was used in Uzbekistan with *Leishmania* parasites isolated from patients to provide high virulence [193]. However, the problem of *Leishmanization* generally stems from safety and standardization issues [193].

Second- and Third-Generation Vaccines

Second generation is vaccination with synthetic or recombinant subunits, purified fractions, recombinant bacteria, or viruses carrying *Leishmania* antigen genes and genetically or otherwise attenuated live parasites [209].

Third-generation vaccines include DNA vaccines and have advantages compared with recombinant protein vaccines. They have a stable structure and comparatively lower cost than recombinant protein vaccines. They also don't need a cold chain for transport, and several genes can be brought together for vaccine purposes [191].

Generally, the DNA of antigens used for recombinant vaccine candidate is also used for DNA vaccine. DNA vaccines can be applied as a single combination of several genes and following vaccination with recombinant proteins and as Vaccinia virus for expression of proteins [191]. Third-generation DNA vaccines showed average values of parasite load reduction of 59% in laboratory animal models, but their success in field trials has not yet been reported [194].

Glycoprotein 63 (gp63), membrane glycoprotein 46 (gp46, also known as M-2), fucose mannose ligand (FML), *Leishmania* homolog of receptors for activated C kinase (p36/LACK), NH36, protein Q chimera, cysteine proteinase [196] B and CPA, GRP78, LD1 antigens, hydrophilic acylated surface protein B1 (HASPB1), LCR1, salivary protein 15 (SP15), promastigote surface antigen 2 (PSA-2), A-2, histone H1, MML, *Leishmania* elongation and initiation factor (LeIF), *L. major* homolog of the eukaryotic stress inducible protein-1 (LmSTI1), *L. major* homologue of the eukaryotic thiol-specific-antioxidant (TSA) and Leish-111f, HSP, SLA, FPA, 1G6, 4H6, GBP, LPG were investigated under the title of second- and third-generation vaccines against *Leishmaniasis* [193, 210-232].

Antigens Used in Vaccine Development Against *Leishmaniasis*

Glycoprotein 63 (gp63)

63 kDa surface metalloprotease gp63 plays an important role in evasion of immune responses in the host and survival and degradation of fibronectin. gp63 is a conserved structure and is largely available on the promastigote surface of all species [189, 233, 234]. Among the defined subunit vaccines, the gp63 antigen has been studied most extensively [235]. gp63 is used in second- and third-generation vaccines with different adjuvant and delivery systems such as *Salmonella typhimurium* BCG pCMV pCMV3ISS and in combination with the other antigens such as KMPII, TRYP, and LACK [194]. The protection effect of gp63 with conflicting results was tested with different animal models (mostly mouse strains) [233].

Immunization with gp63 transformed into *S. Thyphimurium* gp63 expressed in BCG provided resistance against *L. major* or *L. donovani* infection but did not express a delayed-type hypersensitivity response in mice [189]. Three doses of the recombinant antigen were administered with BCG but only partial protection was achieved against virulent *L. major* promastigotes [195]. In contrast, gp63 encapsulated in liposome elicited a strong delayed-type hypersensitivity (DTH) response with a significant rate of protection by the Th1 type of immune response. Also the recombinant gp63 (rgp63) does not elicit a protective response in human T-cell clones [236].

A small-scale vaccine Phase I and II trial of rgp63 was studied in a velvet monkey model against *L. major* infection [233, 237]. It is unfortunate that in humans and animal models, the T-cell responses to gp63 have been variable [187]. With another approach, synthetic gp63 peptides were loaded into dendritic cells (DCs), and results showed that DCs pulsed with some gp63-derived synthetic peptides provide protection, but the others caused exacerbation of disease [193].

This conflicting result can be explained: gp63 is a large protein and may have different epitopes stimulating different types of immune responses [233].

Leishmania Homologue of Receptors for Activated C Kinase Lack

Leishmania homologue of receptors for activated C kinase (LACK) is a highly conserved antigens species and is expressed by the promastigote and amastigote forms of the parasite [238]. LACK has an interest as a vaccine candidate against *Leishmaniasis* owing to its immunopathogenic role in murine *L. major* infection [193]. However, the LACK protein induced early expression of IL-4 and directed immunity to nonhealing Th2-type response in BALB/c mice [239]. Also vaccination with LACK is not accomplished in animal models challenged with *L. amazonensis* and *L. donovani* parasites. Therefore, researchers focused on the LACK DNA after this inefficient approach with LACK proteins [193].

LACK is one the most studied DNA vaccines against CL and VL [240]. DNA vaccination with a plasmid harboring the LACK gene in dogs against *L. infantum* provides 60% protection in dogs [241]. In another study conducted with mice, LACK DNA induced Th1 responses but couldn't protect animals from *L. donovani* infection [242]. The LACK DNA and LACK protein with IL-12 induced protection against *L. major* infection but failed for protection against *L. donovani* [243].

Fucose Mannose Ligand (FML)

FML is a glycoprotein mixture and major immunogenic component of it is gp36 [190]. Fucose mannose ligand (FML) is one of the other most studied antigens of *Leishmania* parasites. FML was patented in Brazil, and its trade name is Leishmune® (patent INPI number: PI1100173-9, Federal University of Rio de Janeiro, Brazil) [244]. Leishmune® was the first commercially licensed vaccine and has been used for the treatment of dogs against VL since 2004 [240]. This formulation contains FML obtained from *L. donovani* and saponin as an adjuvant [245]. It was demonstrated that Leishmune® provides up to 80% protective efficacy in Phase III trials in dogs in Brazil and protection continue up to 3.5 years post-vaccination [190].

Kinetoplastid Membrane Protein-11 (KMP11)

Kinetoplastid membrane protein-11 (KMP-11) is 11 kDa surface membrane protein of promastigote and amastigote form of parasites [234]. KMP-11 was implicated as a potential vaccine candidate in immune-protection experiments [246]. KMP-11 expressed in ts-4 mutants of *Toxoplasma gondii* provided significant protection against *L. major* infection in BALB/c mice [193]. Vaccination with 200 μ g of KMP11 elicited a mixed cytokine TH1/TH2 response in hamsters against VL [194]. In another study, a cocktail of plasmid DNA encoding KMPII, TRYP, LACK, and GP63 did not protect dogs against *L. infantum* virulent challenge [247].

Cysteine Proteinases (CPS)

Cysteine proteinase is one of proteolytic enzymes belonging to the papain superfamily. *Leishmania* cysteineproteinases (CPs) has an important role in host-parasite interaction and in immune evasion [248]. Three classes of CPs have been identified in *Leishmania* (CPA, CPB, CPC); they are involved in parasite survival, replication, and onset of disease [193]. Therefore, CPs is an attractive target for drug and vaccine development [249].

Cysteine proteinases stimulated lymphoproliferative immune responses and production of IFN-γ in patients with CL. Also *L. chagasi* cysteine proteinase 1 plus BCG provided protection in mice [250]. Also DNA forms of cysteine proteinase were investigated as a vaccine against *Leishmaniasis*. The hybrid CPA/B elicits a protective immune response against *L. major* challenge in mice and a cocktail of *Leishmania infantum* CPA/B used in dogs [251].

Lypophosphoglycan (LPG)

Recent studies have focused on the surface glicoconjugates of parasites for vaccine development. LPG is one of the most important surface glycoproteins of *Leishmania*. LPG covers all surfaces of parasites, including flagella, and has an important role for survival of parasites in humans and vectors. The basic LPG structure includes of a 1-O-alkyl-2-lyso-phosphatidyl inositol lipid anchor, a heptasaccharide glycan core, a long phosphoglycan (PG) polymer composed of (Galb1-4Mana1-PO4)n repeat units (n = 10-40), and a small oligosaccharide cap [252].

Recently, many novel and interesting microbial antigens, including mycobacterial glycolipids, can be recognized by T cells; these antigens are presented to T cells by a special subset of MHC class I proteins known as CD147. Therefore, LPG gain importance as a vaccine candidate [187].

A study has shown that intranasal vaccination with lipophosphoglycan of *L. amazonensis* is an important immunomodulatory molecule [253]. Other experiments have shown that LPG provided excellent protection to *L. major* infections in BALB/c mice [254, 255]. However, protection depended on the use of adjuvants such as liposomes or *Corynebacterium parvum* and on the integrity of the molecule. Therefore, LPG can be a good vaccine candidate only when used with appropriate adjuvants.

Biodegradable polymers are being used as adjuvant and carriers because of their biocompatible, nontoxic nature and biodegradable properties. However, to the best of our knowledge, there are no antileishmanial vaccine studies based on polymers. In our research, for the first time, the protective efficacy and immunogenicity of lipophosphoglycan and polyacrylic acid conjugate (LPG-PAA) in *L. donovani* infected BALB/c mice were investigated, and our results suggest that the vaccination with LPG-PAA conjugate resulted in significant protection against a progressive infection with *L. donovani*. The partial protection by an LPG crude antigen against *Leishmaniasis* has been previously reported. However, in most of this study, the antileishmanial efficiency of LPG was investigated in CL models. Our present study showed the antileishmanial effect of LPG and other vaccine formulation containing LPG against VL. As a result, LPG-PAA conjugate provides good protection in mice against *L. donovani* infection (unpublished data).

Histone (H1)

Leishmania histone H1 (LeishH1) is a low-molecular-weight lysine-rich protein [256]. *Leishmania* parasites have only two copies of histone H1, and *L. major* H1 is a small, basic, nuclear protein [257]. In one study, *Leishmania* histone H1 polypeptide induced a level of protection against *L. major* infection in BALB/c susceptible mice [258]. The recombinant histone 1 (H1) provided partial protection assessed in beagle dogs against *L. infantum* challenge and in African green monkeys against *L. major* infection [193]. H1 protein was also used with other antigens as a cocktail vaccine.

Paraflagellar Rod Protein 2 (PFR-2)

PFR are highly conserved among kinetoplastid parasites, including *Leishmania* and *Trypanosoma*. Immunogenicity of *pfr-2* gene and protein of *Leishmania mexicana* was investigated in a hamster model. Lesion development was prevented against *L. panamensis* but was ineffective against *L. mexicana* [259]. Another study showed that PFR-2 DNA vaccines provide protection in mice [260].

Leishmania-Derived Recombinant Polyprotein (LEISH-111F)

Leish-111f is the first antileishmanial human vaccine, which entered Phase I clinical testing. This study was performed in southern Italy [261]. Multisubunit recombinant *Leishmania* polyprotein MML, also known as Leish-111f, and a safe adjuvant, which is promoting Th1 responses, has potential application in the prevention and treatment of *Leishmaniasis* [262].

Heat-Shock Proteins (HSPs)

Heat-shock proteins (HSPs) are highly evolutionary conserved proteins and play essential roles in the immune system [263]. Heat-shock proteins (HSPs) are multifunctional proteins and have a prophylactic and therapeutic effect against cancer and infectious diseases [264]. Studies demonstrate that HSPs are needed to further explore and examine the value of this important molecule in the control of *Leishmaniasis* [265].

Nucleoside Hydrolase (NH36)

The nucleoside hydrolyses (NH36) is a vital enzyme of *Leishmania* parasites. NH36 releases purines or pyrimidines of foreign DNA to be used in the synthesis of parasite DNA [266]. It was shown that DNA vaccine and antigen of *Leishmania donovani* NH36 could provide significant protection against *L. chagasi* and *L. mexicana* [267].

Promastigote Surface Antigen (PSA-2)

The *L. major* parasite surface antigen-2 (PSA-2) is a family of glycoinositol phospholipids anchored glycoprotein that comprises three distinct polypeptides [268]. It has been shown that vaccination with PSA-2 induces a TH1 type of immune response in mice and provides protection against *L. major* infection [269]. Native parasite surface antigen (PSA-2) plus *Corynebacterium parvum* provide significant protection in mice through a Th1 cell-mediated immune response. However, vaccination with recombinant PSA-2 expressed in E. coli along with *C. parvum* failed to protective immunity in mice despite the induction of Th1 responses [270].

Thiol-Specific Antioxidant (TSA)

TSA is homologous to eukaryotic thiol-specific antioxidant proteins. TSA plus murine IL-12 was found to elicit strong T-cell immune responses in mice against

L. major [233]. TSA was also used with the *L. major* stress-inducible protein-1 (LmSTI1) and the *L. braziliensis* elongation and initiation factor (LeIF) [190].

Protein Q Chimera

The capacity of a quimeric protein, formed by the genetic fusion of five antigenic determinants from four *Leishmania* proteins, used with BCG, has shown protection (~90%) in dogs against *Leishmania infantum* infection [271]. Protein Q with CpG-ODN also decreased the parasite load in the liver and spleen of mice approximately 99% and induced high IgG2a/IgG1 ratio, high IFN-γ with low IL-4 production [193].

Soluble Leishmanial Antigen (SLA)

Soluble *Leishmanial* antigen (SLA) plus *Corynebacterium parvum* preparation protected BALB/c mice against a fatal infection with *Leishmania* major. Furthermore, nine purified distinct fractions separated from SLA had protection with cell-mediated immune responses [272].

Hydrophilic Acylated Surface Protein B1 (HASPB1)

Recombinant HASPB1 was used without adjuvant and reduced the parasite (*L. donovani*) number to 60% in mice with specific IFN-gamma producing CD8+ T cells [273]. HASPB1 was also used as a combination with H1 in dogs against *L. infantum* [194].

Glucose-Regulated Protein 78 (GRP78)

GRP78 is one of the members of the 70 kDa heat-shock protein family. GRP78 has a function in the translocation of proteins from the cytoplasm into the endoplasmic reticulum and sequestration of glycoprotein precursors in the endoplasmic reticulum matrix [274]. Recently, *Leishmania donovani* GRP78 has been suggested as a new and promising *Leishmania* vaccine candidate [275]. Studies showed that rGRP78 and a GRP78 DNA vaccine protect different mice models against *L. major* challenge [193].

Salivary Protein 15 (SP-15)

Sand fly salivary protein is suggested as a potential vaccine candidate against CL because it provides strong protection [276]. It has been shown that a protein in the saliva of old world *Phlebotomus papatasi* sand fly (SP-15) of was highly immunogenic for mice [277]. Another result suggests that SP-15 protein provides a uniform immune response as a vaccine [276].

Amastigote-Specific A2 Proteins

A2 proteins are considered to be virulence factors and play an important role in the survival of this protozoan parasite in the macrophages. A2 genes belong to a multigene family and are composed of multiple copies of 10 amino acid repeat sequences [278]. A2 antigens are shared by various *Leishmania* species and induced a potent Th1 immune response in mice models against *L. donovani* infection [279].

In a study, recombinant A2 protein, an amastigote specific antigen, and saponin were investigated as vaccine against *Leishmania* (*Leishmania*) *chagasi* infection in dogs. Results showed that immunization with an rA2 antigen was immunogenic and induced partial protection in dogs [280]. Immunization with recombinant *L. donovani* A2 protein provide significant protection correlating with a mixed Th1/Th2 as well as a humoral response [281]. The protection also correlated with *in vitro* splenocyte proliferation production of IFN-γ in mice [278].

DP72

The DP72 is a native glycoprotein of *Leishmania* parasites [235]. *In vivo* animal studies showed that the dp72 native antigen provides protection against both VL and CL [282]. In addition, some studies have shown that dp72 native antigen demonstrated only partial protection to VL differently from CL [283].

Dendritic Cell-Based Vaccination Strategies

DCs are one of the most important elements of the immune system. They alert T lymphocytes about the type of invading antigen and address their polarization for an efficient immune response [159]. DCs are available in all tissue and serve as a host cell for *Leishmania* parasites. Parasites can enter DC directly or after infection of blood cells [237]. Parasites use DC-SIGN receptors, which are appropriate for amastigotes; then the surface phenotype of DCs mature and change. Infected DCs induce a Th1 response and IL-12, which is important factor for elimination of *Leishmania* parasites [284]. Thus, DC can be used as an effective adjuvant for vaccine attempts against *Leishmaniasis* [285].

With recent developments, antigen-loaded DCs were used for immunization against *Leishmaniasis* [159]. DCs enhance a specific immune response after incubation with specific antigens and phagocytosis.

Heidrun Moll *et al*. demonstrated that epidermal Langerhans cells (LC) are critical for primary immune response to *Leishmania* infection. They ingest the parasite and express MHC class II molecules for a long time to activate naive *L. major* specific Th cells in Balb/c mice. So LCs induce a protective immune response to *L. major* infection based on the initiation of a Th1-like response mediated by IL-12 and [286].

Different studies have shown that *ex vivo* antigen-loaded Langerhans cells, myeloid cells, or DHs provide protection against *L. major* infection in Balb/c mice [287-290].

CURRENT TREATMENT REGIMENS FOR *LEISHMANIASIS*

Chemotherapeutic treatments of *Leishmaniasis* remain the main strategy for managing the disease of all clinic forms. Mainly, there are two common drug therapies: the first therapy includes the antimony (which known as pentavalent antimonials) and meglumine antimoniate; the second therapy includes sodium stibogluconate (pentostam). Additionally, other drugs that are approved for use are pentamidine, amphotericin B, and miltefosine [291, 292]. Most available drugs are costly, require long treatment regimens, and are losing their effectiveness, necessitating the discovery of new drugs. Several new drugs, including miltefosine and sitamaquine (both can be given orally), are in the pipeline; however, their efficacy needs to be further evaluated [181].

There are important disadvantages for all of the available drugs. Each has different toxicity ranging from transient and tolerable to severe and even dangerous. Most require lengthy, expensive, and often painful injections as the route of administration except for miltefosine due to it being orally bioavailable. High cost and rapidly evolved resistance are the major disadvantages of liposomal formulations of amphotericin B. Unfortunately, it is not completely understood how these drugs act against the parasites. In many parts of the world, parasites have developed resistance against these drugs, which reduces the efficiency of conventional medications.

Especially, pentavalent antimony resistance to these drugs has become a significant problem in some regions of India. In the state of Bihar, India, for example, over 65% of the cases of VL cannot be treated with antimony drugs. Resistance necessitates very high drug doses in order to accomplish a cure, or the drug is completely ineffectual. The toxicity of this drug is one of the most dangerous problems. Moreover, the pentavalent antimonials require management by injection over several weeks to months, so that it can be painful, expensive, and prohibitive to some patients in more isolated regions. Another disadvantage is the fact that the bioactive structures of antimony compounds are not well defined. In addition, the mechanism of action of these drugs is not well understood. These compounds are highly toxic and have significant side effects: nausea, anorexia, malaise, headache, lethargy, and more. Side effects are partially due to trivalent antimony accumulations [293].

Amphotericin B is generally used in treating *Leishmania* infections that are resistant to the antimonial drugs. It is also administered by injection over a long period of various weeks. The side effects are fever, chills, renal dysfunction, anemia, nausea, and anorexia. Cardiac death is sometimes reported in patients who were previously treated by antimonial drugs. Liposomal preparations of AmBiosome, Amphocil, and Abelcet are better tolerated and more effective; however, they are intensely more expensive [293]. On the other hand, there are also some studies on developing new formulations in order to decrease the expense of Amphotericin B.

The discovery of miltefosine (trade names Impavido and Miltex) is major progress in *Leishmaniasis* treatment. Approved for use in India, Germany, and Colombia, it is the first available oral treatment for *Leishmaniasis*. It is highly efficient with cure rates up to 98% after a 28-day course of treatment [39]. Side effects are tolerable; however, some significant side effects are nausea, vomiting, and teratogenicity. In spite of the accomplishment of this drug, it still displays available concerns, as miltefosine-resistant parasites have been cultured relatively easily in the laboratory [294, 295]. This may indicate beforehand eventual resistance in the clinic.

Due to the fact that the current treatments of *Leishmaniasis* have significant disadvantages, there is still an immediate need for the development of novel antileishmanial therapies. Various investigational compounds are being assessed for antileishmanial activity reported in the literature and discuss the status of many of these compounds [291, 296-303].

Paromomycin (Phase III), which is injectable for the treatment of VL, and sitamaquine (Phase II), as an alternative oral treatment of VL, are two drugs currently in clinical trials [293].

Drugs Used for *Leishmaniasis* Treatment

Approximately 25 drugs have antileishmanial activity. Some of them are classified as antileishmanial for humans, and most are used parenterally. Choosing the appropriate drug in treatment of *Leishmaniasis* is important because, especially in species such as *L. donovani* and *L. tropica*, it is confronted with drug resistance. In the treatment, the most common drugs, first proposed by the WHO, are pentavalent antimony compounds such as stibogluconate sodium (Pentostam®), meglumine antimoniate (Glucantime®), and ethilstibamine (Neostibosan®). Other pentavalent antimony compounds parenterally used are amphotericin B, liposomal amphotericin B, pentamidine, paromomycin sulphate, and interferon-γ, and, for oral use, ketoconazole, itraconazole, dapsone, and allopurinol. Antimony compounds have disadvantages such as parenteral application, long duration of treatment, and side effects. When drug resistance occurs against antimony compounds, other antileishmanial drugs such as pentamidine, paromomycin, allopurinol, amphotericin B, and oily formulations miltefosine, ketoconazole, itraconazole, fluconazole, terbinafine and metronidazole could be used. However, used drugs in treatment of the disease are toxic. In order to overcome disadvantages of current antileishmanial drugs such as toxicity, resistance, and expensiveness, researches tend toward new alternative therapies.

Pentavalent Antimonials

For more than five decades, pentavalent antimonials, the generic sodium stibogluconate (pentostam, Fig. **1**) and branded meglumine antimoniate (Fig. **2**) are being used in the treatment of *Leishmaniasis*. They are the first-line drugs of choice in which resistance is not reported [304].

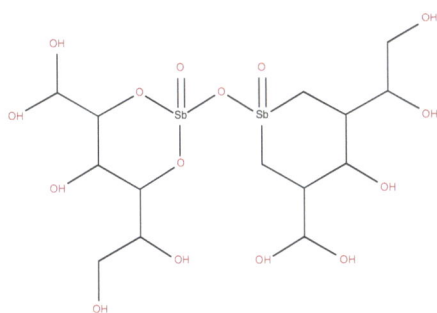

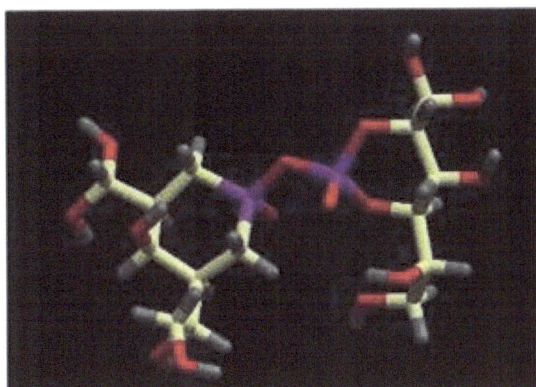

Fig. (1). Two-dimensional (2D) and three-dimensional (3D) molecular structure of sodium stibogluconate. The composition of the salt of sodium antimony gluconate is variable; therefore, its exact molecular weight (MW) cannot be determined. It contains 30% to 34% Sb and is freely soluble in water.

Initially trivalent antimonials (SbIII) were applied for the treatment of *Leishmaniasis*; however, it was soon discovered that pentavalent antimonials (SbV) were more effective and successful to treat VL while also being less toxic. Another clinically used pentavalent antimonial formulation is the meglumine antimoniate (Glucantime). According to recent data, thiol redox potential of the cell is compromised by inducing the efflux of intracellular thiols and by inhibiting

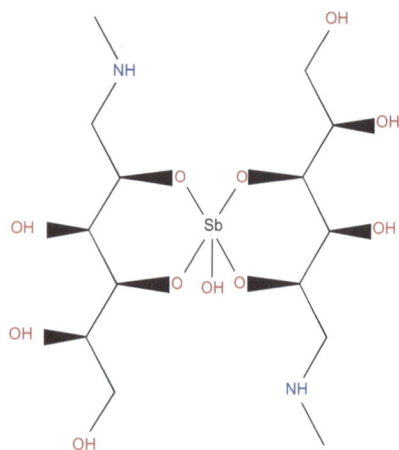

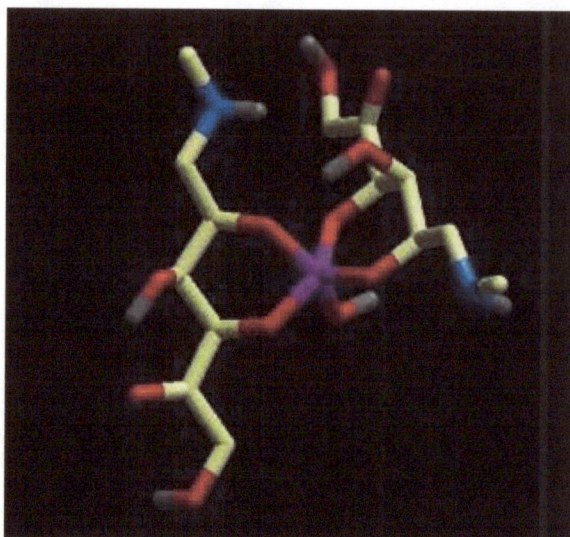

Fig. (2). Two-dimensional (2D) and three-dimensional (3D) molecular structure of meglumine antimonate, MW 366 g/mol and contains 33% Sb. 1 g dissolved in 3 ml of water.

trypanothione reductase [305]. To become active SbV, which is defined as a prodrug, it has to be converted to its trivalent form (SbIII). Also to show its activity against *Leishmania* and other intracellular amastigotes, SbV has to enter the host cell and cross the phagolysosomal membrane. As with bacteria and yeast, enzymes can be used for the metal reduction for the *Leishmania* [306]. The thiol-dependent reductase (TDR1) is a recently found parasitic enzyme, which contains domains similar to omega glutathione transferases, and it takes a role in the catalization of the conversion of SbV to SbIII. In this reaction, glutathione is used as a reductant [307]. ACR2 is a new antimonate reductase characterized in *Leishmania*, and its function is identified such that it causes reduction in the SbV level; this way, it increases the *Leishmania* cells' sensitivity against SbV [308]. There is evidence that, nonenzymatically, some thiols, such as parasite-specific thiols (as trypanothione) and macrophage-specific thiols (as glycylcysteine) [309], can reduce the SbV to SbIII. For drug activation, there is more than one mechanism.

The parasitic aquaglyceroporin, aquaporin 1 transporter is supposed to be responsible for the transport of antimonials into amastigotes [310]. The transport of SbV *via* phosphate transporter is based on penetration of pentavalent arsenate, a complex of SbV into parasitic cells. Both forms of antimonials (Sb III and SbV) kill the *Lesihmania* species by DNA fragmentation, suggesting the role of apoptosis, beta-oxidation of fatty acid and adenosine diphosphate phosphorylation. In addition to this, the antimonials inhibit glycolysis and metabolic pathways and increase efflux of intracellular thiols by a ATP binding cassette [311] transporter, multidrug-resistance protein A (MDRPA) [300, 314, 316]. Pentamonials are also known to inhibit trypanothion reductase, which is an enzyme responsible for protection from host-reactive oxygen and nitrogen species to parasites [305]. In Fig. (**3**), proposed action mechanisms of antimony and resistance process in *Leishmania* spp are shown.

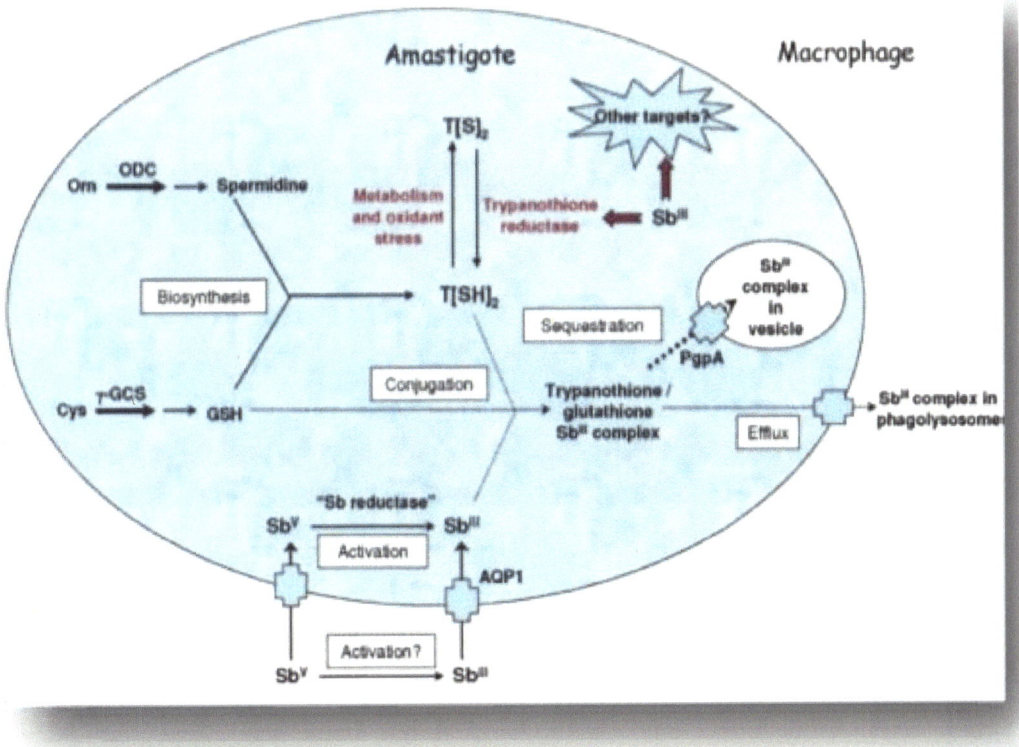

Fig. (3). Proposed action mechanisms of antimony and resistance process in *Leishmania* spp. Levels of ornithine decarboxylase (ODC), γ-glutamylcysteine synthetase (GCS), and an intracellular P-glycoprotein (PgpA) are elevated in some laboratory-derived resistant lines (thick lines), whereas decreased Sb reductase is observed in others. Dotted lines indicate nonenzymatic steps implicated in resistance. The red arrow indicates inhibition of trypanothione reductase and other targets. Uptake of Sb(III) is mediated *via* an aquaglycoporin (AQP1) [312].

Pentamidine

Pentamidine, which is an aromatic diamine, is used to cure *Leishmaniasis* as a second-line drug. Second-line drugs, as the isethionate or methanesulphonate salts of pentamidine, have been used in the treatment of VL refractory and SbV (Fig. **4**). Pentamidine can enter the parasite by using the arginine and polymine transporters and accumulates in the mitochondria. When pentamidine accumulates in mitochondria, it enhances the efficacy of mitochondrial respiratory chain complex II and resistance to pentavalent antimony in *Leishmania* amastigotes [313].

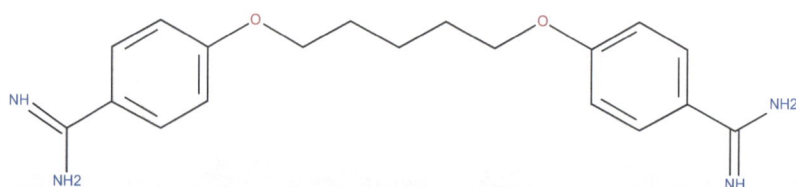

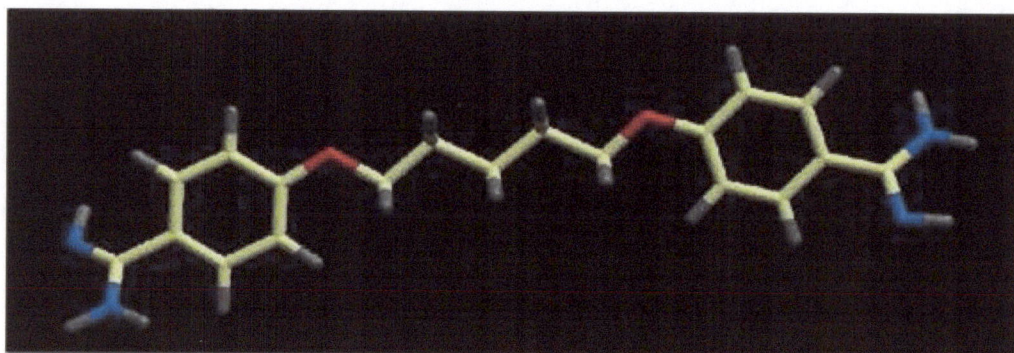

Fig. (4). 2D and 3D molecular structure of pentamidine, MW 341 g/mol, 1 g dissolved in 10 ml of water.

Amphotericin B (AmB)

Amphotericin B is a polyene antifungal that has been used as a second-line treatment for *Leishmaniasis* since the 1960s. The adverse effect of plain AmB had been circumvented with its three clinical formulation, which are liposomal AmB (L-AmB: Ambiosome), Amb colloidal dispersion (ABCD: Amphocil), and AmB lipid complex (ABL: Abelcit). In these three clinical forms of AmB, deoxycholate

Table 2.   Currently Available Antileishmanial Drugs and their Mechanism of Action in *Lesihmania*

Drug	Action Mechanism	Advantage	Disadvantage	References
Amphotericin B (polyene antibiotic)	Increase membrane permeability resulting in cell death; make complexes with 24-substituted sterols, such as ergosterol in the cell membrane, causing pores, which alter ion balance; acts as an inhibitor of ergosterol biosynthesis	Primitive resistance is unknown	Require prolonged hospitalization High cost, high fever with rigor, chills, hypokalemia, renal dysfunction	[298, 314]
Miltefosine (hexadecylphosph-ocholine)	Drug interacts with the cell membrane of *Leishmania* by modulation of cell surface receptors, inositol metabolism and phospholipase activation; cell death being mediated by apoptosis	Effective and harmless	Teratogenic, vomiting and diarrhea. Nephrotoxic	[314]
Pentavalentantimonials: Meglumine antimoniate (Glucantime) or sodium stibogluconate (Pentostam)	Display direct parasitical activity by generation of ROS, depletion of thiols, modulation of bioenergetic pathways (glycolysis, fatty acid beta oxidation, inhibition of ADP phosphorylation, blocking of SH groups of amastigote proteins) and inhibition of topoisomerase II; activated within the amastigote/macrophage after conversion to the trivalent form.	Simply handiness and low cost	Acquired resistance, cardiac arrhythmias, Myalgia, pancreatitis, hepatitis	[298, 312, 314]
Paromomycin (aminoglycoside antibiotic), also known as aminosidine or monomycin	It is proposed to induce respiratory dysfunction in *L. donovani promastigotes*. It also promoted ribosomal subunit association of both cytoplasmic and mitochondrial forms, low Mg+2, which induced dissociation; also in bacteria, inhibits protein synthesis, but in *Leishmania*, the exact mechanism is not yet known.	Remarkable, well tolerated, and relatively affordable; acts synergisticall y with antimonials	Lack of efficacy in East Africa	[325]
Sitamaquine (8-aminoquinoline, originally WR6026)	Unknown, but possibly affects mitochondrial electron transport chain.	Its efficacy and toxicity are not known exactly.	Unknown	[316]

had been replaced by other lipids. It is known that the antileishmanial activity of AmB and its lipid formulation are due to its interaction of sterols, *i.e.*, ergosterol of *Leishmania* and cholesterol of host macrophages [317] (Fig. **5**). The interaction of AmB with ergosterol leads to the formation of transmembrane AmB channels, which enhance membrane permeability, thereby allowing leakage of cytoplasmic components, which eventually leads to cell death [318].

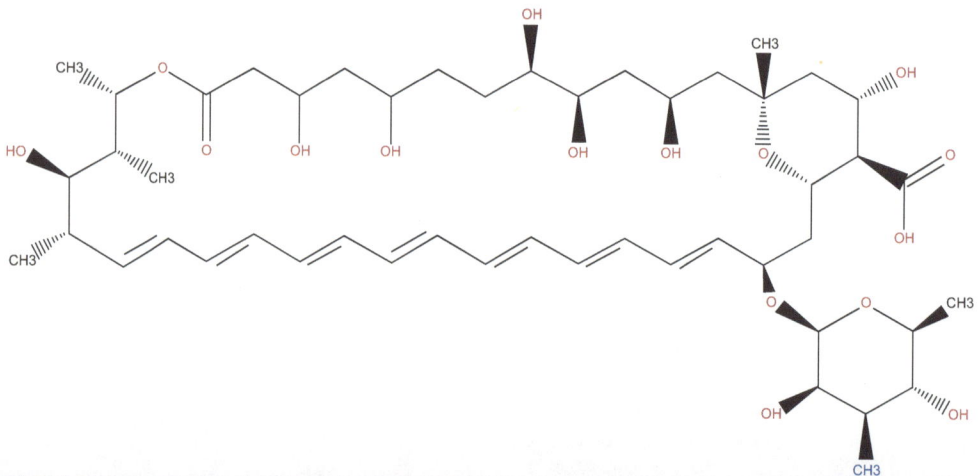

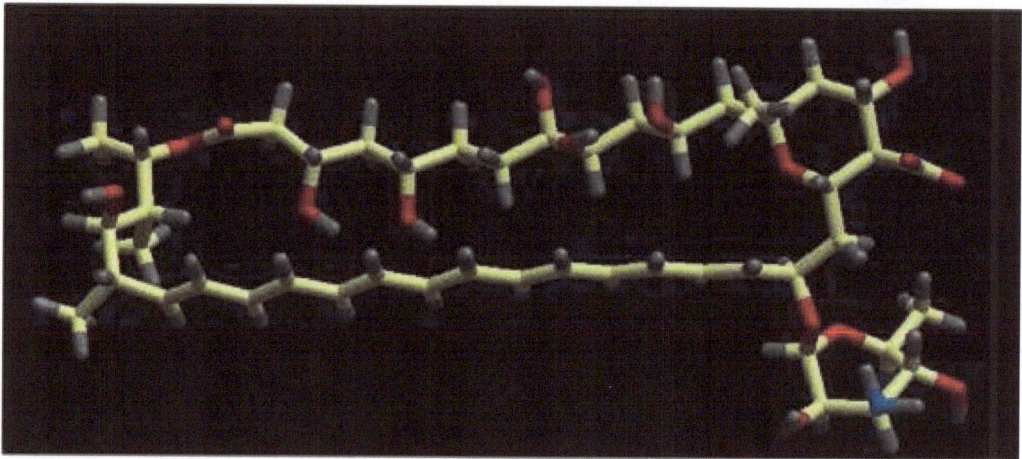

Fig. (5). 2D and 3D molecular structure of amphotericin B, MW 924 g/mole, insoluble in water and amphotericin solutions should be used immediately after preparation.

Miltefosine

Miltefosine, a phosphocholine analogue, was initially developed as an antineoplastic agent (Fig. **6**). It was found to have antileishmanial activity *in vitro* and *in vivo*, probably *via* effects on cell-signaling pathways membrane synthesis [319-321]. Although the exact mode of antileishmanial action of miltefosine is still unknown, it has been found that it causes an apoptosis-like process. Also, miltefosine reduces the lipid content in promastigotes membrane and enhances the phophatidylethonolamine content, suggesting a partial inhibition of phophatidylethonolamine- N- methyltransferase, which leads to decreased parasite proliferation [322].

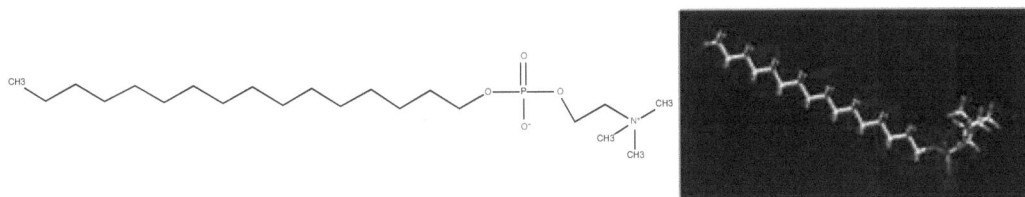

Fig. (6). 2D and 3D molecular structure of miltefosine, MW 407.568 g/mol.

Paromomycin

Paromomycin, an aminoglycoside antibiotic, is a potentially useful antileishmanial topical agent in humans and also is used for treatment of canine *Leishmaniasis* (Fig. **7**) [323]. Recently it has been shown that cationic paromomycin binds to the negatively charged *Leishmanial* glycocalyx, suggesting mitochondria as a primary target [315]. In addition to this, it is known that paromomycin inhibits translocation and recycling of ribosomal subunits and hence protein synthesis. Paromomycin promotes association of 50S and 30S subunits of cytoplasmic and mitochondrial ribosomes and stops their recycling, which eventually inhibits protein synthesis in *Leishmania donovani* [324]. Further exploration came from the study of Hirkoma *et al.*, which proves that paromomycin interacts with 30S and 50S subunits without inhibiting the association of translation initiation factor-3 (IF3) to the 30S ribosomal subunit [333].

Sitamaquine

Sitamaquine has broad-spectrum antiprotozoal activity and affects the parasite motility, morphology, and growth (Fig. **8**). Sitamaquine action mechanism involves electrostatic interaction between a phospholipid anionic polar head group and positively charged sitamaquine and then with phospholipid acyl chains leading to drug insertion within biological membranes [326].

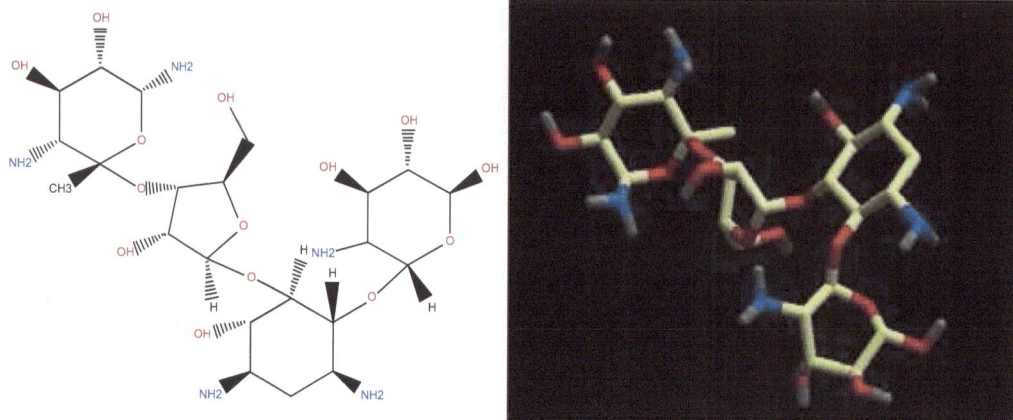

Fig. (7). 2D and 3D molecular structure of paromomycin, MW 615.629 g/mol.

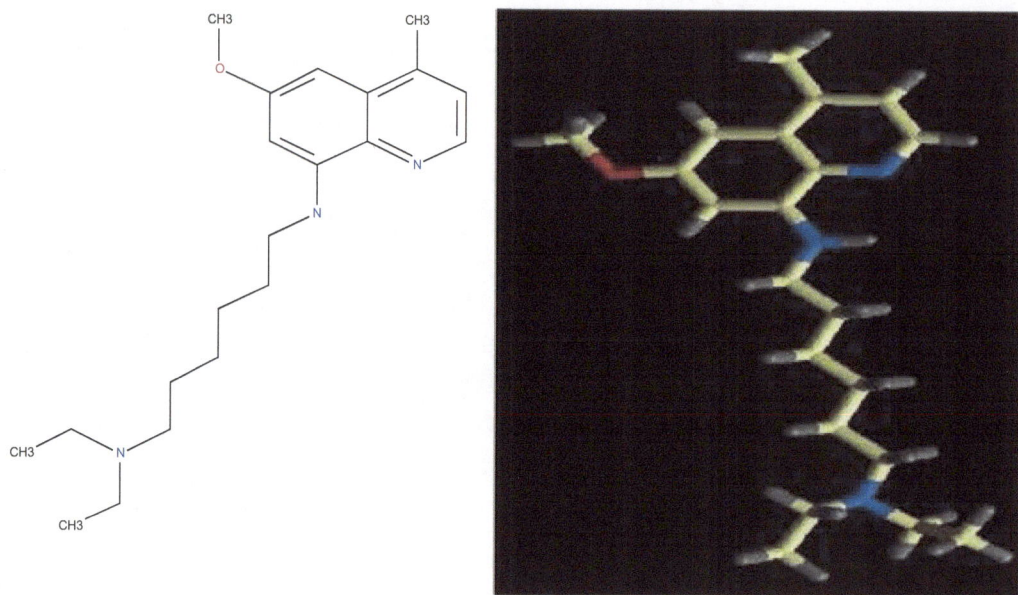

Fig. (8). 2D and 3D molecular structure of sitamaquine, MW 343.506 Da.

Azoles

Azole, as with amphotericin B, targets the sterol biosynthesis. Mainly it is used for systemic fungal infection, but it has shown good chemotherapeutic activity against several kinetoplastid parasites, including *Leishmania*. The activity of the currently used azoles is variable against different *Leishmania* species due to differences in the sterol biosynthetic pathways and sterol requirements among the various *Leishmania* species.

Imidazoles/Triazoles (ketoconazole, Fluconazole, Itraconazole)

The efficacy of the azole compounds has been investigated by a number of researchers in the treatment of New World CL. These antifungal compounds include two different classes: imidazoles (*e.g.*, ketoconazole) and triazoles (*e.g.*, fluconazole, itraconazole). Studies on the use of oral ketoconazole for the treatment of New World CL emphasize the importance of speciation because the efficacy of treatment has been shown to vary according to species.

Nucleoside Analogues

In the 1980s, allopurinol, a pyrazolopyrimidine, entered clinical trials for the treatment of VL and CL, both alone and in combination with antimonials. Though no successful treatment for human disease exists, it is still used in treatment of canine *Leishmaniasis*. Allopurinol (4-hydroxypyrazolo(3,4-d) pyrimidine) is believed to act by prohibiting the *de novo* synthesis of pyrimidines, probably through the formation of allopurinol ribotide, which leads to the inhibition of protein synthesis in the *Leishmania* parasite [327]. In comparative studies, wide variations in sensitivity of the promastigotes of different species to the pyrazolopyrimidines allopurinol and allopurinol riboside were reported to be due to differences in the affinity of the purine salvage pathway enzymes. The allopurinol action mode is thought to involve conversion to ribonucleoside triphosphate analogues and incorporation into RNA, thereby disrupting macromolecular biosynthesis. The pharmacokinetic properties are a major limitation to the use of allopurinol or its derivatives for treatment of human *Leishmaniasis* [328].

Imiquimod

Imiquimod is an immune-response modifier that increases local cytokine production, with subsequent activation of both the innate (rapid, nonspecific) and adaptive (specific, cellular, and humoral) immune systems (Fig. **9**) [329]. The combination therapy with imiquimod and meglumine antimoniate is a promising alternative regimen for the treatment of New World CL.

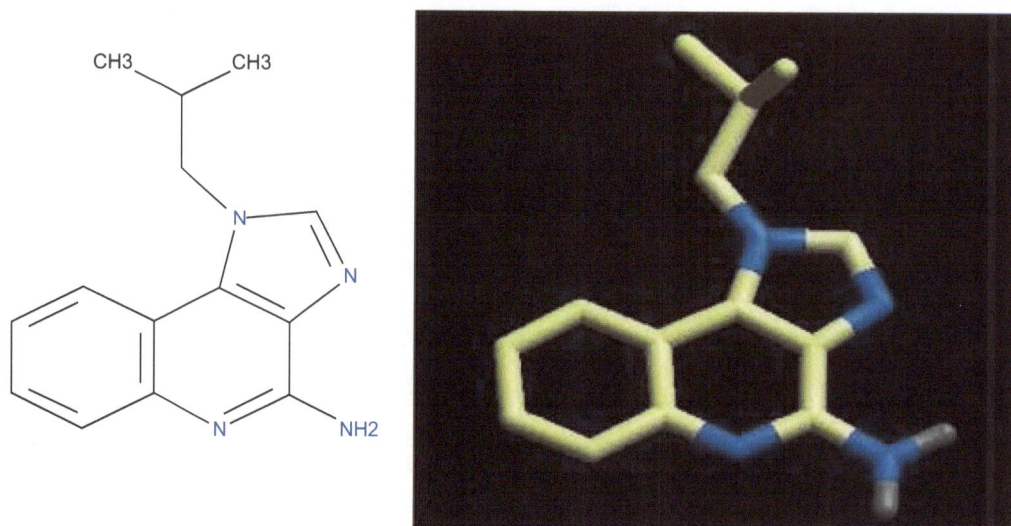

Fig. (9). 2D and 3D molecular structure of imiquimod, MW 240.304 g/mol.

Combinations of Conventional Drugs

It is known that drug resistance is an important problem in the treatment of parasitic diseases. As mentioned below, resistant *Leishmania* strains against conventional treatment regimens have evolved rapidly in all endemic regions of the world. Therefore, the numbers of treatment failures have been intensely increasing in endemic regions. In order to decelerate the spreading speed of drug resistance and develop more successful treatment regimens, scientists have recently started to investigate the effectiveness of combined use of antileishmanial drugs in therapy [330, 331]. Application of combination therapy was first performed in Africa in the late 1980s. In this study, approximately 4000 VL patients were exposed to pentavalent antimonial plus paramomycin treatment, while the control group received only single-dose pentavalent antimonial therapy. Nine months after treatment, it was shown that combination therapy was more effective than antimonial treatment and reduced mortality rates by causing fewer complications [332]. In another study, a combination of sodium stibogluconate with an indolyl-quinolone derivative was used in hamsters with the VL model. It was demonstrated that combination therapy achieved 100% success in the clearance of the liver and spleen of animals from parasite evasion, while indolyl-quinolone and sodium stibogluconate therapy each alone exhibited 93% and 80% success, respectively [333]. Also, in different studies, paromomycin-pentostam combinations achieved more than 82% success in treatment of VL patients in Sudan and India [334]. In a new study, Sundar *et al.* combined single-dose amphotericin B with oral miltefosine or paromomycin with various dosages and applied this treatment regimen on 226 patients in the Bihar region of India, which is an endemic place for *Leishmaniasis*, where drug resistance is intensely observed. According to the results, nine months after treatment, healing rates of patients, who suffered from VL, reached 95%; these results were accepted as successful and promising [335]. As noted, combination therapy can be determined as encouraging for fighting against drug resistance. However, a number of studies are still expected, and such studies must be reliably supported.

Other Drugs

Leishmaniasis is the only tropical disease being treated by non-*Leishmanial* drugs. Moreover, the exact mechanisms of drugs are not known. Scientists try to find new drugs, drugs combinations, and new drug targets (Tables **2** and **3**). Agents such as rifampicin, isoniazid, dapsone, chloroquine, cyclosporine, recombinant interferon, nifurtimox, and monoclonal antibodies, which have found some favor in human and animal studies involving Old World CL, have not been investigated for their efficacy against New World disease [336, 337]. In addition, several novel compounds have demonstrated *Leishmanicidal* activity, such as antimicrobial peptides, and a diverse number of plant extracts, such as chalcones, alkaloids, terpenes, and phenolics [293]. There is still much more to learn about the activity of these agents. They are still on an experimental platform and have not yet been evaluated in clinical trials.

Treatment Regimens for VL and HIV Co-Infections

Co-infection of VL with human immunodeficiency virus (HIV) is one of the most dangerous forms of *Leishmania* disease. Especially in endemic regions for both

Table 3.   New Drug Targets for *Leishmaniasis*

Drug Target	Drug Target Mechanism	References
Peptidases	There are 154 peptidase in *Leishmania major* genome. T proteasome, which is responsible for degradation of ubiquitinated proteins in cytosol, is a multi-subunit, multi-catalytic peptidase. Benzamidine and TPKC(N-tosyl-l-lysyl-chloromethylketone) reduce the viability and induce morphological changes.	[317, 338-344]
Enzymes of polyamine biosynthesis	As with polyamine, putrescin, spermidine, and spermine play an important role in growth and differentiation from promastigote to amastigote; also polyamines down-regulates lipid peroxidation generated by oxidants compounds and makes the environment compatible for survival.	[317, 345-351]
Enzymes of glycosomal machinery	Takes a role in many metabolic activities such as glycolysis, oxidation of fatty acid, lipid biosynthesis, and purine salvage pathways *etc.*	[317, 352, 353]
Enzymes of thiol metabolic	Scientists designed specific inhibitors against TR (triptophan reductase); it may be an ideal drug, which will stop parasite growth without altering host glutathione reductase (GR) activity	[317, 356, 359]
Cyclin dependent kinases	The chemical inhibitor of Cdk related kinase3 (CRK3) impairs the parasite viability within macrophage, thus validating CRK3 as a potential drug target. The CRK3 and LdGSK3 (*Leishmania donovani* glycogen synthesis kinase) combination play a role in cell cycle control and apoptosis and play a role in cell division cycle, transcription, apoptosis, and differentiation	[317, 360-363]
Mitogen activates proteins kinases (MAPK),	MAPK gene deleted promastigotes after differentiation amastigote *Leishmania* spp. mislay proliferate capacity	[317, 363-365]
Enzymes of sterol biosynthesis	Shows its effects the cell membrane structure	[317, 366]
Dihydrofolate Reductase (DHFR)	A key enzyme in folate metabolism linked to the production of thymidine, inhibition of dihydrofolate reductase (DHFR); anticipates biosynthesis of thymidine and DNA biosynthesis	[317, 367- 373]
Topoisomerases	Topoisomerase II is needed due to the presence of a complex intercatenated network of thousands of mini-circles as well as maxi-circles in kinetoplastids mitochondria	[317, 373-376]
Metacaspases	It is essential for the proper segregation of the nucleus and kinetoplast, parasite survival. It also plays a role in apoptosis	[317, 377-381]

VL and HIV, such as India, these two infections come into contact and constitute this big problem. VL/HIV co-infections are seen not only in endemic regions but also in nonendemic regions of the world. VL/HIV co-infections have been reported in 35 countries until now; this includes four southwestern Europe countries (Spain, Italy, Portugal, France), which are not endemic for VL or HIV [382-384]. Since global distributions of both diseases all over the world have tremendously increased, it is estimated that the number of VL/HIV co-infection cases will rapidly augment in the near future. This is a bad news because treatment of VL patients co-infected with HIV is difficult. In the initial phase of this epidemic, physicians applied high dosages of pentavalent antimonials, which ultimately led to high mortality rates and enhanced toxicity [385-389]. Combined use of pentavalent antimonials and amphotericin B was successful on HIV negative patients, but treatment failed in HIV-positive patients [330]. Furthermore, regardless of which antileishmanial drug is used, there is a relapse risk at the rate of nearly 60% in the first year of treatment. In order to diminish relapse rates, antiretroviral therapy can be used, especially at high dosages. On the other side, this therapy is too expensive to be applied in developing countries such as India [388, 389]. Instead of antiretroviral therapy, second-line antileishmanial therapy applications are performed, but this usually causes secondary resistance against these drugs. Sinha *et al.* performed amphotericin B treatment in a combination with antiretroviral therapy on 55 patients with a VL/HIV co-infection. Survival rates for patients exposed to combination therapy for two years were evaluated at 85%. During this period, treatment succeeded to prevent HIV infection in 83% of co-infected patients. Another good result was that large amounts of patients initially responded to therapy against VL. However, two years after treatment, relapses of VL were observed in nearly half the treated patients [390]. As seen, although initial treatment is successful, there is a maximum risk of VL relapse. Therefore, new and comprehensive researchers are required for accurate treatment of infection without relapses.

Potential Drug Targets in *Leishmania* Parasites

The glycolytic enzymes of the parasites, which are potential drug targets, are found partially separated into compartments in both promastigotes and amastigotes. The first enzymes of the glycolytic pathway are consumed in a special organelle called a glycosome, which includes all *Leishmania* spp. [390], the 3D structure of a bifunctional DHFR-thymidylate synthase from *Leishmania* major on the basis of the trypanosomal glycolysis inhibition. One study designed a compound -2'-deoxy- 2'-(3-methoxybenzamido) adenosine that was 45-fold more potent than adenosine and, therefore, had more affinity for the trypanosomal enzyme than the human equivalent of glyceraldehyde-3-phosphate dehydrogenase (GADPH) [391].

The other interesting drug target for chemotherapeutic agents is the synthesis of sterols in *Leishmania* spp. Lanosterol, which is demethylation, produces cholesterol as the major sterol in mammalian hosts. On the contrary, *Leishmania* has ergostane sterols-episterol and 5- OH-dehydroepisterol. The similtude of these sterols to the fungus major sterol, which is episterol, has created the basis of the fungicidal drugs such as azoles and polyene antibiotics. The major disadvantage of this kind of treatment is the inclusion of the host cholesterol by the amastigote, which can lead to parasite resistance to the drug.

Purine metabolism of the parasite is different from its mammalian equivalent and has taken advantage of another target for chemotherapy in *Leishmaniasis*. Their incompetence to synthesize from the beginning the purine ring from metabolic precursors has led them to obtain it from the host. Hypoxanthine guanine phosphoribosyl transferase, which is the *Leishmania* amastigotes enzyme, enormously uses the abnormal inosine allopurinol as substrate and converts it into its comparable nucleoside. This leads to the action of allopurinol being able to block the purine salvage pathway, which caused purine famishment and death of the parasite cell. On the other site, *Leishmania* parasites again synthesize pyrimidine. Thymidylate synthase, which also presents the activity of dihydrofolate reductase, has been targeted by the anticancer drug methotrexate, the antimalarial agent pyrimethamine, and aromatic diamidines.

To protect the organism against oxidative stress, trypanosomatids have evolved a unique system, which is called trypanothione metabolizing. Among the potential drug targets for the diseases caused by the group trypanosomatidae, probably trypanothione reductase is one of the best investigated. Trypanothione reductase, which is the enzyme responsible for maintaining trypanothione in its reduced form, is ideal to be central to the redox defense systems of trypanosomatids. Trypanosomes lacking trypanothione reductase showed increased sensitivity to oxidative stress [392]. In a study, TR created knockouts in *L. donovani* and *L. major* to study the physiological role of TR in *Leishmania*. Their attempts to obtain TR-null mutants failed [393]. Trivalent arsenic drugs, substituted naphthoquinones, nitrofurans and 1,3-bis-2 (chloroethylnitrosourea) have been reported as powerful inhibitors of trypanothione reductase [394]. Polyamine synthesis inhibitors also inhibit trypanothione synthesis by reducing parasite spermidine pools.

Cysteine proteases, which is another target for the synthesis of anti-trypanosomal drugs, plays an important role in parasitic infections and lacks superfluity compared with mammalian systems [395, 396]. *Leishmania* parasites have three cysteine protease gene families [397]. Various cysteine protease inhibitors have been studied in tissue culture models of parasite growth. Eventually, the mechanism of parasite bioactivity and virulence will reveal potential targets for therapeutic drugs and vaccines [9].

Drug-Resistance Mechanism of *Leishmania* Parasites

Drug-resistant parasites are a major problem in the field since *Leishmaniasis* management relies on drugs [312]. Unfortunately, limited information is available on the biochemical and molecular mechanism that contributes to drug resistance in *Lesihmania* spp. However, the mechanistic reasons for drug resistance are only partially understood.

Pentavalent Antimony Resistance

Since SbV-containing drugs are still the treatment of choice against all forms of *Leishmaniasis*, it is likely that resistance will increase and spread more rapidly. Antimonial resistance has been found to be associated with overexpression of a heat shock protein (HSP70) gene [405]. Transporters of an ABC family, MRPA and pentamidine, resistant protein 1 (PRP1), which act as an efflux pump for antimonials, are also linked to antimony resistance (Fig. **10**) [399].

SbIII resistance mutants selected for the related metal arsenide have pinpointed the crucial role of drug transporters and of trypanothione. Trypanothione is the major reduced thiol of *Leishmania* cells consisting of a spermidine and a bis-glutathionel conjugate [401]. The role of the transporters, including ABC transporters, and of enzymes modulating trypanothione metabolism in the context of oxyanion metal resistance, has recently been reviewed. Similarly to arsenide resistance, resistance to SbV is multifactorial. Novel genes involved in antimony resistance have recently been isolated [402].

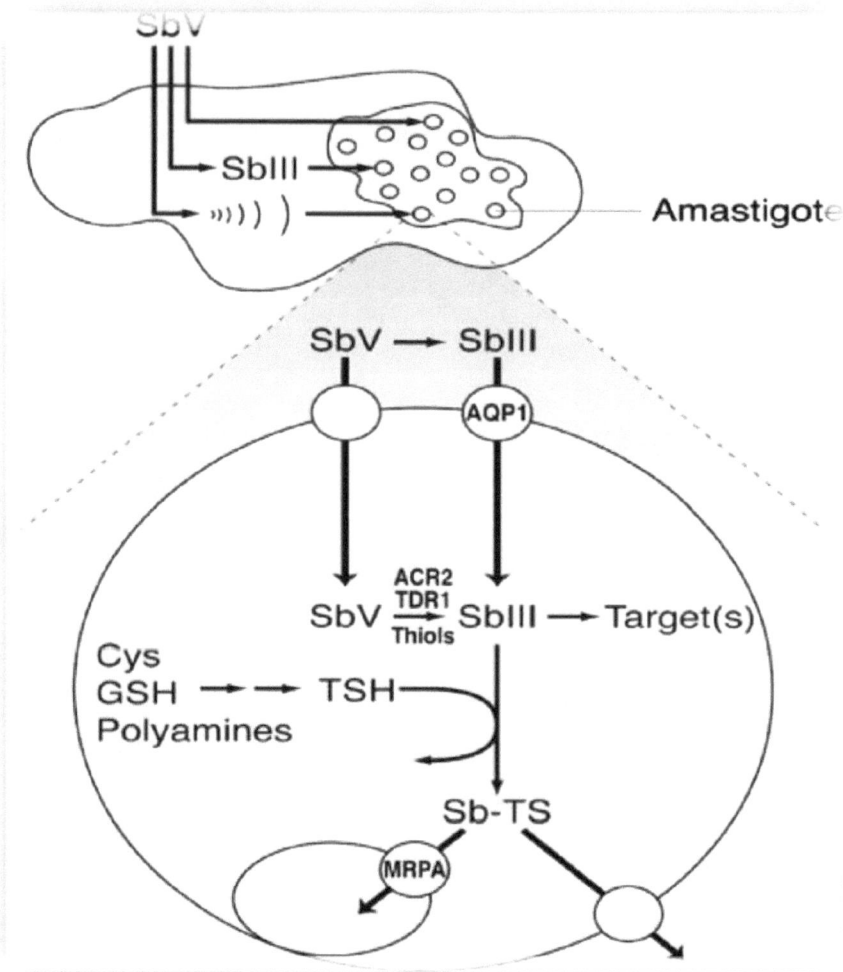

Fig. (10). Resistance mechanisms to pentavalent antimonials in *Leishmania* amastigotes. Pentavalent antimony (SbV) is first converted to SbIII and then enters the macrophages in the amastigote parasite within the phagolysosome, or it can be reduced to a trivalent form in the cytosol (or within the phagolysosome). Besides the direct effect on parasite, SbV also can cause cell death by affecting cell signaling. SbV can enter the amastigotes by an unknown transporter or by an aquaglyceroporin AQP1 transporter in its SbIII form. Inside the parasite thiols or the other, the novel ACR2 and TDR1 reductases play a role in the conversion of SbV to SbIII. İnside the cell, SbIII may interact with some cellular targets and also can make conjugation with various thiols, including cysteine, glutathione, and trypanothione. It is not clear if conjugation formation is mediated enzymatically or not. The trypanothione level is increased in antimony-resistant cell lines; this increase causes the conjugation efficiency to metal. By using the ABC transporter, MRPA metal-thiol conjugate can be either sequestered into an organelle or by using an efflux system, possibly corresponding to another ABC transporter, which can be extruded out of the cell [400].

Amphotericin B Resistance

Clinical AmB resistance cases of *Leishmania* have not yet been reported, but AmB-resistant strains have been selected *in vitro*. Due to recent studies, it is thought that the reason for the AmB resistance is improved by a gene [403]. Changes in membrane fluidity and an ergosterol precursor rather than ergosterol found in a sensitive parent are correlated to the emergence of resistance. Binding affinity of sterol to the sterol-modified membranes is decreased due to these changes (Fig. **11**). Analysis of *L. donovani* cells selected for AmB resistance revealed that an ergosterol precursor is the predominant membrane sterol instead of ergosterol itself. This may change membrane fluidity and permeability, resulting in decreased AmB uptake and increased efflux in the mutants [404]. Collateral resistance to a number of unrelated drugs was observed in the AmB mutants and could be attributable to altered permeability.

Miltefosine Resistance

Broadly, the main reason for miltefosine resistance in *Leishmania* is drug efflux decrease, although many mechanisms are reported for this decreased intracellular drug concentration. It has been discovered that single-point mutation at LdMT and LDRos3 in experimental *Leishmaniasis* may lead to resistance. In addition to LdMT, overexpression of a multidrug-resistant MDR1 gene, which encodes a glycoprotein, is also responsible for drug resistance [406]. Furthermore, miltefosine resistance is also correlated with lipid content in parasite membrane. It has been observed that the amount of unsaturated phospholipid alkyl chains was lower in miltefosine-resistance parasites [411]. The possible resistance mechanisms for the reduction in drug uptake are differences in the plasma membrane permeability, faster drug metabolism, and drug efflux mechanism on the membrane. A recent study has shown that overexpression of the P-glycoprotein gene MDR1 causes resistance to the daunomycin, which is an anticancer agent for *Leishmania*. P-glycoproteins are ABC transporters, which are responsible for multidrug resistance in cancer cells. P-glycoprotein-overexpressed *Leishmania* cells were resistant against miltefosine. Miltefosine cross resistance

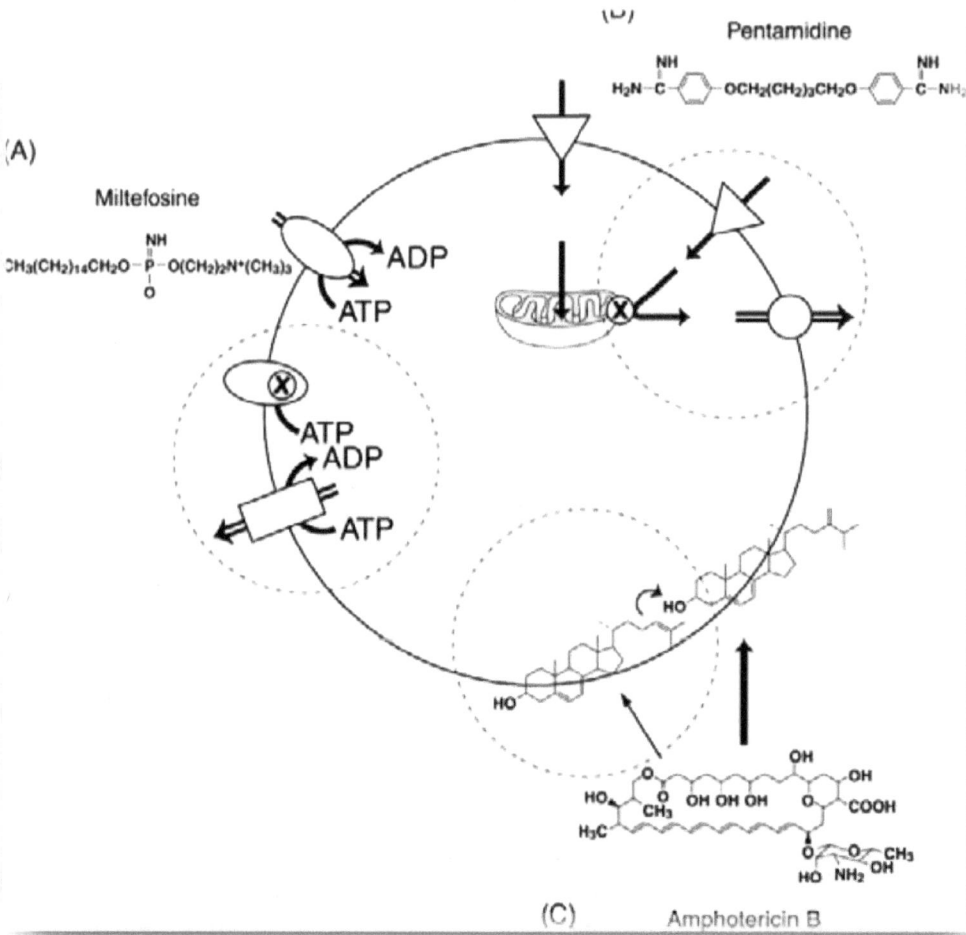

Fig. (11). Action mechanisms of some antileishmanial drugs and resistance process in *Leishmania* parasites against these drugs. (**A**) Miltefosine is a drug that is taken up by an aminophospholipid P-type ATPase [411] transporter system, and, if a point mutation occurs in this system, accumulation of the drug decreases and resistance improves [405]. It is possible that miltefosine can be extruded from the cell by the ABC transporter [406]. (**B**) Transporter system has not been identified for the pentamidine. Pentamidine is active in a resistant cell, and, in the sensitive cell, it accumulates in the mitochondria but not in the resistance cells [407]. The ABC transporter system is responsible for extradition of cytosol-accumulated drugs in the resistant cells [408]. (**C**) Amphotericin B interacts with ergostane-based sterols, which are found on the membrane. The most abundant sterol is ergosta-5,7,24(241)-trien-3-ol [409]. Amphotericin B resistance is linked to the buildup of ergosterol precursors such as cholesta-5,7,24-trien-3-ol (structure on the left) for which the drug has lower affinities [404, 410].

can be decreased by some compounds, which convert the multidrug resistance by interacting with the P-glycoprotein [412]. MDR1 is a p-glycoprotein gene that plays a role in miltefosine resistance.

Recently, subcellular localization of MDR1 was elucidated. It has been clarified that this p-glycoprotein gene had been found in a number of secretory and endocytic compartments and transports substrates into these secretory compartments before exported from the parasite by the exocytosis [413]. Drug-resistance mechanism studies against the miltefosine for *L. donovani* cells have revealed a correlation between the resistance and reduction of accumulation of this drug. Reduction of the drug accumulation was caused by deficiency in the inward translocation, which is clarified as the movement from the outer to the inner leaflet of the plasma membrane. A novel P-type of ATPase, aminophospholipid translocase subfamily LdMT protein has been newly described [405]. Two different point mutations on the protein were implicated in loss of translocation of both drugs and glycerophospholipids. Miltefosine is a major drug for the control of *Leishmania* infections. However, it does not prevent resistant mutants. In laboratory conditions, miltefosine-resistant parasites can be generated; however, the scenario in the field is not the same as with the laboratory, and parasites may be less virulent because of destroyed phospholipid translocations. Miltefosine can be combined with the other drugs to prevent drug resistance. Further studies will show the effects of these novel drugs against *Leishmania* infections.

Paromomycin Resistance

Possible mechanisms of resistance in *Leishmania* could be related to the effect of paromomycin on RNA synthesis and to modifications of membrane polar lipids and membrane fluidity, leading to altered membrane permeability [414]. In *Leishmania* transfection, the bacterial neomycin phosphotransferase gene is used as a selectable marker, which confers resistance to paromomycin [415]. As scientists attempt to generate live attenuated parasite strains for vaccine development using gene-targeting technologies, it will be important that recombinant strains do not contain markers conferring resistance against conventional antileishmanial drugs.

Sitamaquine Resistance

Although resistance against this drug has not been reported in clinical practice, *in vitro* resistance against *Lesihmania donovani* promastigote has been reported by selecting drug pressure 160 πm concentration [416]. In one study conducted on CL caused by *Leishmania* major on BALB/c mice, sitamaquine dihydrochloride did not reduce the parasite burden, and lesion progression was continued [417]. In order to reveal success of this novel drug, further investigations are required.

Azoles Resistance

Resistance to azoles has not been elaborated in *Leishmania* but has been studied extensively in the yeast *Candida albicans*. It can be mediated by overexpression of efflux pumps [418], mutations in the lanosterol 14a-demethylase gene, or overexpression of the latter gene. Modulation in the activity of enzymes involved in sterol metabolism also may induce azole resistance in fungi. Indeed, azole-resistant mutants of *C albicans* had membrane sterol changes consistent with a mutation in the delta 5, 6-sterol desaturase gene. The lack of ergosterol in the cytoplasmic membrane of fluconazole-resistant strains also imparted resistance to AmB. Similarly, ketoconazole decreases drastically the level of ergosterol in *Leishmania*, which leads to increased resistance to AraB [419].

Pentamidine Resistance

Pentamidine resistance against different *Leishmania* species was discovered in laboratory investigations. Recent studies have suggested that pentamidine could enter through the arginine and polyamine transporter system, and intracellular concentration of the arginine and polyamines has a role in the drug-resistance mechanism [420]. According to recent studies, many of the common polyamines, amino acids and nucleobases, sugars, or other metabolites could not inhibit the transport by themselves [407].

According to recent studies, pentamidine accumulates in the mitochondria and greatly enhances the efficacy of mitochondrial respiratory chain complex II inhibitors. Due to pentamidine *in vitro* studies, it does not accumulate in the mitochondria of the resistant mutants and is extruded from the cell. A calcium channel blocker, verapamil, could reverse some of the multidrug resistance and reduce the pentamidine efflux [408].

Purine Analog Resistance

Resistance to nucleoside analogs has been induced in *Leishmania in vitro*. Two separate mutations, leading to decreased accumulation of purines, were characterized in *Leishmania* spp: the first involved transport of inosine, guanosine, and their analogues; the second implicated the transport of adenosine and its analogues [421]. Mutants lacking both transporters have been obtained by selecting parasites with two toxic analogues, suggesting that other purine transporters also must be present in *Leishmania*. *Leishmania* also can respond to purine analogues by amplifying specific portions of its genome. *Leishmania* selected for inosine dialdehyde or tubercidin resistance had mutations in transporter activity, but also had a 55 kb amplified extrachromosomal circle [422]. Resistance to mycophenolic acid, which is an inhibitor of the inosine monophosphate dehydrogenase (IMPDH), an enzyme involved in the synthesis of guanine nucleotides, has been induced in *Leishmania*. Resistance has been associated to the amplification of the *impdh* gene as part of a linear stable amplicon. Selection of *Trypanasoma gambiense* for mycophenolic acid also led to the amplification of the *impdh* gene, but in this case the whole chromosome was amplified [426].

Antifolates Resistance

Mainly two mechanisms are responsible for the antifolat resistance in *Lesihmania* spp. The first mechanism is the overexpression of the target enzyme DHFR-TS (102). This overexpression was mediated by *dhfr-ts* gene amplification (103). Amplification of *dhfr-ts* following MTX (methotrexate) resistance only has been described in *L. major* mutants, but when a preferred resistance mechanism was disrupted in *L. tarentolae*, *dhfr-ts* was amplified upon MTX selection, and, in at least one case, the DHFR (dihydrofolate reductase) overproduced *in L. major* had a point mutation in a position known to correlate with MTX resistance in mammalian DHFRs. Amplification of the *dhfr-ts* gene is also observed in bacteria resistant to trimethoprim and in cancer cells resistant to MTX. Mutations in the target gene constitute a common mechanism of resistance to MTX in cancer cells and the main mechanism of pyrimethamine resistance in the malaria parasite *Plasmodium* [424]. In addition to *dhfr-ts,* another locus was shown to be frequently amplified in different species of *Leishmania* selected for MTX resistance. It corresponds to the H locus, and the mechanism by which it confers resistance remained elusive for several years. Transfection studies led to the isolation of the gene, and its characterization indicated that its gene product, named PTR1, belongs to the family of short-chain dehydrogenases (a14). Gene disruption studies and PTR1 biochemical characterization indicated that PTR1 is involved in the salvage of oxidized pterins and also is capable of reducing folates into dihydrofolates and into tetrahydrofolates. PTR1, therefore, confers resistance by bypassing the need for DHFR. To be effective against *Leishmania*, antifolate-based chemotherapy would therefore need to target DHFR-TS and PTR1, and, indeed, such an inhibitor recently has been shown to be effective against *Leishmania.*

Physical Methods for Treatment of Cutaneous *Leishmaniasis*

Cryotherapy

Currently cryotherapy has been only used in *Leishmania* species causing cutaneous disease in the Old World (such as *L. tropica* and *L. infantum*) [425]. In one study among 461 patients in Turkey, 415 [(90%) probably infected with *L. tropica* promastigotes] had been cured by at least one lesion with the cryotherapy method by using liquid nitrogen [426]. There have been increasing reports of hypopigmentation associated with the use of treatment by cryotherapy. However, onset of repigmentation occurred as early as two to three months of treatment in most patients. The optimal period time of each application and the time intervals between application periods are not well defined; for example, in a study in Greece, two cycles of 10-30 seconds freezing time are enough for *L. tropica* lesions [427]; on the contrary, in Jordan, one to three periods of two applications 15-20 second freezing time with a thaw of 1 minute between periods are used for *L. major* or *L. tropica* infection [428].

Cryotherapy was used together with intralesional meglumine antimoniate against *L. major* and *L. tropica* infections in Iran; cure ratios of cryotherapy plus meglumine antimoniate were approximately 90% [429].

Heat Therapy in Cutaneous Leishmaniasis

ThermoMed® (ThermoSurgery Technologies, Inc., Phoenix, Arizona) has developed a device for treatment of CL, which has been FDA-approved. Principles of this device work by radio-frequency-generated heat directly to a lesion region, which includes amastigotes [425]. Generation of heat can be controlled locally. Local anesthetic is required because the treatment method is painful. Guatemalan *L. mexicana* infected CL patients have been treated by heat therapy, which proved effective as meglumine antimoniate [430].

CO_2 Laser

A carbon dioxide laser has been used to convert into vapor CL lesions for treatment in Turkmenistan and Iran [431, 432]. Principles of carbon dioxide laser methods, based on power of 30W (maximum 100W) and a pulse width of 0.5-5 seconds, until the ulcer bed turned brown and the hemostasis was performed, provided 94% curing. First, CL lesions were anesthetized by local injection of 1-2% lidocaine [425].

Plants Used for *Leishmaniasis* Treatment

For the treatment of *Leishmaniasis*, scientists try to find new methods, new drugs, drug target, and a new source of antileishmanial compounds. For this reason, plant products are potential sources of new and selective agents for the treatment of important tropical diseases caused by protozoans and other parasites. The chemical diversity present in plants and the promising leads, which have already been demonstrated significant against parasitic diseases, also are needed to be addressed against *Leishmania* parasites. The diverse chemical groups for the plant extracts has been assigned as alkaloids, flavonoids, pheylpropanoids, steroids, and terpenoids [433]. Different strategies can be employed to plants to improve herbal medicine and isolate different active compounds from them. These strategies could include the investigation of traditional usage, considering the chemical composition and toxicity of the plants [434]. For the extraction process, scientists have used different plant parts and solvents. Usually, extraction of solvents with different polarities is employed. In the bioactivity-guided fractionation method, sequentially, active plant extracts are fractionated, and each fraction and/or pure compound is evaluated for biological activity and toxicity for the purification and isolation. This fractionation method is simple, reproducible, rapid, and low cost. To screen the biologically active plant substances in the *Leishmania* promastigote, axenic amastigote and intracellular amastigote forms of the parasite can be used. Due to the results of standard *in vitro* drug tests done on axenic, amastigotes are more significant and easy to manipulate and quantify than the *in vitro* tests done on promastigotes [297]. *In vitro* tests on *Leishmaniasis* can be achieved by using different methods such as cell counting, colorimetric method with Alamar blue or acid phosphatase activity, MTT-based method, which evaluates the viability of the cell population and determines ornithine decarboxylase activity, or using a fluorescent dye such as a propidium iodide and a fluorescence-activated cell sorter (FACS) [435]. Green fluorescent protein (GFP) or luciferase-derived reporters are the new alternatives for the development of drug-screening tests on the *Leishmania*. To screen the potential of new antileishmanial drugs on the intracellular forms of parasites isolated from patients, a lactamase assay has been used [436]. For the application of medicinal plants in the treatment of *Leishmaniasis*, *in vitro* screenings are only the first steps to prove the efficacy and safety. The efficacy of anti-*Leishmaniasis* drugs varies due to the *Leishmania* species, the immune status of the patient, or the pharmacokinetic properties of the drugs. Researchers around the world have become aware of the great effort of antileishmanial activity of natural products such as crude plant extracts, fractions, and essential oils and many compounds isolated from plants. Pentavalent antimonials such as meglumine antimoniate and sodium stibogluconate are the drugs used for first-line therapy against *Leishmaniasis*.

The developments of antileishmanial plant products or their analogs and to understand their action mechanism have a dramatic positive impact on the treatment of *Leishmaniasis*. A safe, nontoxic, and cost-effective drug is urgently required to eliminate this problem from every corner of world. Safer, shorter, and cheaper treatments, such as the identification of the most cost-effective surveillance system and control strategies and a suitable vector control approach, are among the important aspects for the control and complete eradication of this deadly disease. In the ongoing search, the chemotherapeutic properties and action mechanism of approximately 250,000 plant species have been studied (Table **4**).

Table 4.   Plants and their Extract Used to Treatment of *Leishmania Species*

Leishmania Species	Family/Plant Species	Active Extracts from Plants	References
Aloeaceae			
L. major	Aloe nyeriensis	Methanolic extract	[437]
L. major		Aqueous extract	[437]
Asteraceae			
L. amazonensis	Achillea millefolium	Essential oil	[438]
L. Donovani	Anthemis auriculata	Anthecotulide	[439]
L. donovani		4-Hydroxyanthecotulide	[439]
L. donovani		4-Acetoxyanthecotulide	[439]
L. donovani	Baccharis dracunculifolia	Crude extract	[440]
L. donovani		Hautriwaic acid lactone	[440]
L. donovani		Ursolic acid	[440]
L. donovani		Uvaol	[440]
L. donovani		2a-Hydroxy-ursolic acid	[440]
L. amazonensis	Calea montana	Ethanolic extract	[441]
L. donovani	Elephantopus mollis	Dichloromethane extract	[442]
L. amazonensis	Tanacetum parthenium	Plant powder	[443]
L. amazonensis		Dichloromethane extract	[443]
L. amazonensis		Parthenolide	[444]
L. amazonensis		Guaianolide	[445]
L. amazonensis	Vernonia polyanthes	Methanolic extract	[446]
Annonaceae			
L. chagasi	Annona coriacea	Total alkaloids extract	[447]
L. chagasi	Annona crassiflora	Total alkaloids extract	[447]
L. amazonensis	Annona muricata	Ethyl acetate extract	[448]
L. chagasi	Guatteria australis	Total alkaloids extract	[447]
L. infantum	Polyalthia suaveolens	Methanolic extract	[449]
L. amazonensis	Pseudomalmea boyacana	Ethyl acetate extract	[448]
L. amazonensis	Rollinia exsucca	Hexane extract	[448]
L. amazonensis	Rollinia pittieri	Hexane extract	[448]
L. amazonensis	Xylopia aromatica	Methanolic extract	[448]
Apocynaceae			
L. amazonensis	Himatanthus sucuuba	Ethanolic extract	[450]
L. amazonensis	Pagiantha cerifera	Dichloromethane extract	[451]

(Table 4) contd.....

Leishmania Species	Family/Plant Species	Active Extracts from Plants	References
Caricaceae			
L. amazonensis	Carica papaya	Ethanolic extract	[441]
Celastraceae			
L. major	Maytenus putterlickoides	Methanolic extract	[437]
Clusiaceae			
L. amazonensis	Calophyllum brasiliense	(-) Mammea A/BB	[452]
Crassulaceae			
L. amazonensis	Kalanchoe pinnata	Quercetin diglycoside	[453]
Flacourtiaceae			
L. amazonensis	Laetia procera	Casearlucine A	[454]
L. amazonensis		Caseamembrol A	[454]
L. amazonensis		Laetiaprocerine A	[454]
L. amazonensis		Laetiaprocerine D	[454]
L. amazonensis		Butanolide	[454]
Fabaceae			
L. major	Acacia tortilis	Aqueous extract	[437]
L. major	Albizia coriaria	Aqueous extract	[437]
L. amazonensis	Copaifera reticulata	Oleoresin	[455]
Goodeniaceae			
L. amazonensis	Scaevola balansae	Dichloromethane extract	[456]
Ginkgoaceae			
L. amazonensis	Ginkgo biloba	Isoginkgetin	[457]
Menispermaceae			
L. chagasi	Cissampelos ovalifolia	Total alkaloids extract	[447]
Malpighiaceae			
L. amazonensis	Lophanthera lactescens	LLD3	[458]
Meliaceae			
L. donovani	Dysoxylum binectariferum	Chloroform fraction	[459]
L. donovani		Rohitukine	[459]
Olacaceae			
L. donovani	Minquartia guianensis	Dichloromethane extract	[442]
Papaveraceae			
L. donovani	Bocconia integrifolia	n-Hexane extract	
L. donovani		Dichloromethane extract	[442]
L. donovani		Methanol extract	[442]

(Table 4) contd.....

Leishmania Species	Family/Plant Species	Active Extracts from Plants	References
Rutaceae			
L. panamensis	Galipea panamensis	Coumarin compound 1	[460]
L. panamensis		Coumarin compound 2	[460]
L. panamensis		Phebalosin	[460]
L. panamensis		Artifact murralongin	[460]
L. panamensis		Murrangatin acetonide	[460]
Rhamnaceae			
L. donovani	Gouania lupuloides	Dichloromethane extract	[442]
L. donovani		Methanol extract	[442]
Solanaceae			
L. donovani	Brugmansia sp	Dichloromethane extract	[86]
Scrophulariaceae			
L. donovani	Scoparia dulcis	Dichloromethane extract	[442]
L. donovani	Scrophularia cryptophila	Crypthophilic acid A	[461]
L. donovani		Crypthophilic acid C	[461]
L. donovani		Harpagide	[461]
L. donovani		Acetylharpagide	[461]
L. donovani		Buddlejasaponin III	[461]
Umbelliferae			
L. major	Ferula szowitsiana	Auraptene	[462]
L. major		Umbelliprenin	[462]
Verbenaceae			
L. amazonensis	Lantana sp	Ethanolic extract	[441]
Zingiberaceae			
L. amazonensis	Hedychium coronarium	Ethanolic extract	[441]

Mechanisms of Action of Herbal Compounds

For the development and understanding of the action mechanism of new plant-based antileishmanial drugs, it is important to know drug targets, metabolic differences, and the mode of action. For example, since there is a structural difference between DNA topoisomerases of human and parasites, targeting of *Leishmanial* kinetoplastid topoisomerases has been mostly applied in recent studies by the use of chemotherapeutic agents, which can impair the structure of mentioned enzymes. Topoisomerase inhibitors can be classified into two groups: Class I and Class II inhibitors. Class I inhibitors include compounds that induce the generation of covalent enzyme-DNA complexes or topoisomerase poisons, while Class II inhibitors prevent the molecular functions of the enzymes [463]. Parasitic mitochondrion is another substantial target for chemotherapeutics since they possess different structures and functions when compared with its analogs in mammalians. Since retention of mitochondrial transmembrane potential is one of key factors for survival of *Leishmania* parasites, in some studies, researchers target to change this potential with various chemotherapeutics in order to cause apoptosis-dependent parasite death [464]. Many of compounds such as enzymes, sterols, purines, and pyrimidines, which play active roles in metabolisms of *Leishmania* parasites, are being targeted in approaches to develop new antileishmanial drugs, since these compounds display lots of metabolic and structural variations in parasites as distinct from humans. It is expected that these mentioned antileishmanial agents inhibit macromolecules of parasites but not mammalian hosts [465]. Different from host cells, *Leishmania* parasites have a relatively weak and *Leishmania*-specific antioxidant system, which is composed from trypanothione (T(SH)2) and trypanothione reductase (TryR) instead of a glutathione/glutathione reductase system. In this system, glutathione generates a molecule named dithiol trypanothione, and this molecule is responsible for DNA precursor synthesis, evacuation of thiol conjugates, and detoxification of hydroperoxides [466]. In biosynthesis of glutathione and spermidine, rate-limiting enzymes such as γ-glutamylcysteine synthase (γ-GCS), Ornithine decarboxylase (ODC), and trypanothione synthase play active roles. Therefore, a mentioned rate to limit enzymes can be selectively targeted by chemotherapeutic agents for inhibition of the parasites. Trypanothione reductase is known as another important enzyme in the redox metabolism of *Leishmania* parasites. This enzyme performs the transition of reducing equivalents from the NADP+/NADPH to T(SH)2 enzymes.

Hence, enzymes serve in a trypanothione-dependent antioxidant system and are considered appropriate targets of antileishmanial drug candidates [467]. Additionally, due to lack of enzymes such as catalase and glutathione peroxidases,

Leishmania parasites do not resist the negative effects of free radicals, which leads to oxidative stress, and then apoptosis occurs [468]. Despite the fact that *Leishmania* parasites can easily disrupt functions of T cells, macrophages, and NK cells in order to provide more suitable conditions to survive, recent studies demonstrated that use of some plant-derived antileishmanial drugs directly stimulated the production of nitric oxide, which is capable of restoring the immune response of the hosts [469]. In various studies performed in different regions of the world, it was shown that plant products such as aurones, terpenes, lignans, chalcones, isoflavonoids, saponins, flavonoids, quinones, alkaloids, tannins, terpenoids, iridoids, and oxylipins indicated strong antileishmanial activity. For example, *Chalcones Licochalcone A*, which is isolated from the roots of Chinese plant liquorice, exhibited disruption of mitochondrial dehydrogenase enzymes and specifically impaired the respiratory chains of the parasites by inhibiting fumarate reductase [470, 471].

Flavonoids

Luteolin, which is isolated from vitex negundo and quercetin derived from *Fagopyrum esculentum*, are products rich in flavonoids. It has been demonstrated that luteolin prevented the linearization process of kDNA mini-circles, which caused arresting of the cell cycle and suppression of DNA synthesis [472]. Quercitin (aglycone) has the same mode of action mechanism. This molecule carries out iron-chelating, which is a process that decreases the performance of ribonucleotide reductase, an enzyme necessary for parasitic DNA synthesis. Furthermore, its combined use with SSG induces parasite clearance. Another extract, rich of flavonoids, is *Kalanchoe pinnata* (KP). Its significant antileishmanial activity has been indicated in recent years. The basis of this antiparasitic efficacy depends on production of huge amounts of free nitrogen radicals [473]. In *in vivo* studies, KP decreased delayed-type hypersensitivity (DTH) responses in mice infected with *Leishmania* parasites. An EtOH extract of *Piper betle L.* and a methanolic extract of eugenol rich PB-BM indicated high antileishmanial effectiveness by inducing mitochondria-mediated apoptosis [474] and by activating reactive oxygen species dependent apoptosis [475]. When IC_{50} concentrations were applied on *Leishmania* parasites, guaianolide isolated from

Tanacetum parthenium (L.), Schultz Bip also triggered morphological changes [440].

Saponins

Research with the α-hederin, β-hederin, and hederagenin, obtained from the leaves of *Hedera helix* (araliaceae), exhibited strong antiproliferative activity on *L. infantum* and *L. tropica* promastigotes. Researchers observed that treatment with these molecules leads to reduction in parasitic membrane potential and, consequently, remarkable loss in membrane coherence [476]. Among these, the metabolite also showed significant activity against the amastigote forms and exhibited strong antiproliferative activities on human monocytes. The saponins appear to inhibit growth of *Leishmania* promastigotes by acting on the membrane of the parasite with induction of a drop in membrane potential. The hederecolchiside-A1, isolated from *Hedera colchica*, shows strong activity against the promastigotes and amastigotes of *L. infantum*, but also shows notable activity on human monocytes. The saponin, mimengoside-A, which is isolated from the leaves of *Buddleja madagascariensis* (loganiaceae), displays activity against promastigotes of *L. infantum*. Muzanzagenin, obtained from the roots of *Asparagus africanus* (liliaceae), displays activity with an IC$_{50}$ value 31 μ g/mL against the *L. major* promastigotes. However, it is known that the metabolite also inhibits the proliferation of human lymphocytes [447, 478].

Quinones

Plumbagin, one of secondary metabolite, isolated from Pera benensis showed antileishmanial activity by generating significant amounts of reactive oxygen intermediates, but it was also established that this molecule can be cytotoxic for mammalian hosts since it exacerbates topoisomerase II dependent DNA cleavage [479]. Another napthoquinone obtained from *D. montana Roxb.* (ebenaceae), named as diospyrin, showed significant antileishmanial effectiveness against *L. donovani* promastigotes with a MIC of 1.0 µg/mL. Generation of free radicals, inhibition of DNA topoisomerase I, and causing apoptosis composed the promastigote-killing mechanism of this extract. But its activity against amastigotes has not been considered so far [480]. Primin 2-methoxy-

6pentylcyclohexa -2,5-1,4-dione, present in *Primulaobconica* and primulaceae, shows significant *Leishmanicidal* activity against *L. donovani* with an IC_{50} of 0.711 µM.

Alkaloids

For *Leishmaniasis* treatment, alkaloids have been abundantly used. Berberine chloride, which is an alkaloid obtained from *Berberis aristata*, directly targets mitochondrial enzymes of amastigotes. This results in breakdown of the respiratory system. It also ceases macromolecular biosynthesis of the parasites [481]. A parasite-killing mechanism of this extract is stage-specific. In promastigotes, erberine chloride drives parasites to caspase-independent, but oxidative stress mediated apoptosis-like death [482]. Berberine chloride caused oxidative-burst-mediated parasite death in *Leishmania*-infected neutrophils, while it triggered apoptosis and inflammation by activating mitogen-activated protein kinases (MAPKs). This extract leads to phosphorylation of p38 MAPK and declines the levels of extracellular-signal-related kinase, ERK1/2 [482]. An EtOH extract of *Tabernaemontana catharinensis* leaves, including alkaloids such as coronaridine (7%) and voacangine (53%), was demonstrated to possess *Leishmanicidal* efficacy, independently from NO production in macrophages [483]. On the other hand, alkaloid fractions extracted from *Nuphar Lutea*, showed an antileishmanial effect by activating macrophages to produce high levels of NO [484]. Julocrotine, an alkaloid extracted from *Croton pullei var. glabrior*, leads to comprehensive morphological changes such as chromatin condensation, appearance of vesicular, swelling of the mitochondrion *etc.* in *L. Amazonensis* promastigotes instead of killing the infectious agents [485].

Naphthyl Isoquinoline Alkaloids

For all naphthylisoquinoline alkaloids, ancistroealaine-A, which is isolated from *Ancistrocladus ealaensis* (ancistrocladaceae), exhibits activity against *L. Donovani* promastigotes with an IC_{50} value 4.10 μ g/mL. Ancistrocladinium A and B isolated from yet undescribed *Congolese Ancistrocladaceae* species, require 2.61 and 1.52 μ g/mL concentrations, respectively, to reach the IC_{50}

toward *L. major* promastigotes. The possible mode of antileishmanial action of ancistrocladinium A and B is an apoptosis-like death pathway [175].

Bisbenzyl Isoquinolinic Alkaloids

Daphanandrine, which is isolated from *Albertisia papuana* obaberine, obtained from *Pseudoxandra sclerocarpa* (annonaceae), gyrocarpine produced by *Gyrocarpus americanus* (hernandiaceae) and limacine isolated from *Caryomene olivasans* (menispermaceae), shows antileishmanial activity against *L. donovani*, *L. braziliensis*, and *L. amazonensis* with an IC100 of approximately 50 μ g/mL. SAR studies show that, among these alkaloids, alkaloids with methylated nitrogen are more active than those with nonsubstituted or aromatic nitrogens, while quaternization of one or more nitrogen atoms upshots in the loss of antileishmanial activity [486].

Steroidal Alkaloids

Of all the alkaloids, holamine, which is 15-α hydroxyholamine, holacurtine and *N*-desmethylholacurtine obtained from *Holarrhena curtisii* (apocynaceae), the metabolite holamine, offers the strongest activity against *L. donovani* $(1.56 > IC_{50} > 0.39 \mu$ g/mL) compared with holacurtine and *N*-desmethyl holacurtine $(6.25 > IC_{50} > 1.56 \mu$ g/mL) [487].

Benzoquinolizidine Alkaloids

Klugine, cephaeline, isocephaeline, and emetine have been isolated from *Psychotria klugii* (rubiaceae), and they show significant *Leishmanicidal* activities against *L. donovani*. Among these metabolites, klugine (IC$_{50}$ of 0.40 μ g/mL) and isocephaline (IC$_{50}$ 0.45 μ g/mL) exhibit <13- and <15-fold less potent activity in relation to cephaline with IC$_{50}$ of 0.03 μ g/mL proves >20- and >5-fold more *in vitro* activity against *L. donovani* when compared with pentamidine and amphotericin-B, respectively. Emetine exhibits activity against *L. donovani* with an IC$_{50}$ value 0.03 μ g/mL; however, it produces toxicity in the treatment of *L. major* based CL [488].

Diterpene Alkaloids

Azitine, isoazitine, 15, 22-*O*-Diacetyl- 19-oxo-dihydroatisine isolated from aconitum, delphinium, and consolida species, display significant *Leishmanicidal* activities. The metabolite isoazitine exhibits the strongest activity against promastigotes of *L. infantum* with IC_{50} values of 44.6, 32.3, and 24.6 μ M at 24, 48, and 72 h of culture, respectively. Azitine with IC_{50} values of 33.7 and 27.9 μ M at 72 h of culture, respectively, exhibit activity against promastigotes of *L. infantum* [488].

Pyrrolidinium Alkaloid

Phlomis brunneogaleata includes (2*S*,4*R*)-2-carboxy-4-(*E*)- *p*coumaroyloxy-1,1-dimethylpyrrolidin salt. This salt displays activity with an IC_{50} of 9.1 μ g/mL against axenic amastigotes of *L. donovani*.

Acridone Alkaloids

The gravacridonediol and rhodesiacridone isolated from *Thamnosma rhodesica* (rutaceae) exhibit 69% and 46% inhibition at 10 μ M concentration, respectively, against promastigote of *L. major*. The compounds also showed activity against *L. major* amastigotes and cause over 90% and 50% inhibition at 10 and 1 μ M concentration, respectively.

β-Carboline Alkaloids

The harmaline, which is isolated from *Peganum harmala* (nitrariaceae), shows amastigotespecific activity (IC_{50} of 1.16 μ M). Harmine, isolated from same plant species, decreases spleen parasite load by approximately 40%, 60%, 70%, and 80% in free liposomal, niosomal, and nanoparticular forms, respectively, in mice models. In BALB/c mice model canthin-6-one and 5-methoxycanthin-6-one occurring in plant species of rutaceae and simaroubaceae, demonstrate *in vivo* activity against *L. amazonensis*. *N*-hydroxyannomontine and annomontine, isolated from *Annona foetida* (annonaceae), exhibit effective *Leishmanicidal* potentials.

Alkaloids from Marine Source

Marine sponges such as *Amphimedonviridis*, *Acanthostrongylophora* species, *Neopetrosia* species, *Plakortis angulospiculatus*, and *Pachymatisma johnstonii* serve as rich sources of alkaloids with significant antileishmanial potentials. Renieramycin A extracted from the *Neopetrosia* species is a La/egfp (expressing enhanced green fluorescent protein) inhibitor, which exhibits effective antileishmanial activity against *L. amazonensis* with IC_{50} 0.2 μ g/mL. *Araguspongin C*, which is isolated from a marine sponge *Haliclona exigua*, shows *Leishmanicidal* activity against promastigotes as well as amastigotes at 100 μ g/mL concentrations [489]. Among the ciliatamides A-C isolated from *Aaptos ciliate*, the peptide ciliatamides at 10.0 μ g/mL concentrations inhibit 50% growth in *L. major* promastigotes [490]. The lipopeptides, almiramides A-C isolated from cyanobacterium *Lyngbya majuscule,* displays significant *in vitro* antileishmanial activity against *L. donovani*. Dragonamide A, E, and herbamide B, isolated from the same cyanobacterium strain, shows *in vitro* activity against *L. donovani* with EC50 values of 6.5, 5.1, and 5.9 μ M, respectively. Viridamide A, isolated from oscillatory *nigro-viridis*, displayed activity against *L. mexicana* with EC50 of 1.5 μ M. Venturamides A and B, obtained from cyanobacterium *Oscillatoria* species, exhibits activity against *L. Donovani* with EC50>19.0 μ M. *valinomycin*, adodecadepsipeptide, isolated from *Streptomyces* strains, exhibits activity against promastigotes of *L. major* with EC50 < 0.11 μ M, but also cytotoxicity to 293T kidney epithelial cells and J774.1 macrophages [491].

Lignans

Diphyllin obtained from *Haplophyllum bucharicum* (rutaceae) demonstrated antileishmanial effects on promastigotes. Due to addition of effective dosages of this extract, cell cycles of *Leishmania* promastigotes were observed to arrest in the S-phase. On the other hand, when its effectiveness is investigated on amastigotes, it was shown that Diphyllin prevented the attachment of parasites to macrophage surfaces, so this avoids the entrance of the promastigotes into their hosts, which is essential for their survival [492]. Among the lignans (+)-medioresinol, (-)-lirioresinol B and (+) - nyasol, display activity against the amastigotes of *L.*

amazonensis, but it is known that lignans also exhibit high selectivity in their activity against the promastigotes of *L. major* [493].

Tannins

According to enhanced expression of proinflammatory cytokines such as tumor necrosis factor-alpha (TNFα) and interferon gamma (IFNγ), and also the lifted release of nitric oxide in host cells of *Leishmania* parasites, it was determined that proanthocyanidins and its structural analogs had immunomodulatory features. Also, phenol including extracts and flavan-3-olgallocatechin tannins stimulated the expressions of different cytokines such as IFNγ, TNFα, IL-1, IL-12, and IL-18, which are responsible from the development of Th1 immune responses [494, 495].

Terpenoids

Terpenoids, divided into five different categories, are named as iridoids, monoterpenes, sesquiterpenes, triterpenes, and diterpenes. Linalool, which is one of the monoterpenes, is obtained from leaves of *Croton cajucara* (euphorbiaceae) and abundantly enhanced the production of NO in host macrophage cells infected with *Leishmania* parasites. Moreover, it directly targeted the amastigotes in the host, which was proved by swelling of parasitic mitochondrion and disorders in nuclear and kinetoplast chromatin [496]. In researches, performed with sesquiterpene lactones including artemisinin and its derivatives, it was demonstrated that their inhibition mechanisms on parasites precisely depends on formation of large amounts of free radicals in *Leishmania* [497]. Artemisinin also serves as an immunomodulator since it exacerbates the immune response by enhancing expressions of iNOS and the other cytokines [455, 498]. Triterpene such as dihydrobetulinic acid indicated antileishmanial efficacy on *L. donovani* by disrupting DNA topoisomerases I and II, which leads to apoptotic cell deaths [499]. Ursolic and oleanolic acids, which are found in the terpenes group obtained from *Pourouma guinensis* plants, also prevented the growth of parasites, but did not stimulate NO production from host macrophage cells. However, they caused a decline in phagocytic performance of macrophages. 18β-glycyrrhetinic acid (GRA), which is an extract isolated from *Glycyrrhizza glabra L.* (licorice), again showed *Leishmanicidal* effectiveness by enhancing Th1 cytokine response and

NO production [500]. Similarly, an ethanolic extract of a diterpene named as 16α-Hydroxycleroda-3,13(14)Z-dien-15,16-olide, isolated from *Polyalthia longifolia*, impaired the DNA topoisomerase I enzyme and lead to apoptosis-mediated parasite death [501].

Oxylipin

One type of oxylipins, called 3(S)-16,17-didehydrofalcarinol, which is obtained from *Tridax procambens* (asteraceae), directly inhibited *Leishmania* parasites without providing production of NO within macrophages [502]. Another oxylipin, called momordicatin, which is an aqueous extract of *Momordica charantia*, impaired the functions of the *Leishmanial* superoxide dismutase enzyme, while it did not harm the host SOD [503]. Since SOD is an important enzyme, which is responsible for mediating oxidative stress, inhibition of this enzyme leads to enhanced release of free radicals, which is harmful for the parasite [504]. Again, an EtOH extract of Tinospora sinensis inhibited parasites by causing oxidative burst by stimulating ROS and NO production in macrophages [505]. *Himatanthus sucuuba Latex* (apocynaceae) increased release of TNF-α and NO and, on the other side, decreased the levels of TGF-β within macrophages [506].

Miscellaneous

G3, obtained from *Withania somnifera*, demonstrated an antileishmanial effect by dysfunctioning protein kinase C (PKC) and stabilizing topoisomerase I-DNA complex. These events resulted in apoptosis. An extract gained from *Allium sativum L.* (garlic) was exhibited to target different regions in parasites. This extract was observed to impair thiol metabolism and plasma membrane integrity, while it promoted generation of Th1 inflammatory cytokines at the same time [507]. Application of garlic extract together with SSG generated a synergistic effect and increased the immunomodulatory features of the extract alone [508]. Ajoene, an isolated extract, leads to parasite death by inducing morphological changes in the nuclear envelope, causing large autophagic vacuoles and megasomes formation. In another study, it was demonstrated that an extract, which is isolated from aloe vera leaves, stimulated the generation of reactive oxygen species within *Leishmania*-infected macrophages; this resulted in arrest of the parasitic cell cycle [509, 510]. An extract obtained from *Chenopodium ambrosiodes L.* enhanced the generation of NO in lymph nodes [511]. Similarly, ascaridol, which is a compound found in the essential oils of *Chenopodium ambrosiodes*, shows its antileishmanial efficacy *via* inducing the formation of free oxygen radicals [512]. Physalins B and F, which are extracted from *Physalis angulate*, demonstrated an antileishmanial effect independent of NO production [513]. One of extracts, peganine hydrochloride dehydrate, which is obtained from *Peganum harmala*, impaired the functions of DNA topoisomerase I enzyme and lead to apoptosis-mediated cell death [514]. In another study, antileishmanial effectiveness of calceolarioside A, which is isolated from *N. arbortristis* (night jasmine), was shown to increase when applied together with SSG [515]. Amarogentin, an extract isolated from *Swertia chirata*, lead to parasitic cell death *via* adhering to DNA topoisomerase I and dysfunctioning the binary complex formed between topoisomerase I enzyme and DNA [516]. In another study, researchers observed that the EtOH extract of *Desmodium gangeticum* provided removal of *Leishmania* parasites from macrophages due to its immunostimulant properties [516]. Quassin, an extract obtained from *Quassia amara*, displayed an antileishmanial effect by stimulating an immune response according to abundant NO production and upregulation of proinflammatory cytokines such as TNF-α and IL-12 [517]. Despite the fact that it showed no antileishmanial efficacy, picroliv, one of the plant extracts obtained from *Picrorhiza kurroa*, exhibited enhanced *Leishmanicidal* effectiveness of conventional antileishmanial drugs such as SAG and miltefosine [518].

Plants and Microorganism-Based New Drugs for *Leishmaniasis*

Scientists try to develop new medicinal drugs based on plants and microorganisms (Table **5**) considering the limited repertoire of existing antileishmanial compounds. At the same time in improving these compounds, it is important to understand their molecular and biochemical characteristics; it is equally important to moderate chances of drug resistance, and, in this regard, using herbal compounds in combination with conventional drugs is an attractive chemotherapeutic option worthy of future consideration [519].

Table 5.   New Drugs for *Leishmaniasis*

Drug	Isolated Plants or Microorganism	Mechanisms of Action	Affected Parasite	Refs.
Afidicoline	Isolated from fungus *Nigrospora sphaerica*	Affecting cellular division and also DNA polymerase inhibitor	Promastigote and amastigote *Leishmania donovani*	[520]
Hypocrellins A and B Pigments	Isolated from fungus *Hipocrella bambusae*	More active than AmB and pentamidine against parasite	*Leishmania donovani*	[521]
Nerolidol	Essential oil of some plants	It inhibits the first step of ergosterol and dolical synthesis	*Leishmania amazonensis, L. Chagasi, L. braziliensis*	[522]
Tanacetum parthenium	Plant extract	Decreases the parasite internalization in macrophages up to 84%	*L. amazonensis*	[431]
Croton cajucara	Essential oil	Reduces the parasitic infection and increases the nitric-oxide production and leads parasitic defense	*L. amazonensis*	[483]
Peschiera australis	Plant extract	Has an important role in parasitic defense	*L. amazonensis*	[522]

Photodynamic Therapy

Photodynamic therapy (PDT) can be considered a noninvasive therapeutic modality, which uses a photosensitizer, visible light, and oxygen for treatment of cancerous and premalignant diseases [523-525]. PDT has been used for therapeutic purposes since the late 1970s, and it has potential application in various areas of medicine, such as against malignant and nonmalignant indications. PDT was first developed for treatment of malignant tumors. More recently, it has been started to be used in the treatment of other dermatological diseases such asactinic keratosis (AK) lesions, basal cell carcinoma, Bowen's disease, and, finally, CL [526, 529]. This treatment application includes a two-stage technique in which the administration of a sensitizing drug is followed by visible light irradiation. After the administration of the sensitizing drugs into the targeted cells, the unhealthy region is irradiated by the light, which leads to transfer of energy to molecular oxygen, resulting in generation of reactive oxygen species (ROS), which cause cell death [528, 529]. PDT can be applied to patients by two different ways: topical and systemic. In systemic PDT, the photosensitive drug is administered to humans by injecting the photosensitizing drug into a vein and the drug; thanks to its special properties, it is expected to find cancer cells in a short period. On the other hand, the drug is subcutaneously administered to lesion sides in topical treatment [530]. After administration, the drug reaches cancer cells, where it accumulates. Following irradiation with visible light, cancer cells can be eliminated by oxidative stress bound to production of free radicals.

Properties of Photosensitizers

For clinical applications of PDT, the characteristics of used photosensitizers are important. An ideal photosensitizer must be chemically pure, target neoplastic tissue, reach the highest accumulation into target cells in a short span of time after administration, have a short half-life, be nonhazardous for normal tissues and generate a large amount of cytotoxic oxygen derivatives. Lipophilicity of the photosensitizers is another significant point for PDT treatment. It is know that, generally, penetration of the lipophilic drugs into cells through membranes is easier than using lipophobic drugs. Lipophilic sensitizers can be taken directly into target cells through the cell membrane. There is a direct proportion between lipophilicity and uptake amounts of photosensitizers, in such a way that uptake of the drug increases due to enhancement in lipophilicity. However, until now, target cell selection mechanisms of photosensitizers have not been clearly identified. There are some hypotheses that include differences in permeability of tumor cell membrane, an increase in the number and permeability of blood vessels, and decreased lymphatic drainage. Additionally, the low pH in the interstitial fluid of the tumors contributes to the selective distribution of the photosensitizing drugs in treatment [531, 532].

Effect Mechanism of Photosensitizing Drugs

Today the most commonly used photosensitizing agents in PDT are δ-5-aminolaevulinic acid (ALA) or methyl ester (MAL) [533-535]. ALA is the first product in the heme biosynthesis pathway, which is maintained in mitochondria. This compound is naturally synthesized from glycine and succinate by the catalization activity of the ALA synthetase (ALAS) enzyme [536]. Following its synthesis, ALA reaches cytosol where a condensation reaction has occurred. This reaction undergoes with the help of zinc-dependent aminolevulinate dehydratase enzyme, and, subsequently, it induces the formation of porphobilinogen (PBG) from two molecules of ALA [537, 538]. In the next step of the heme biosynthesis pathway, four molecules of PBG combine and form tetrapyrolle - hydroxymethylbilane (HMB) with the help of the porphobilinogen deaminase enzyme (PBDG). After that, four different molecules of PBG attach to PBDG, resulting in the formation of hexapyrolle. Afterward, hemolytic cleavage of hexapyrolle leads to the release of HMB. Finally, HMB can enter into the spontaneous pathway and form uroporphyrinogen I [539, 540]. This molecule is converted into coproporphyrinogen, and coproporphyrinogen is converted into protoporphyrinogen IX inside the mitochondria. Protoporphyrinogen IX is then converted into protoporphyrine (Pp IX). This reaction is catalyzed by protoporphyrinogen oxidase. Pp IX is a porphyrinic compound that can emit intense fluorescence and demonstrate photodynamic activity when it is irradiated by light. PpIX is a strong photosensitizer, which accumulates in the mitochondria of tumor cells, causing damage of these cells following light exposure. In the heme biosynthetic pathway, ALAS1 and ferrochelatase enzymes are considered rate-limiting. In general, the activity of the ALAS1 enzyme is controlled by the heme molecule through the negative feedback mechanism. When heme is synthesized sufficiently, it binds to the heme-regulatory motif in ALAS sequence, which targets mitochondria and hence prevents the transfer of ALAS1 precursor into mitochondria. Furthermore, it was proved that heme attenuates transcription of ALAS1 besides regulating its mitochondrial import. Normally bound to a feedback mechanism, PpIX is produced in sufficient amounts, which provides for their effective conversion to heme by ferrochelatase. On the other hand, exogenously administered ALA bypasses these natural regulation mechanisms, which results in enhanced production of PpIX. In this situation, effectiveness of the ferrochelatase enzyme then becomes too low and cannot convert excessively produced PpIX to heme. Finally, this leads to heavy accumulation of PpIX within cells. Nearly four to six hours later, following administration of ALA, PpIX is synthesized and accumulated within target cells. Irradiation of these cells causes excitation of the photosensitizer and production of singlet oxygen, which exhibits cytotoxic effects [541-544]. PpIX may be produced locally by all the nucleated cells and is detected in the epidermis within three to eight hours after systemic administration of the photosensitizer. Studies on animals and human volunteers have proved that PpIX can be eliminated from the organism between 24 and 48 hours after administration of

ALA or MAL by any way. Hence the risks of prolonged photosensitivity reduces in this therapy [545].

Clinical Trials of Photodynamic Therapy

Topical use of PDT with ALA for the treatment of AK was approved by the US Food and Drug Administration (US FDA) in 1999, and this technique has been applied on patients since that date. Moreover, in different studies, it has been reported that dermatological diseases such as acne and photorejuvenation can be successfully treated with PDT; however, these applications have not yet been approved by the FDA. The only limiting factor in the use of ALA is its transport rate; therefore, accumulation amounts within target cells. The temperature- and pH-dependent transportation system for ALA requires energy and accumulation of porphyries and does not change significantly in tumors in contrast with healthy body cells. 10% to 20% ALA are the concentrations at which the best therapeutic results are obtained [546, 547]. MAL, which is the esterified form of ALA, is more lipophilic than ALA and can more easily select neoplastic cells. Higher lipophilicity of MAL may enhance the phototoxicity induced by PpIX. MAL can penetrate into target cells by using active transportation and also passive diffusion through the cell membrane. Energy is not required for passive diffusion, and this mechanism is not saturable. Moreover, it can be principally effective in neoplastic cells. It is believed that MAL has higher potential for selectively reaching into tumor cells than ALA owing to its significant ability to penetrate cell membranes. Following penetration, MAL is converted to ALA; the subsequent metabolic steps in order to produce intramitochondrial Pp IX remain the same. In Europe, MAL has been used in the treatment of AK and BCC since 2001. After that, it was approved for the treatment of AK in 2004 in the USA, and it was approved in Brazil for AK and for superficial and nodular BCC in 2006. Currently, MAL has been approved in many countries of Europe, Asia, and the Americas for the treatment of AK, BCC, and Bowen's disease. Recently, in 2009, MAL was approved in Brazil for treatment of Bowen's disease [547, 548].

Photodynamic Therapy in *Leishmaniasis*

As described previously, in antileishmanial therapy, the first choice to treat a *Leishmaniasis* case is the application of chemotherapy by using current antileishmanial drugs. Pentavalent antimonials such as meglumine antimoniate and sodium stibogluconate are the first-line drugs used in the treatment of CL. However, these drugs include a stibium element, which is toxic for humans. Clinical manifestations, such as nephrotoxicity and cardiotoxicity induced by the use of pentavalent antimonials, can be seen in patients with CL. Hence, this situation restricts the use of these drugs in treatment. Recently developed drug resistance includes the other disadvantages of the drugs. It was demonstrated that parasites have generated resistance against antileishmanial drugs while vectors have developed resistance against insecticides. This situation decreases the effectiveness of applied antileishmanial drugs. Furthermore, the regions that are affected from *Leishmaniasis* may be expected to spread all around the world, since global warming has been rapidly increasing. Because of these reasons, researchers have recently gone toward developing new approaches in order to cope with the disease. These approaches include development of new antileishmanial compounds, cryotherapy, and physical treatment techniques. Among them, photodynamic therapy (PDT) constitutes one of the most promising treatment approaches, especially against CL. PDT has been clinically used in treatment of patients for approximately 10 years, and successful results have been obtained until now.

The first use of PDT against CL was reported in 2003. Girdle *et al.* maintained the treatment and healing of multiple CL lesions of a 34-year-old man from Libya by using PDT. The patient had been treated by systemic administration of sodium stibogluconate (Pentostam®). However, according to the authors, treatment remained insufficient, and there was no healing observed in the lesions of the patient. Clinicians applied MAL onto lesions by the help of Tegaderm® self-adhesive dressings. Lesions were irradiated with a red light (75 J/cm^2) 28 times for the initial three months, twice weekly, and afterward once a week for one month. The healing process of multiple lesions started after four to six PDT sessions, and, at the end of 20 sessions, all the lesions were successfully treated. During treatment sessions, some side effects such as local erythema and a burning sensation following irradiation were reported. Histologic analysis of biopsy materials demonstrated no *Leishmania* parasites existing within treated tissues at the end of the treatment sessions [549].

After this first successful trial, Enki *et al*. tried to treat 11 Israelis who had totally 32 CL lesions caused by *L. major* infection by using PDT. Lesions had occurred approximately 2.5 months before applications of patients for treatment. Lesions were exposed to 10% of ALA, and lesion sides were irradiated with a red light (100 J/cm^2). After two treatment sessions, only slight post-inflammatory hyperpigmentation and superficial crusting were observed, but the lesions had not completely healed. In some patients, side effects such as mild to temporary burning sensations were reported. It was determined that one patient did not report any side effects, lesions of this patient healed at a rate of 50% after three treatment sessions. However, amastigote forms of parasites were determined in direct preparations of this patient. The patient did not maintain his treatment process after three sessions. Therefore, healing of the lesions could not have been further followed up [550].

In 2004, Gardlo *et al*. reported the successful treatment of a 19-year-old Turkish male with CL. His lesion was on his left shoulder recognized three months prior. The *Leishmania* species that caused the lesions were not detected. The diameter of the lesion was nearly 5 cm, and its surface was crusted. Before the treatment, crusted tissue was removed superficially, and MAL was applied onto the lesion sides. Afterward, in five treatment sessions, the region was illuminated with a red light (75 J/cm^2) in seven-day periods. Erythema and mild burning sensations were reported on the shoulder of the patient for several days after treatment sessions. At the end of the therapy, the lesion was completely cured, and only slight hypopigmentation and local hair loss were seen on the treated region as minimal side effects of the treatment [551].

In 2006, Asilian and Davami reported the first placebo-controlled, randomized study in order to demonstrate the efficacy of PDT. In this study, 20 patients with a total of 31 lesions were treated with PDT, while 15% paromomycin ointment was applied to 19 patients with a total of 34 lesions, and the effectiveness of these two therapies were compared. In the placebo group, a white paraffin-based ointment was applied to 18 patients with a total of 30 lesions. PDT was carried out by the administration of 10% Alan lesion sides, covered for four hours. Thereafter, lesions were irradiated with a red light (100 J/cm^2) once a week for one month. The results showed that 29 lesions (94%), which were treated with PDT, were completely healed within three months after therapy, while two lesions (6%) were determined as "partially improved." On the other hand, 41% experienced complete healing, and a 29% "partial improvement" was observed when patients were exposed to paramomycin ointment. Moreover, in the placebo group, 13% experienced complete healing, and 40% partial improvement was determined, indicating that the best results were achieved in treatment of patients with PDT. On the other side, in histological analysis of biopsy materials that was obtained from patients after treatment, no *Leishmania* amastigote was detected in the PDT group, while amastigotes were detected in 65% and 20% biopsy samples of patients for paramomycin and placebo groups, respectively. According to another evaluation, deep and/or disfiguring scars were determined in eight (42%) patients in the paromomycin group and two (11%) in the placebo group on the surface of treated regions. No scarcity was observed on the skins of patients in the PDT group during nine months after the beginning of the study [552].

In 2006, Ghaffarifar *et al.* performed the treatment of five patients from Iran with seven CL lesions caused by *L. major*. Lesions occurred one to three months prior to the treatment session. For treatment, a 10% solution of ALA was topically administered into the lesions for four hours. The treatment lasted four sessions. In every session, lesions were illuminated by using a red light (100 J/cm^2). Different from the previous studies, selective accumulation of PpIX in the lesions of patients was determined. In histological samples, no *Leishmania* amastigotes were observed following one or two treatment sessions. Five of seven lesions (71%) were completely healed within two weeks after completing the treatment session. It was indicated that the size of the remained lesions reduced more than 95%. Patients were followed up for four months and no rehearsal was observed in treated patients during this period. The authors report excellent cosmetic results [553].

In 2007, Sohl *et al.* reported a study that demonstrated the successful treatment of a 57-year-old male who caught CL caused by *Leishmania tropica* during travel to Italy. The patient was first presented in the dermatology department due to an erythematous papule on his left cheek for four months. The patient initially was suspected with pyoderma; therefore, he was treated with oral amoxicillin for four weeks and doxicyline for another four weeks. However, when skin biopsy and polymerase chain reaction were directly investigated, the disease of the patient was diagnosed as CL whose causative agent was *L. tropica*. Following the correct diagnosis, the patient was first exposed to 15% paromomycin ointment and additionally with oral itraconazole for two months. However, this technique failed to heal the lesions. Then pentamidine was administered to the patient in an intramuscular method, and this treatment was supplemented with five sessions of cryotherapy. Eight months after the origin of the lesions, the man was treated with three session of MAL-PDT (100 J/cm^2) with intervening periods of consecutive one and four months. The lesion healed rapidly with good cosmesis [554].

Despite all successful results obtained in clinical trials, Akilov *et al.*, in 2007, reported a first study, which demonstrated that PDT application had no sufficient efficacy when performed in *in vitro* and *in vivo* assessments. In this study, researchers investigated the antileishmanial effectiveness of ALA-dependent PDT on *in vitro* culture of *L. major* promastigotes and amastigotes and then *in vivo* murine models with CL. In *in vitro* study, PpIX levels, which were generated within parasites, were assessed in order to better understand the conversion rates of ALA to toxic PIX. At first, authors incubated *L. major* promastigotes with 0.1 mM ALA, but the PpIX concentration remained at very low levels, indicating that conversion did not occur successfully. On the other hand, when parasites were exposed to 0.1 mM of exogenous PpIX, its accumulated level within parasites was determined as 100-fold higher than ALA. It also was demonstrated that ALA treatment did not exhibit significant antileishmanial effects on *L. major* amastigotes, and generated PpIX levels after exposure to ALA were nearly same both for *Leishmania*-infected and noninfected host J774.2 cells. On the other hand, when ALA-based PDT was topically applied on a murine CL model, a significant decrease in the number of parasites in lesions was shown; however, markedly tissue destruction also was observed in mice. Following treatment with ALA, the numbers of macrophages in lesion sides were substantially decreased, while levels of interleukin-6 in the infected skin were increased. According to these results, this study revealed that *in vitro* antileishmanial effects of ALA-based PDT were insufficient, but this application demonstrated great efficacy on murine models with CL; however, this treatment may be toxic due to decrease in the number of macrophages [555].

In 2007, the same group investigated *in vitro* and *in vivo* activity of two different photosensitizers: 5-ethylamino-9-diethylaminobenzo(a)phenoselenazinium chloride (EtNBSe) and (3,7-Bis(N,N-dibutylamino) phenothiazinium bromide (PPA904) for their applications in PDT. In this study, antileishmanial effectiveness of these drugs was also compared, and the results demonstrated that inhibitory effects of these photosensitizers changed due to application type. EtNBSe had more *in vitro* antileishmanial activity, while the efficacy of PPA904 was markedly higher on *in vivo* murine models. In this study, cytotoxic effects of these two dyes also were investigated, and it was indicated that the macrophages are more sensitive to photodynamic therapy than *L. major* parasites independent from type of photosensitizer. According to long-term observation, the numbers of parasites in the lesions were determined to be on increase on days two to four and on decrease between days five and seven. Additional treatment sessions were suggested within an interval of five to seven days by the authors. Moreover, it was also shown that PDT by using PPA904 could work as an immunomodulatory, since its dose dependently induced the production of IL-12p70. This stimulation was thought to provide rapidly healing mice treated with PPA904-PDT. Authors in this study exhibited that these new applied photosensitizing drugs demonstrated significant *in vivo* antileishmanial effects against CL; these findings may contribute to curative PDT approaches for further clinical trials [556].

In 2009, Akilov *et al.* reported another study to optimize topical PDT with PPA904 for its therapeutic usage against CL. In order to establish the optimal conditions for this application, authors compared two distinct methods: (1) changing the duration of topical application with PPA904 cream (500 mM) and (2) administration of several consecutive PDT regimens. An initial regimen recommended by the manufacturer (Photopharmica Co. Ltd., Leeds, UK) was used as a control. In experiments, the cream, whose final concentration was 500 microM, was applied topically into lesions for 30 minutes, and then the lesion side was irradiated with a light source [50 J/cm(2)] at 665+/-15 nm. The best results were obtained when PPA904-based PDT was applied with a long time (90 minutes). Furthermore, three consecutive treatment regimens with four-day intervals provided the best healing effect. In this study, the mechanisms responsible for kinetics of drug penetration, depth of necrosis in the CL lesions after PDT, and daily changes in the parasitic load following therapy have been discussed [557].

Gardner *et al.*, in 2010, demonstrated the efficacy of acenaphthoporphyrins within liposomes in PDT of CL. It was known that acenaphthoporphyrins were good photosensitizers; however, their hydrophobicity restricts their potential for use in PDT. Therefore, authors developed a system that used liposomes in order to transfer this hydrophobic drug into target cells. In this study, acenaphthoporphyrins were delivered by liposomes made up of dimyristoyl phosphatidylcholine (DMPC) and to liposomes made up of a mixture of DMPC, cholesterol (Chol), and distearoyl phosphatidylglycerol (DSPG) in a 2:1:0.8 molar ratios. According to the confocal microscope image, it was determined that the DMPC liposomes delivered photosensitizer drugs into promastigotes of *Leishmania tarentolae*. It was also evaluated that DMPC:Chol:DSPG liposomes were effective against axenic and intracellular amastigotes of the pathogenic *L. panamensis in vitro*. According to the results, this efficacy was bound to increase exposure time of *Leishmania* cultures to visible light [558].

In 2010, Latorre-Esteves *et al.* reported another study that demonstrated the efficacy of an antimicrobial photodynamic therapy, which can be monitored in a murine model of CL by using *L. major* expressing green fluorescence protein (GFP). In this study, the antileishmanial effect of PPA904-based PDT was investigated in a mice model infected with GFP expressing *L. major* parasites. Antileishmanial efficacy was evaluated by the measurement of fluorescence intensity of GFP and PPA904. It was determined that fluorescence values of GFP and PPA904 were proportionally on decay by the time indicating that parasitic load in lesions of mice decreased following exposure to PDT. According to fluorescence measurement, it also was demonstrated that, in two days after treatment, there was an approximately 80% reduction in the numbers of parasites in lesions when compared with fluorescence intensity before treatment. The authors suggested that this monitoring model might provide optimization of determining efficacy of PDT as a therapy in treatment of CL [559].

In 2010, Peloi *et al.* investigated the effectiveness of PDT using methylene blue (MB) as the photosensitizing compound and a light-emitting diode (LED) against

ACL. Hamsters were experimentally infected with *L. amazonensis* for composing a CL model. After occurrence of the lesions in the footpad of hamsters, the animals were exposed to MB three times a week for three months. The lesions were illuminated with LED for 1 hour and 10 minutes later after each application with MB. Evaluation of success of the treatment was performed by the measurement of the hamster lesion thickness every week. Furthermore, the parasitic load in the regional lymph node of the hamsters was measured at the end of the treatment. According to the results, it was determined that thickness of lesion in the footpad significantly decreased, and the number of parasites in the regional lymph node of the hamsters were reduced when they were treated with MB+LED. Results indicated that PDT by using MB+LED against ACL possessed strong antileishmanial efficacy. This therapy was evaluated as promising, since it is an inexpensive technique, and the patient can apply it in his/her wound without requiring technical assistance [560].

In 2011, Song *et al.* tried to investigate *in vitro* and *in vivo* antileishmanial efficacies of PDT by using methylene blue; they also used this technique in order to treat a patient with CL. In this study, an effect of the application of PDT together with pentavalent antimony (SbV) was compared with the use of SbV alone. In *in vitro* tests, the cell viability of *Leishmania amazonensis* parasites was evaluated after exposure to different concentrations of MB by using MTT colorimetric assay. In *in vivo* analysis, PDT was used to treat two lesions of a patient with CL. A low dose of SbV was applied systematically to a patient, while PDT was used for treating one of the lesions. It was observed that IC_{50} values ranged between 20 and 100 μM, according to use of different concentrations of MB for PDT in *in vitro* tests. Combined use of SbV and PDT provided rapid wound healing when it was compared with the use of SbV alone. These results demonstrated that application of PDT by using MB may be used to treat CL caused by *L. amazonensis*, and its combined use with pentavalent antimonials can be a further promising method for treatment of CL in clinical cases [561].

Different from the aforementioned, in our recent study, we investigated the effects of visible light on various cell parameters of *L. tropica* parasites such as morphology, proliferation, infectivity, cell cycle, and glucose consumption, *in vitro*. The results demonstrated that the morphology of parasites changed; the cell cycle was affected from exposure to light, and this caused parasites to remain at the G0/G1 phase. Moreover, the proliferation, infectivity, glucose consumption, and mitochondrial dehydrogenase activities of parasites were decreased. Thus, for the first time, in this study, the effects of light on biological activities of *Leishmania* parasites were shown. It is thought that results obtained in this study are important in terms of demonstrating that visible light possesses antileishmanial efficacy alone, and this effect must be taken into account in the treatment of patients with CL with PDT. Furthermore, this study also reveals out that antileishmanial activity of PDT depends on not only the production of cytotoxic compounds during conversion of heme to porphrines but also changes in biological parameters of parasites following irradiation with visible light [562].

All this data indicate that the success of PDT in treatment of CL reveals that PDT can be an alternative therapy technique instead of current antileishmanial applications and can enhance the efficacy of conventional antileishmanial drugs while reducing their toxic effects when applied together. The only point, which puts a question mark in the minds about PDT, is the toxic effects of photosensitizing drugs used during application. It is thought that PDT can be a more promising treatment model for CL when this toxicity problem is overcome.

Immunotherapy for *Leishmaniasis*

Over the last 20 years, immune-based therapies (immunotherapy), either alone or combined with chemotherapy, have been improved as additional approaches in the treatment of *Leishmaniasis*. Immunotherapy has been used to accelerate the specific immune response in immunologically responsive patients and has been found an effective reaction in those who are nonresponsive.

Immunotherapy includes using biological agents to modulate and modify immune responses to achieve prophylactic and therapeutic goals. It is based on the simple concept that our body's defense systems have the talent to protect us against some diseases. It is thought that disease occurs when there is either a failure or a suboptimal or excessive immune reaction. This could be removed simply by appropriate immune modulation or interventions using immunomodulatory agents or biological response modifiers. So immunotherapeutic agents can apply their effect by directly or indirectly increasing the host's natural defenses; thereby the restoration of the impaired effector functions or decreasing host excessive and harmful responses to the use of chemical and biological compounds to modulate immune responses has been under active investigation for over 30 years. In spite of positive results in animal models, the types of chemicals, bacterial extracts, and viruses used as nonspecific immunomodulators have proved not effective in clinical trials [39]. However, recent advances in gene manipulations, including translational techniques, have led to the availability of highly purified biological compounds, which are being evaluated in preclinical models and in clinical trials [182].

Treatment for *Leishmaniasis* includes sodium stibogluconate (SSG) [173], amphotericin B [174], paramycin sulphate [175], and meglumine antimoniate [176]. In CL, the most frequently used drugs are topical paromomycin sulphate with methylbenzethonium chloride (MBCL) or urea.

In 1940, pentavalent antimonials such as SSG have been the major drugs for treatment of *Leishmaniasis* [177, 178]. The generally accepted dose of antimonials is 20 mg/kg intravenously or intramuscularly for 20 days [179]. Lipid formulation of amphotercin B is acute VL and effective in children and adults in all endemic areas.

Several factors determine and influence treatment options, which include the size, number, appearance, and location of the lesions; duration of clinical disease prior to first treatment; frequency of relapses and reinfections; presence and severity of either mucosal or diffuse cutaneous involvement; immunosuppression; co-infections and prior anti-*Leishmania* treatment; and age of the patient [180].

In general, systemic antimonials are given to patients with multiple large lesion(s) or lesion(s) on the face, over joints, or close to vital organs, while patients with small lesion(s), which are not at cosmetically important sites, are treated intralesionally or left untreated if the patients are from CL-endemic areas [180]. Diagnosis of VL is always followed by treatment due to the high morbidity and mortality related to the disease. In Bihar, India (where 45% of the world VL occurs), resistance has made use of antimonials redundant. Lipid formulation of amphotericin B is efficacious and requires short-term treatment duration [181]; the rediscovery of paromomycin and identification of miltefosine has driven the therapeutic advancement for VL [182].

The disease is characterized by the development of ulcerative skin lesions lasting for months and, in most cases, is resolved by Th1 T cell activity. Although in patients with a defective cellular immune response, a long-lasting chronic disease (recurrent CL orDCL) may develop [183]. Most patients recover from the disease after primary exposure to the parasite, but a small percentage may develop severe secondary life-persisting lesions in the mucocutaneous tissue (MCL). The disease is well developed in the presence of Th2 T-cell-mediated immunity. The visceral form caused by *L. donovani*, *L. infantum* is characterized by systemic infection of the reticuloendothelial system.

Until recently, only two vaccines (one live and one killed) were licensed for use in humans and one for prophylaxis in dogs. Also, the number of available drugs for treating the disease is limited, and most of the parasites develop drug resistance. In the last 20 years, immunotherapy has been developed as an additional treatment of *Leishmaniasis*. Immunotherapy has been used to accelerate the specific immune response in immunologically responsive patients and to establish an effective reaction in those who are nonresponsive [183].

It is clear from both murine and human studies, there are promising choices to conventional chemotherapy, especially in patients with refractive *Leishmaniasis*. Although different studies utilize different *Leishmania* antigens, which are received for different treatment durations, there is a significant need to standardize immunotherapeutic protocols use in treatment of *Leishmaniasis* [184, 185].

Nanotechnologic Approaches

Nanotechnology is the creation of functional materials, devices, and systems at atomic and molecular scales (1-100 nm), where properties differ significantly from those at a larger scale. The importance of nanoscience comes from the changes in physical rules and different properties of material and energy at the nanoscale. Nanoscaled materials have different and novel properties than do their bulk counterparts. One of the most important features is their broad surface area with respect to their volumes. A wide surface area affects the interactions between elements and nanoparticles. Nanotechnology has already been used in broad fields of life, such as cosmetics, sunscreens, textiles, paints, electronics, materials engineering, agriculture, optics, industry *etc.* Moreover, nanotechnology is thought to be a future technology with several opportunities for application. One of the most important nanotechnologic application areas, which hold the expectation of providing great benefits for humanity in the future, is medicine. The use of nanotechnology and nanomaterials in medical research is growing rapidly. Recently, nanotechnologic developments in microbiology have gained importance in the field of chemotherapy [563-565]. In several studies, it was demonstrated that metal oxide nanoparticles such as TiO_2 and Ag_2O nanoparticles had antimicrobial activities on different kinds of microbial agents. Generally, effect mechanisms of these metal oxide nanoparticles depend on generating ROS resulting in oxidative stress, breakdown of ATP production, and, finally, apoptosis within the cells. It has been shown in the literature that activation of these nanoparticles by illuminating different kinds of light such as UV and visible light or with the effect of magnetic waves, amounts of free radicals produced from nanoparticles condensely increased. On the other hand, some nanoparticles, such as silver nanoparticles, possess an additional effect mechanism in order to enhance the elimination of microbial agents. These nanoparticles can easily penetrate cell membranes and compose strong interactions with sulphur- and phosphor-containing molecules within the cells. These interactions lead to impairment of proteins, enzymes, and DNA of infectious agents, and respiration within these cells stops. All of this causes death of microbial cells [566-570].

Until now, metal oxide nanoparticles, especially TiO_2 and Ag_2O, thanks to their unique properties, described above were repeatedly shown to have the potential to eliminate several kinds of bacteria, virus, and fungi. However, no study demonstrates their antileishmanial effects on *Leishmania* parasites in the literature. It has been known for a long time that *Leishmania* parasites are susceptible to ROS, and a new treatment strategy dependent on production of these oxygen derivatives may eliminate the restrictions in the treatment of the disease. Considering this data, the effects of nanoparticles on *Leishmania* parasites have, for the first time, been investigated in our preliminary studies, and it was found that both TiO_2 and Ag_2O nanoparticles had antileishmanial effects under different conditions.

We first investigated the effects of TiO_2 nanoparticles on the proliferation of *Leishmania* parasites in the dark and under UV light. It was observed that, under dark conditions, TiO_2 nanoparticles (100 µg/ml) decreased the proliferation of parasites, but this effect was not significantly different to the effect that UV light had demonstrated alone on parasites. Conversely, TiO_2 nanoparticles (100 µg/ml) under UV light were observed to show a significant effect on parasites and inhibit the proliferation of parasites in contrast to a control group and an experiment group, which were only exposed to UV light. This result indicates that TiO_2 nanoparticles have great potential to show antileishmanial effects [571].

Similar to TiO_2 nanoparticles, antileishmanial effects of Ag_2O nanoparticles (100 µg/ml) were also investigated under dark conditions and under UV light. In this study, the efficacies of Ag_2O nanoparticles were examined by determination of biological parameters of *L. tropica* such as morphology, metabolic activity, proliferation, infectivity, and survival in host cells, *in vitro* after their exposure to Ag_2O nanoparticles in the dark and under UV light. Obtained results indicate that parasite morphology and infectivity were impaired in comparison with the control in the presence and absence of UV light. However, enhanced effects of Ag_2O nanoparticles were determined on the morphology and infectivity of parasites under UV light. On the other hand, Ag_2O nanoparticles exhibited great antileishmanial effects by inhibiting the proliferation and metabolic activity of *L. tropica* promastigotes by 1.5- to threefold, respectively, in the dark, and 2- to 6.5- fold, respectively, under UV light. Moreover, Ag_2O nanoparticles inhibited the survival of amastigotes in macrophages, and this effect was more substantial in the presence of UV light. This study was the first time that Ag-NPs were determined to possess antileishmanial effects on *L. tropica* parasites through investigating their effects on various cellular biological parameters of promastigote and amastigote forms. Results demonstrate that use of Ag_2O may represent a future alternative to current antileishmanial drugs. Since *Leishmaniasis* is spreading rapidly worldwide, and because antileishmanial drugs have several disadvantages, it can be thought that treatment based on Ag_2O may has an important role in overcoming *Leishmaniasis*. Determination of the antileishmanial effects of Ag_2O is also important for the further development of new compounds containing nanoparticles in *Leishmaniasis* treatment [572].

What is the Future of antileishmanial Drug Discovery?

Because of the disseminated location and intracellular nature of the *Leishmania*, *Leishmaniasis* is a significant global burden and a great challenge for drug discovery. Mainly, due to their versatile nature and attractive advantages in the context of parasitic diseases, emulsions, liposomes, and nanoparticles are the potential colloidal drug carriers. Nanoparticles (NPs) used in drug delivery systems may improve the controlled release index of drugs. They are very small and intelligent particles with a magnetic core, therapeutic load, and recognition layer. NPs are made of inorganic or organic materials, and they can be biodegradable [573]. Biodegradable nanoparticles such as PLGA, PLA, chitosan, gelatin, polycaprolactone, and polyalkylcyanoacrylates are used as drug delivery vehicles due to their therapeutic value and decreasing the risks of toxicity of some medicinal drugs. They also help to increase the bioavailability, solubility, and retention time of many potent drugs, which are difficult to deliver orally [574].

Some macrophage-mediated diseases can be functionally treated by using nanoparticles. It is known that mononuclear phagocyte cells engulf *Leishmania* parasites, but also they remove drug particles from body circulation. Also macrophages can identify the cell-surface ligands exploited in nanoparticulate systems by anchoring specific entities to ensure their internalization into the cells [575]. Liposomal amphotericin B is an antileishmanial drug, which is a combination of liposomes and nanoparticles. It has been shown that they improve the efficacy and tolerability of drugs. Due to better stability and easy commercialization, a second generation of colloidal carriers such as solid lipid nanoparticles and nanostructured lipid carriers represent a good manner [576]. Amphotericin B must be administered by slow intravenous injection because it is not absorbed in the gastrointestinal tract, and it has poor solubility. Recent studies are aimed to develop an oral delivery system that will evaluate the absorption of nanosuspensions [577]. Oral delivery of a nanosuspension form of amphotericin B was tested on an *L. donovani* infected Balb/c mouse model [57].

Hydrophobic drugs such as amphotericin B can be delivered by novel lipid particle-based delivery systems such as cochleates. The cochleate system assists in the uptake of amphotericin B from the gastrointestinal tract, and the effectiveness of this system has been displayed on a mouse model infected with systemic candidiasis. This system may have potential for therapeutic application [579]. Mendoza *et al.* have developed a novel formulation for edelfosine with a lipid nanoparticulate system to decrease the systemic toxicity and improve the therapeutic potential of the drug [580]. The lipid-employed Compritoll has advantages *in vitro* because it used asmatrix material for nanoparticle development and takes a role in the controlled release of edelfosine. Nonspecific lipid transfer proteins are small basic proteins extracted from plants.

Due to their molecular weight, there are two different nonspecific lipid transfer proteins: nsLTP1 (10 kDa) and nsLTP2 (7 kDa) [581]. NsLTPs can bind a broad range of lipid molecules; they also have high potential for drug-carrier systems. These proteins have been purified from a variety of plants, barley seeds, hops, rice, tomato, the *pandan pandanus amaryllifolius*, and *cumin cuminum cyminum* [582]. Transfer activity of these carriers should make them useful when drugs must cross through lipid membranes. Combination studies with nsLTP1 and several drugs can be used for additional pharmaceutical applications. A study done by Pato *et al.* showed that wheat nsLTP1 can bind ether phospholipid analogues such as edelfosine, ilmofosine, and an antifungal conazole derivative (BD56) with similar affinity [583]. Pato and co-workers also displayed an interaction between amphotericin B and nsLTP1; however, the authors could not prove any affinity between them. As a result of their study, nsLTPs can be used as part of antileishmanial drug-carrier systems. The combination of drugs and chemotherapy has upgraded prospects for curbing the emergence of drug resistance and has proven to increase activity through the use of compounds with synergistic or additive activity, reducing the needed doses and toxic side effects. In a recent study, a topical formulation containing 15% paromomycin and 0.5% gentamicin was evaluated in a Phase II trial in Tunisia and France [584]. It demonstrated that a 20-day cure with this combination was safe and effective against CL caused by *L. major*. The effectiveness of drug combinations in chemotherapy is measured by the interaction index. The combination and individual drug-dose effect data, their isobolar analysis, and fractional inhibitory concentrations (FIC) can be calculated due to this methodology [585]. Monzote and his friends showed that a combination of essential oil extracted from *Chenopodium ambrosioides* and pentamidine had a synergic effect against promastigotes of *L. amazonensis*, but they had no effect when combined with meglumine antimoniate or amphotericin B [586]. In traditional medicine, to increase the effect of drug combinations, antibiotics or synthetic drugs with natural products such as plants are used. The aim of new projects for scientists around the world is to develop a new generation of phytochemicals, which can be used alone or in combination with antibiotics or synthetic drugs. With the help of these new formulations, they will try to cure the disease.

ACKNOWLEDGEMENTS

Declared none.

CONFLICT OF INTEREST

The authors confirm that this chapter contents have no conflict of interest.

REFERENCES

[1]   Singh S. New developments in diagnosis of leishmaniasis. Indian J Med Res. 2006 Mar; 123(3): 311-30.
[2]   Organization. WH. Expert Committee on the Control of Leishmaniases, Technical Report Series 949. 2010.
[3]   Desjeux P. Human leishmaniases: epidemiology and public health aspects. World Health Stat Q. 1992; 45(2-3): 267-75.
[4]   Dey A, Singh S. Transfusion transmitted leishmaniasis: a case report and review of literature. Indian J Med Microbiol. 2006 Jul; 24(3): 165-70.
[5]   Herwaldt BL. Leishmaniasis. Lancet. 1999 Oct 2; 354(9185): 1191-9.
[6]   Sundar S, Rai M. Laboratory diagnosis of visceral leishmaniasis. Clin Diagn Lab Immunol. 2002 Sep; 9(5): 951-8.
[7]   Chiodini PL, Moody AH, Manser DW, Jeffrey HC. Atlas of medical helminthology and protozoology: Churchill Livingstone; 2001.
[8]   Mosser DM, Miles SA. Avoidance of Innate Immune Mechanisms by the Protozoan Parasite, Leishmania spp. In: Gazzinelli EYDaRT, editor. Protozoon in macrophage2007. p. 118-28.
[9]   Roberts LJ, Handman E, Foote SJ. Science, medicine, and the future: Leishmaniasis. BMJ. 2000 Sep 30; 321(7264): 801-4.

[10]   Cardo LJ. Leishmania: risk to the blood supply. Transfusion. 2006 Sep; 46(9): 1641-5.

[11]   Mathur P, Samantaray JC. The first probable case of platelet transfusion-transmitted visceral leishmaniasis. Transfus Med. 2004 Aug; 14(4): 319-21.

[12]   Chung H, Chow H, Lu J. The first two cases of transfusion kala-azar. Chin Med J. 1948; 66: 325-6.

[13]   Kostman R, Barr M, Bengtsson E, Garnham P, Hult G, editors. Kala-azar transferred by exchange blood transfusion in two Swedish infants1963.

[14]   Mauny I, Blanchot I, Degeilh B, Dabadie A, Guiguen C, Roussey M. [Visceral leishmaniasis in an infant in Brittany: discussion on the modes of transmission out endemic zones]. Pediatrie. 1993; 48(3): 237-9.

[15]   Singh S, Chaudhry VP, Wali JP. Transfusion-transmitted kala-azar in India. Transfusion. 1996 Sep; 36(9): 848-9.

[16]   Kubar J, Quaranta JF, Marty P, Lelievre A, Le Fichoux Y, Aufeuvre JP. Transmission of L. infantum by blood donors. Nat Med. 1997 Apr; 3(4): 368.

[17]   Caldas AJ, Costa JM, Gama ME, Ramos EA, Barral A. Visceral leishmaniasis in pregnancy: a case report. Acta Trop. 2003 Sep; 88(1): 39-43.

[18]   Symmers WS. Leishmaniasis acquired by contagion: a case of marital infection in Britain. Lancet. 1960 Jan 16; 1(7116): 127-32.

[19]   Cruz I, Morales MA, Noguer I, Rodriguez A, Alvar J. Leishmania in discarded syringes from intravenous drug users. Lancet. 2002 Mar 30; 359(9312): 1124-5.

[20]   Manson-Bahr PEC. Diagnosis, Late of Overseas Development Administrastion. London 1987.

[21]   Meinecke CK, Schottelius J, Oskam L, Fleischer B. Congenital transmission of visceral leishmaniasis (Kala Azar) from an asymptomatic mother to her child. Pediatrics. 1999 Nov; 104(5): e65.

[22]   Zuk PA. Viral transduction of adipose-derived stem cells. Methods Mol Biol. 2011; 702: 345-57.

[23]   Kotton CN, Lattes R. Parasitic infections in solid organ transplant recipients. Am J Transplant. 2009 Dec; 9 Suppl 4: S234-51.

[24]   le Fichoux Y, Quaranta JF, Aufeuvre JP, Lelievre A, Marty P, Suffia I, *et al.* Occurrence of Leishmania infantum parasitemia in asymptomatic blood donors living in an area of endemicity in southern France. J Clin Microbiol. 1999 Jun; 37(6): 1953-7.

[25]   Riera C, Fisa R, Udina M, Gallego M, Portus M. Detection of Leishmania infantum cryptic infection in asymptomatic blood donors living in an endemic area (Eivissa, Balearic Islands, Spain) by different diagnostic methods. Trans R Soc Trop Med Hyg. 2004 Feb; 98(2): 102-10.

[26]   Otero AC, da Silva VO, Luz KG, Palatnik M, Pirmez C, Fernandes O, *et al.* Short report: occurrence of Leishmania donovani DNA in donated blood from seroreactive Brazilian blood donors. Am J Trop Med Hyg. 2000 Jan; 62(1): 128-31.

[27]   Colomba C, Saporito L, Polara VF, Barone T, Corrao A, Titone L. Serological screening for Leishmania infantum in asymptomatic blood donors living in an endemic area (Sicily, Italy). Transfus Apher Sci. 2005 Nov; 33(3): 311-4.

[28]   Silva LA, Romero HD, Nogueira Nascentes GA, Costa RT, Rodrigues V, Prata A. Antileishmania immunological tests for asymptomatic subjects living in a visceral leishmaniasis-endemic area in Brazil. Am J Trop Med Hyg. 2011 Feb; 84(2): 261-6.

[29]   Sharma MC, Gupta AK, Das VN, Verma N, Kumar N, Saran R, *et al.* Leishmania donovani in blood smears of asymptomatic persons. Acta Trop. 2000 Sep 18; 76(2): 195-6.

[30]   Cattand P, Desjeux P, Guzman MG, Jannin J, Kroeger A, Medici A, *et al.* Tropical Diseases Lacking Adequate Control Measures: Dengue, Leishmaniasis, and African Trypanosomiasis. 2006.

[31]   Banuls AL, Hide M, Prugnolle F. Leishmania and the leishmaniases: a parasite genetic update and advances in taxonomy, epidemiology and pathogenicity in humans. Adv Parasitol. 2007; 64: 1-109.

[32]   Lines J, Harpham T, Leake C, Schofield C. Trends, priorities and policy directions in the control of vector-borne diseases in urban environments. Health Policy Plan. 1994 Jun; 9(2): 113-29.

[33]   Patz JA, Daszak P, Tabor GM, Aguirre AA, Pearl M, Epstein J, *et al.* Unhealthy landscapes: policy recommendations on land use change and infectious disease emergence. Environmental Health Perspectives. 2004; 112(10): 1092.

[34]   Myers SS, Patz JA. Emerging threats to human health from global environmental change. Annual Review of Environment and Resources. 2009; 34: 223-52.

[35]   Quinnell RJ, Courtenay O. Transmission, reservoir hosts and control of zoonotic visceral leishmaniasis. Parasitology. 2009 Dec; 136(14): 1915-34.

[36]   Ostyn B, Vanlerberghe V, Picado A, Dinesh DS, Sundar S, Chappuis F, *et al.* Vector control by insecticide-treated nets in the fight against visceral leishmaniasis in the Indian subcontinent, what is the evidence? Tropical medicine & international health: TM & IH. 2008 Aug; 13(8): 1073-85.

[37]   Nigro L, Montineri A, La Rosa R, Zuccarello M, Iacobello C, Vinci C, *et al.* Visceral leishmaniasis and HIV co-infection: a rare case of pulmonary and oral localization. Infez Med. 2003 Jun; 11(2): 93-6.

[38]   Biglino A, Bolla C, Concialdi E, Trisciuoglio A, Romano A, Ferroglio E. Asymptomatic Leishmania infantum infection in an area of northwestern Italy (Piedmont region) where such infections are traditionally nonendemic. J Clin Microbiol. 2010 Jan; 48(1): 131-6.

[39]   Murray HW, Berman JD, Davies CR, Saravia NG. Advances in leishmaniasis. Lancet. 2005 Oct 29-Nov 4; 366(9496): 1561-77.

[40]   Sharifi I, Fekri AR, Aflatoonian MR, Khamesipour A, Mahboudi F, Dowlati Y, *et al.* Leishmaniasis recidivans among school children in Bam, South-east Iran, 1994-2006. Int J Dermatol. 2010 May; 49(5): 557-61.

[41]   Michel G, Pomares C, Ferrua B, Marty P. Importance of worldwide asymptomatic carriers of Leishmania infantum (L. chagasi) in human. Acta Trop. 2011 Aug; 119(2-3): 69-75.

[42]   Berman J. Current treatment approaches to leishmaniasis. Curr Opin Infect Dis. 2003 Oct; 16(5): 397-401.

[43]   Bailey MS, Lockwood DN. Cutaneous leishmaniasis. Clin Dermatol. 2007 Mar-Apr; 25(2): 203-11.

[44]   Boelaert M, Criel B, Leeuwenburg J, Van Damme W, Le Ray D, Van der Stuyft P. Visceral leishmaniasis control: a public health perspective. Trans R Soc Trop Med Hyg. 2000 Sep-Oct; 94(5): 465-71.

[45]   Berman JD. Human leishmaniasis: clinical, diagnostic, and chemotherapeutic developments in the last 10 years. Clin Infect Dis. 1997 Apr; 24(4): 684-703.

[46]   Miles MA, Lainson R, Shaw JJ, Povoa M, de Souza AA. Leishmaniasis in Brazil: XV. Biochemical distinction of Leishmania mexicana amazonensis, L. braziliensis braziliensis

and L. braziliensis guyanensis--aetiological agents of cutaneous leishmaniasis in the Amazon Basin of Brazil. Trans R Soc Trop Med Hyg. 1981; 75(4): 524-9.

[47]   Osorio LE, Castillo CM, Ochoa MT. Mucosal leishmaniasis due to Leishmania (Viannia) panamensis in Colombia: clinical characteristics. Am J Trop Med Hyg. 1998 Jul; 59(1): 49-52.

[48]   Santrich C, Segura I, Arias AL, Saravia NG. Mucosal disease caused by Leishmania braziliensis guyanensis. Am J Trop Med Hyg. 1990 Jan; 42(1): 51-5.

[49]   Salotra P, Sreenivas G, Pogue GP, Lee N, Nakhasi HL, Ramesh V, *et al*. Development of a species-specific PCR assay for detection of Leishmania donovani in clinical samples from patients with kala-azar and post-kala-azar dermal leishmaniasis. J Clin Microbiol. 2001 Mar; 39(3): 849-54.

[50]   Schallig HD, Oskam L. Molecular biological applications in the diagnosis and control of leishmaniasis and parasite identification. Trop Med Int Health. 2002 Aug; 7(8): 641-51.

[51]   Ak M, Özbel Y, Özensoy S, Turgay N. Visseral Leishmaniasis immun yetmezlikte Önemi Artan Parazit Hastalıkları. Türkiye Parazitoloji Dernegi. 1995.

[52]   Garcia LS. Diagnostic medical parasitology. 4th ed. Washington, D.C.: ASM Press; 2001.

[53]   James WD, Berger TG, Elston DM, Odom RB, ScienceDirect. Andrews' diseases of the skin: clinical dermatology: Saunders Elsevier; 2006.

[54]   Markle WH, Makhoul K. Cutaneous leishmaniasis: recognition and treatment. Am Fam Physician. 2004 Mar 15; 69(6): 1455-60.

[55]   Cabello I, Caraballo A, Millan Y. Leishmaniasis in the genital area. Rev Inst Med Trop Sao Paulo. 2002 Mar-Apr; 44(2): 105-7.

[56]   Desjeux P. Leishmaniasis. Nat Rev Microbiol. 2004 Sep; 2(9): 692.

[57]   Organization. WH. Control of leishmaniasis: Report of a WHO Expert Committee, Technical Report Series 793. World Health Organization; 1990.

[58]   Convit J, Pinardi ME, Rondon AJ. Diffuse cutaneous leishmaniasis: a disease due to an immunological defect of the host. Trans R Soc Trop Med Hyg. 1972; 66(4): 603-10.

[59]   Barral A, Costa JM, Bittencourt AL, Barral-Netto M, Carvalho EM. Polar and subpolar diffuse cutaneous leishmaniasis in Brazil: clinical and immunopathologic aspects. Int J Dermatol. 1995 Jul; 34(7): 474-9.

[60]   Zijlstra EE, Musa AM, Khalil EA, el-Hassan IM, el-Hassan AM. Post-kala-azar dermal leishmaniasis. Lancet Infect Dis. 2003 Feb; 3(2): 87-98.

[61]   Ramesh V, Mukherjee A. Post-kala-azar dermal leishmaniasis. Int J Dermatol. 1995 Feb; 34(2): 85-91.

[62]   Thakur CP, Kumar K. Post kala-azar dermal leishmaniasis: a neglected aspect of kala-azar control programmes. Annals of tropical medicine and parasitology. 1992 Aug; 86(4): 355-9.

[63]   Landau M, Srebrnik A, Brenner S. Leishmaniasis recidivans mimicking lupus vulgaris. Int J Dermatol. 1996 Aug; 35(8): 572-3.

[64]   Gama ME, Costa JM, Gomes CM, Corbett CE. Subclinical form of the American visceral leishmaniasis. Mem Inst Oswaldo Cruz. 2004 Dec; 99(8): 889-93.

[65]   Riera C, Fisa R, Lopez-Chejade P, Serra T, Girona E, Jimenez M, *et al*. Asymptomatic infection by Leishmania infantum in blood donors from the Balearic Islands (Spain). Transfusion. 2008 Jul; 48(7): 1383-9.

[66] Romero HD, Silva Lde A, Silva-Vergara ML, Rodrigues V, Costa RT, Guimaraes SF, *et al.* Comparative study of serologic tests for the diagnosis of asymptomatic visceral leishmaniasis in an endemic area. Am J Trop Med Hyg. 2009 Jul; 81(1): 27-33.

[67] Pittaluga G. Enfermedades de los países cálidos y parasitología general: Jiménez y Molina; 1923.

[68] Badaro R, Jones TC, Carvalho EM, Sampaio D, Reed SG, Barral A, *et al.* New perspectives on a subclinical form of visceral leishmaniasis. J Infect Dis. 1986 Dec; 154(6): 1003-11.

[69] Jeronimo SM, Teixeira MJ, Sousa A, Thielking P, Pearson RD, Evans TG. Natural history of Leishmania (Leishmania) chagasi infection in Northeastern Brazil: long-term follow-up. Clin Infect Dis. 2000 Mar; 30(3): 608-9.

[70] Alvar J, Canavate C, Gutierrez-Solar B, Jimenez M, Laguna F, Lopez-Velez R, *et al.* Leishmania and human immunodeficiency virus coinfection: the first 10 years. Clin Microbiol Rev. 1997 Apr; 10(2): 298-319.

[71] Marty P, Lelievre A, Quaranta JF, Rahal A, Gari-Toussaint M, Le Fichoux Y. Use of the leishmanin skin test and Western blot analysis for epidemiological studies in visceral leishmaniasis areas: experience in a highly endemic focus in Alpes-Maritimes (France). Transactions of the Royal Society of Tropical Medicine and Hygiene. 1994; 88(6): 658-9.

[72] Pineda JA, Gallardo JA, Macias J, Delgado J, Regordan C, Morillas F, *et al.* Prevalence of and factors associated with visceral leishmaniasis in human immunodeficiency virus type 1-infected patients in southern Spain. J Clin Microbiol. 1998 Sep; 36(9): 2419-22.

[73] Ates SC, Bagirova M, Allahverdiyev AM, Baydar SY, Koc RC, Elcicek S, *et al.* Detection of antileishmanial antibodies in blood sampled from blood bank donors in Istanbul. Future Microbiol. 2012 Jun; 7: 773-9.

[74] Kubba R, Al-Gindan Y, El-Hassan A, Omer A. Clinical diagnosis of cutaneous leishmaniasis (oriental sore). Journal of the American Academy of Dermatology. 1987; 16(6): 1183-9.

[75] Rosenblatt JE. Laboratory diagnosis of infections due to blood and tissue parasites. Clin Infect Dis. 2009 Oct 1; 49(7): 1103-8.

[76] Scarisbrick JJ, Chiodini PL, Watson J, Moody A, Armstrong M, Lockwood D, *et al.* Clinical features and diagnosis of 42 travellers with cutaneous leishmaniasis. Travel Med Infect Dis. 2006 Jan; 4(1): 14-21.

[77] Allahverdiyev AM, Uzun S, Bagirova M, Durdu M, Memisoglu HR. A sensitive new microculture method for diagnosis of cutaneous leishmaniasis. Am J Trop Med Hyg. 2004 Mar; 70(3): 294-7.

[78] Chang K, Fong D, Bray R. Biology of Leishmania and leishmaniasis. Leishmaniasis(Human Parasitic Diseases Vol 1). 1985: 1-30.

[79] Gholamhosseinian A, Vassef A. Superiority of hemoglobin to hemin for cultivation of Leishmania tropica promastigotes in serum-free media. J Protozool. 1988 Nov; 35(4): 446-9.

[80] Daneshbod Y, Oryan A, Davarmanesh M, Shirian S, Negahban S, Aledavood A, *et al.* Clinical, histopathologic, and cytologic diagnosis of mucosal leishmaniasis and literature review. Arch Pathol Lab Med. 2011 Apr; 135(4): 478-82.

[81] Pastorino AC, Jacob CM, Oselka GW, Carneiro-Sampaio MM. Visceral leishmaniasis: clinical and laboratorial aspects. J Pediatr (Rio J). 2002 Mar-Apr; 78(2): 120-7.

[82]   Aydenizöz M, Yağcı BB, Özkan AT, Duru SY, Gazyağcı AN. Kırıkkale'deki Köpeklerde Mikrokültür Yöntemi ve IFAT ile Visseral Leishmaniosisin Prevalansının Araştırılması.

[83]   Allahverdiyev AM, Bagirova M, Uzun S, Alabaz D, Aksaray N, Kocabas E, *et al*. The value of a new microculture method for diagnosis of visceral leishmaniasis by using bone marrow and peripheral blood. Am J Trop Med Hyg. 2005 Aug; 73(2): 276-80.

[84]   Ihalamulla RL, Rajapaksa US, Karunaweera ND. Microculture for the isolation of Leishmania, modified to increase efficacy: a follow-up to a previous study. Ann Trop Med Parasitol. 2006 Jan; 100(1): 87-9.

[85]   Boggild AK, Miranda-Verastegui C, Espinosa D, Arevalo J, Adaui V, Tulliano G, *et al*. Evaluation of a microculture method for isolation of Leishmania parasites from cutaneous lesions of patients in Peru. J Clin Microbiol. 2007 Nov; 45(11): 3680-4.

[86]   Hide M, Singh R, Kumar B, Banuls AL, Sundar S. A microculture technique for isolating live Leishmania parasites from peripheral blood of visceral leishmaniasis patients. Acta Trop. 2007 Jun; 102(3): 197-200.

[87]   Boggild AK, Miranda-Verastegui C, Espinosa D, Arevalo J, Martinez-Medina D, Llanos-Cuentas A, *et al*. Optimization of microculture and evaluation of miniculture for the isolation of Leishmania parasites from cutaneous lesions in Peru. Am J Trop Med Hyg. 2008 Dec; 79(6): 847-52.

[88]   Ihalamulla RL, Rajapaksa US, Karunaweera ND. Microculture for the isolation of Leishmania parasites from cutaneous lesions -- Sri Lankan experience. Ann Trop Med Parasitol. 2005 Sep; 99(6): 571-5.

[89]   Grimaldi G, Jr., Tesh RB, McMahon-Pratt D. A review of the geographic distribution and epidemiology of leishmaniasis in the New World. Am J Trop Med Hyg. 1989 Dec; 41(6): 687-725.

[90]   Singh S, Dey A, Sivakumar R. Applications of molecular methods for Leishmania control. Expert Rev Mol Diagn. 2005 Mar; 5(2): 251-65.

[91]   Tavares CA, Fernandes AP, Melo MN. Molecular diagnosis of leishmaniasis. Expert Rev Mol Diagn. 2003 Sep; 3(5): 657-67.

[92]   Liarte DB, Mendonca IL, Luz FC, Abreu EA, Mello GW, Farias TJ, *et al*. QBC for the diagnosis of human and canine american visceral leishmaniasis: preliminary data. Rev Soc Bras Med Trop. 2001 Nov-Dec; 34(6): 577-81.

[93]   Navin TR, Arana BA, Arana FE, Berman JD, Chajon JF. Placebo-controlled clinical trial of sodium stibogluconate (Pentostam) *versus* ketoconazole for treating cutaneous leishmaniasis in Guatemala. J Infect Dis. 1992 Mar; 165(3): 528-34.

[94]   Degrave W, Fernandes O, Campbell D, Bozza M, Lopes U. Use of molecular probes and PCR for detection and typing of Leishmania--a mini-review. Mem Inst Oswaldo Cruz. 1994 Jul-Sep; 89(3): 463-9.

[95]   Wilson SM. DNA-based methods in the detection of Leishmania parasites: field applications and practicalities. Ann Trop Med Parasitol. 1995 Dec; 89 Suppl 1: 95-100.

[96]   Rodriguez N, Guzman B, Rodas A, Takiff H, Bloom BR, Convit J. Diagnosis of cutaneous leishmaniasis and species discrimination of parasites by PCR and hybridization. J Clin Microbiol. 1994 Sep; 32(9): 2246-52.

[97]   Fernandes O, Bozza M, Pascale JM, de Miranda AB, Lopes UG, Degrave WM. An oligonucleotide probe derived from kDNA minirepeats is specific for Leishmania (Viannia). Mem Inst Oswaldo Cruz. 1996 May-Jun; 91(3): 279-84.

[98]   Marfurt J, Nasereddin A, Niederwieser I, Jaffe CL, Beck HP, Felger I. Identification and differentiation of Leishmania species in clinical samples by PCR amplification of the miniexon sequence and subsequent restriction fragment length polymorphism analysis. J Clin Microbiol. 2003 Jul; 41(7): 3147-53.

[99]   de Bruijn MH, Barker DC. Diagnosis of New World leishmaniasis: specific detection of species of the Leishmania braziliensis complex by amplification of kinetoplast DNA. Acta Trop. 1992 Sep; 52(1): 45-58.

[100]   Cupolillo E, Grimaldi Junior G, Momen H, Beverley SM. Intergenic region typing (IRT): a rapid molecular approach to the characterization and evolution of Leishmania. Mol Biochem Parasitol. 1995 Jul; 73(1-2): 145-55.

[101]   Noyes HA, Reyburn H, Bailey JW, Smith D. A nested-PCR-based schizodeme method for identifying Leishmania kinetoplast minicircle classes directly from clinical samples and its application to the study of the epidemiology of Leishmania tropica in Pakistan. J Clin Microbiol. 1998 Oct; 36(10): 2877-81.

[102]   de Andrade AS, Gomes RF, Fernandes O, de Melo MN. Use of DNA-based diagnostic methods for human leishmaniasis in Minas Gerais, Brazil. Acta Trop. 2001 Mar 30; 78(3): 261-7.

[103]   Ashford DA, Bozza M, Freire M, Miranda JC, Sherlock I, Eulalio C, *et al*. Comparison of the polymerase chain reaction and serology for the detection of canine visceral leishmaniasis. Am J Trop Med Hyg. 1995 Sep; 53(3): 251-5.

[104]   Lachaud L, Dereure J, Chabbert E, Reynes J, Mauboussin JM, Oziol E, *et al*. Optimized PCR using patient blood samples for diagnosis and follow-up of visceral Leishmaniasis, with special reference to AIDS patients. J Clin Microbiol. 2000 Jan; 38(1): 236-40.

[105]   Singh DP, Goyal RK, Singh RK, Sundar S, Mohapatra TM. In search of an ideal test for diagnosis and prognosis of kala-azar. J Health Popul Nutr. 2010 Jun; 28(3): 281-5.

[106]   Kumar R, Pai K, Pathak K, Sundar S. Enzyme-linked immunosorbent assay for recombinant K39 antigen in diagnosis and prognosis of Indian visceral leishmaniasis. Clin Diagn Lab Immunol. 2001 Nov; 8(6): 1220-4.

[107]   Sundar S, Maurya R, Singh RK, Bharti K, Chakravarty J, Parekh A, *et al*. Rapid, noninvasive diagnosis of visceral leishmaniasis in India: comparison of two immunochromatographic strip tests for detection of anti-K39 antibody. J Clin Microbiol. 2006 Jan; 44(1): 251-3.

[108]   Teran-Angel G, Schallig H, Zerpa O, Rodriguez V, Ulrich M, Cabrera M. The direct agglutination test as an alternative method for the diagnosis of canine and human visceral leishmaniasis. Biomedica. 2007 Sep; 27(3): 447-53.

[109]   La Placa M, Pampiglione S, Borgatti M, Zerbini M. Complement fixation and intradermal skin test with partially purified "proteic" and "polysaccharidic" antigens from Leishmania donovani. Trans R Soc Trop Med Hyg. 1975; 69(4): 396-8.

[110]   Haldar JP, Saha KC, Ghose AC. Serological profiles in Indian post kala-azar dermal leishmaniasis. Trans R Soc Trop Med Hyg. 1981; 75(4): 514-7.

[111]   Salotra P, Raina A, Ramesh V. Western blot analysis of humoral immune response to Leishmania donovani antigens in patients with post-kala-azar dermal leishmaniasis. Trans R Soc Trop Med Hyg. 1999 Jan-Feb; 93(1): 98-101.

[112]   Mettler M, Grimm F, Capelli G, Camp H, Deplazes P. Evaluation of enzyme-linked immunosorbent assays, an immunofluorescent-antibody test, and two rapid tests (immunochromatographic-dipstick and gel tests) for serological diagnosis of symptomatic

and asymptomatic Leishmania infections in dogs. J Clin Microbiol. 2005 Nov; 43(11): 5515-9.

[113]   Alexander J, Russell DG. The interaction of Leishmania species with macrophages. Adv Parasitol. 1992; 31: 175-254.

[114]   Peters NC, Egen JG, Secundino N, Debrabant A, Kimblin N, Kamhawi S, *et al*. In vivo imaging reveals an essential role for neutrophils in leishmaniasis transmitted by sand flies. Science. 2008 Aug 15; 321(5891): 970-4.

[115]   Woelbing F, Kostka SL, Moelle K, Belkaid Y, Sunderkoetter C, Verbeek S, *et al*. Uptake of Leishmania major by dendritic cells is mediated by Fcgamma receptors and facilitates acquisition of protective immunity. J Exp Med. 2006 Jan 23; 203(1): 177-88.

[116]   Laufs H, Muller K, Fleischer J, Reiling N, Jahnke N, Jensenius JC, *et al*. Intracellular survival of Leishmania major in neutrophil granulocytes after uptake in the absence of heat-labile serum factors. Infect Immun. 2002 Feb; 70(2): 826-35.

[117]   Aga E, Katschinski DM, van Zandbergen G, Laufs H, Hansen B, Muller K, *et al*. Inhibition of the spontaneous apoptosis of neutrophil granulocytes by the intracellular parasite Leishmania major. J Immunol. 2002 Jul 15; 169(2): 898-905.

[118]   von Stebut E, Udey MC. Requirements for Th1-dependent immunity against infection with Leishmania major. Microbes Infect. 2004 Oct; 6(12): 1102-9.

[119]   Ajdary S, Alimohammadian MH, Eslami MB, Kemp K, Kharazmi A. Comparison of the immune profile of nonhealing cutaneous Leishmaniasis patients with those with active lesions and those who have recovered from infection. Infect Immun. 2000 Apr; 68(4): 1760-4.

[120]   Louzir H, Melby PC, Ben Salah A, Marrakchi H, Aoun K, Ben Ismail R, *et al*. Immunologic determinants of disease evolution in localized cutaneous leishmaniasis due to Leishmania major. J Infect Dis. 1998 Jun; 177(6): 1687-95.

[121]   Convit J, Ulrich M, Fernandez CT, Tapia FJ, Caceres-Dittmar G, Castes M, *et al*. The clinical and immunological spectrum of American cutaneous leishmaniasis. Trans R Soc Trop Med Hyg. 1993 Jul-Aug; 87(4): 444-8.

[122]   Ghalib HW, Piuvezam MR, Skeiky YA, Siddig M, Hashim FA, el-Hassan AM, *et al*. Interleukin 10 production correlates with pathology in human Leishmania donovani infections. J Clin Invest. 1993 Jul; 92(1): 324-9.

[123]   Karp CL, el-Safi SH, Wynn TA, Satti MM, Kordofani AM, Hashim FA, *et al*. In vivo cytokine profiles in patients with kala-azar. Marked elevation of both interleukin-10 and interferon-gamma. J Clin Invest. 1993 Apr; 91(4): 1644-8.

[124]   Kenney RT, Sacks DL, Gam AA, Murray HW, Sundar S. Splenic cytokine responses in Indian kala-azar before and after treatment. J Infect Dis. 1998 Mar; 177(3): 815-8.

[125]   Sundar S, Reed SG, Sharma S, Mehrotra A, Murray HW. Circulating T helper 1 (Th1) cell- and Th2 cell-associated cytokines in Indian patients with visceral leishmaniasis. Am J Trop Med Hyg. 1997 May; 56(5): 522-5.

[126]   Babaloo Z, Kaye PM, Eslami MB. Interleukin-13 in Iranian patients with visceral leishmaniasis: relationship to other Th2 and Th1 cytokines. Trans R Soc Trop Med Hyg. 2001 Jan-Feb; 95(1): 85-8.

[127]   Afonso LC, Scharton TM, Vieira LQ, Wysocka M, Trinchieri G, Scott P. The adjuvant effect of interleukin-12 in a vaccine against Leishmania major. Science. 1994 Jan 14; 263(5144): 235-7.

[128] Park AY, Hondowicz BD, Scott P. IL-12 is required to maintain a Th1 response during Leishmania major infection. The Journal of Immunology. 2000; 165(2): 896-902.

[129] Park AY, Hondowicz B, Kopf M, Scott P. The role of IL-12 in maintaining resistance to Leishmania major. J Immunol. 2002 Jun 1; 168(11): 5771-7.

[130] Himmelrich H, Parra-Lopez C, Tacchini-Cottier F, Louis JA, Launois P. The IL-4 rapidly produced in BALB/c mice after infection with Leishmania major down-regulates IL-12 receptor beta 2-chain expression on CD4+ T cells resulting in a state of unresponsiveness to IL-12. J Immunol. 1998 Dec 1; 161(11): 6156-63.

[131] Louis JA, Conceicao-Silva F, Himmelrich H, Tacchini-Cottier F, Launois P. Anti-leishmania effector functions of CD4+ Th1 cells and early events instructing Th2 cell development and susceptibility to Leishmania major in BALB/c mice. Adv Exp Med Biol. 1998; 452: 53-60.

[132] Louis J, Himmelrich H, Parra-Lopez C, Tacchini-Cottier F, Launois P. Regulation of protective immunity against Leishmania major in mice. Curr Opin Immunol. 1998 Aug; 10(4): 459-64.

[133] Scott P, Pearce E, Cheever AW, Coffman RL, Sher A. Role of cytokines and CD4+ T-cell subsets in the regulation of parasite immunity and disease. Immunol Rev. 1989 Dec; 112: 161-82.

[134] Scott P. The role of TH1 and TH2 cells in experimental cutaneous leishmaniasis. Exp Parasitol. 1989 Apr; 68(3): 369-72.

[135] Reiner SL, Locksley RM. The regulation of immunity to Leishmania major. Annu Rev Immunol. 1995; 13: 151-77.

[136] Himmelrich H, Launois P, Maillard I, Biedermann T, Tacchini-Cottier F, Locksley RM, *et al*. In BALB/c mice, IL-4 production during the initial phase of infection with Leishmania major is necessary and sufficient to instruct Th2 cell development resulting in progressive disease. J Immunol. 2000 May 1; 164(9): 4819-25.

[137] Kane MM, Mosser DM. The role of IL-10 in promoting disease progression in leishmaniasis. J Immunol. 2001 Jan 15; 166(2): 1141-7.

[138] Groux H, Cottrez F, Rouleau M, Mauze S, Antonenko S, Hurst S, *et al*. A transgenic model to analyze the immunoregulatory role of IL-10 secreted by antigen-presenting cells. J Immunol. 1999 Feb 1; 162(3): 1723-9.

[139] Allenbach C, Launois P, Mueller C, Tacchini-Cottier F. An essential role for transmembrane TNF in the resolution of the inflammatory lesion induced by Leishmania major infection. Eur J Immunol. 2008 Mar; 38(3): 720-31.

[140] Li J, Hunter CA, Farrell JP. Anti-TGF-beta treatment promotes rapid healing of Leishmania major infection in mice by enhancing in vivo nitric oxide production. J Immunol. 1999 Jan 15; 162(2): 974-9.

[141] Padigel UM, Farrell JP. Control of infection with Leishmania major in susceptible BALB/c mice lacking the common gamma-chain for FcR is associated with reduced production of IL-10 and TGF-beta by parasitized cells. J Immunol. 2005 May 15; 174(10): 6340-5.

[142] Xu G, Liu D, Fan Y, Yang X, Korner H, Fu YX, *et al*. Lymphotoxin alpha beta 2 (membrane lymphotoxin) is critically important for resistance to Leishmania major infection in mice. J Immunol. 2007 Oct 15; 179(8): 5358-66.

[143] Alexander CE, Kaye PM, Engwerda CR. CD95 is required for the early control of parasite burden in the liver of Leishmania donovani-infected mice. European journal of immunology. 2001 Apr; 31(4): 1199-210.

[144] Liew FY, O'Donnell CA. Immunology of leishmaniasis. Advances in parasitology. 1993; 32: 161-259.

[145] Cotterell SE, Engwerda CR, Kaye PM. Leishmania donovani infection initiates T cell-independent chemokine responses, which are subsequently amplified in a T cell-dependent manner. Eur J Immunol. 1999 Jan; 29(1): 203-14.

[146] Kaye PM, Svensson M, Ato M, Maroof A, Polley R, Stager S, *et al*. The immunopathology of experimental visceral leishmaniasis. Immunological reviews. 2004 Oct; 201: 239-53.

[147] Stanley AC, Engwerda CR. Balancing immunity and pathology in visceral leishmaniasis. Immunology and cell biology. 2007 Feb-Mar; 85(2): 138-47.

[148] Rodrigues OR, Marques C, Soares-Clemente M, Ferronha MH, Santos-Gomes GM. Identification of regulatory T cells during experimental Leishmania infantum infection. Immunobiology. 2009; 214(2): 101-11.

[149] Smelt SC, Engwerda CR, McCrossen M, Kaye PM. Destruction of follicular dendritic cells during chronic visceral leishmaniasis. J Immunol. 1997 Apr 15; 158(8): 3813-21.

[150] Engwerda CR, Ato M, Cotterell SE, Mynott TL, Tschannerl A, Gorak-Stolinska PM, *et al*. A role for tumor necrosis factor-alpha in remodeling the splenic marginal zone during Leishmania donovani infection. Am J Pathol. 2002 Aug; 161(2): 429-37.

[151] Tripathi P, Singh V, Naik S. Immune response to leishmania: paradox rather than paradigm. FEMS Immunol Med Microbiol. 2007 Nov; 51(2): 229-42.

[152] Bottrel RL, Dutra WO, Martins FA, Gontijo B, Carvalho E, Barral-Netto M, *et al*. Flow cytometric determination of cellular sources and frequencies of key cytokine-producing lymphocytes directed against recombinant LACK and soluble Leishmania antigen in human cutaneous leishmaniasis. Infect Immun. 2001 May; 69(5): 3232-9.

[153] Ribeiro-de-Jesus A, Almeida RP, Lessa H, Bacellar O, Carvalho EM. Cytokine profile and pathology in human leishmaniasis. Braz J Med Biol Res. 1998 Jan; 31(1): 143-8.

[154] Ezra N, Ochoa MT, Craft N. Human immunodeficiency virus and leishmaniasis. J Glob Infect Dis. 2010 Sep; 2(3): 248-57.

[155] Peters N, Sacks D. Immune privilege in sites of chronic infection: Leishmania and regulatory T cells. Immunol Rev. 2006 Oct; 213: 159-79.

[156] Belkaid Y, Piccirillo CA, Mendez S, Shevach EM, Sacks DL. CD4+CD25+ regulatory T cells control Leishmania major persistence and immunity. Nature. 2002 Dec 5; 420(6915): 502-7.

[157] Engwerda CR, Ato M, Kaye PM. Macrophages, pathology and parasite persistence in experimental visceral leishmaniasis. Trends in parasitology. 2004 Nov; 20(11): 524-30.

[158] Bekeredjian-Ding I, Jego G. Toll-like receptors--sentries in the B-cell response. Immunology. 2009 Nov; 128(3): 311-23.

[159] Brandonisio O, Spinelli R, Pepe M. Dendritic cells in Leishmania infection. Microbes Infect. 2004 Dec; 6(15): 1402-9.

[160] Sacks D, Noben-Trauth N. The immunology of susceptibility and resistance to Leishmania major in mice. Nat Rev Immunol. 2002 Nov; 2(11): 845-58.

[161] Nylen S, Maurya R, Eidsmo L, Manandhar KD, Sundar S, Sacks D. Splenic accumulation of IL-10 mRNA in T cells distinct from CD4+CD25+ (Foxp3) regulatory T cells in human visceral leishmaniasis. J Exp Med. 2007 Apr 16; 204(4): 805-17.

[162] Wilson ME, Jeronimo SM, Pearson RD. Immunopathogenesis of infection with the visceralizing Leishmania species. Microb Pathog. 2005 Apr; 38(4): 147-60.

[163] Zaph C, Uzonna J, Beverley SM, Scott P. Central memory T cells mediate long-term immunity to Leishmania major in the absence of persistent parasites. Nat Med. 2004 Oct; 10(10): 1104-10.

[164] Akira S, Takeda K, Kaisho T. Toll-like receptors: critical proteins linking innate and acquired immunity. Nat Immunol. 2001 Aug; 2(8): 675-80.

[165] Dempsey PW, Vaidya SA, Cheng G. The art of war: Innate and adaptive immune responses. Cell Mol Life Sci. 2003 Dec; 60(12): 2604-21.

[166] Medzhitov R. Toll-like receptors and innate immunity. Nat Rev Immunol. 2001 Nov; 1(2): 135-45.

[167] Medzhitov R, Janeway C, Jr. Innate immune recognition: mechanisms and pathways. Immunol Rev. 2000 Feb; 173: 89-97.

[168] Inohara N, Nunez G. NODs: intracellular proteins involved in inflammation and apoptosis. Nat Rev Immunol. 2003 May; 3(5): 371-82.

[169] Gomes IN, Palma LC, Campos GO, Lima JG, TF DEA, JP DEM, *et al.* The scavenger receptor MARCO is involved in Leishmania major infection by CBA/J macrophages. Parasite Immunol. 2009 Apr; 31(4): 188-98.

[170] Dabbagh K, Lewis DB. Toll-like receptors and T-helper-1/T-helper-2 responses. Curr Opin Infect Dis. 2003 Jun; 16(3): 199-204.

[171] Hemmi H, Kaisho T, Takeuchi O, Sato S, Sanjo H, Hoshino K, *et al.* Small anti-viral compounds activate immune cells *via* the TLR7 MyD88-dependent signaling pathway. Nat Immunol. 2002 Feb; 3(2): 196-200.

[172] Oldham RK, Smalley RV. Immunotherapy: the old and the new. J Biol Response Mod. 1983; 2(1): 1-37.

[173] Solomon M, Baum S, Barzilai A, Pavlotsky F, Trau H, Schwartz E. Treatment of cutaneous leishmaniasis with intralesional sodium stibogluconate. J Eur Acad Dermatol Venereol. 2009 Oct; 23(10): 1189-92.

[174] Sundar S, Mehta H, Suresh AV, Singh SP, Rai M, Murray HW. Amphotericin B treatment for Indian visceral leishmaniasis: conventional *versus* lipid formulations. Clin Infect Dis. 2004 Feb 1; 38(3): 377-83.

[175] Sundar S, Jha TK, Thakur CP, Sinha PK, Bhattacharya SK. Injectable paromomycin for Visceral leishmaniasis in India. N Engl J Med. 2007 Jun 21; 356(25): 2571-81.

[176] Munir A, Janjua SA, Hussain I. Clinical efficacy of intramuscular meglumine antimoniate alone and in combination with intralesional meglumine antimoniate in the treatment of old world cutaneous leishmaniasis. Acta Dermatovenerol Croat. 2008; 16(2): 60-4.

[177] Berman JD. Primary agent for leishmaniasis. Am J Trop Med Hyg. 1988 May; 38(3): 652.

[178] Berman JD. Chemotherapy for leishmaniasis: biochemical mechanisms, clinical efficacy, and future strategies. Rev Infect Dis. 1988 May-Jun; 10(3): 560-86.

[179] Herwaldt BL, Berman JD. Recommendations for treating leishmaniasis with sodium stibogluconate (Pentostam) and review of pertinent clinical studies. Am J Trop Med Hyg. 1992 Mar; 46(3): 296-306.

[180] Gonzalez U, Pinart M, Reveiz L, Alvar J. Interventions for Old World cutaneous leishmaniasis. Cochrane Database Syst Rev. 2008(4): CD005067.

[181] Olliaro PL, Guerin PJ, Gerstl S, Haaskjold AA, Rottingen JA, Sundar S. Treatment options for visceral leishmaniasis: a systematic review of clinical studies done in India, 1980-2004. Lancet Infect Dis. 2005 Dec; 5(12): 763-74.

[182] Sundar S, Rai M, Chakravarty J, Agarwal D, Agrawal N, Vaillant M, *et al.* New treatment approach in Indian visceral leishmaniasis: single-dose liposomal amphotericin B followed by short-course oral miltefosine. Clin Infect Dis. 2008 Oct 15; 47(8): 1000-6.

[183] El-On J. Current status and perspectives of the immunotherapy of leishmaniasis. The Israel Medical Association journal: IMAJ. 2009; 11(10): 623.

[184] Murray HW. Progress in the treatment of a neglected infectious disease: visceral leishmaniasis. Expert Rev Anti Infect Ther. 2004 Apr; 2(2): 279-92.

[185] Badaro R, Lobo I, Munos A, Netto EM, Modabber F, Campos-Neto A, *et al.* Immunotherapy for drug-refractory mucosal leishmaniasis. J Infect Dis. 2006 Oct 15; 194(8): 1151-9.

[186] Nicolle C. Cultures des corps de Leishman isoles de la rate dans trois cas d'anemic sptenique infantile. Bull Soc Pathol Exot. 1908; 1(121): 199-212.

[187] Handman E. Leishmaniasis: current status of vaccine development. Clin Microbiol Rev. 2001 Apr; 14(2): 229-43.

[188] Birnbaum R, Craft N. Innate immunity and Leishmania vaccination strategies. Dermatol Clin. 2011 Jan; 29(1): 89-102.

[189] Modabber F. Leishmaniasis vaccines: past, present and future. Int J Antimicrob Agents. 2010 Nov; 36 Suppl 1: S58-61.

[190] Kedzierski L. Leishmaniasis vaccine: where are we today? Journal of global infectious diseases. 2010; 2(2): 177.

[191] Allahverdiyev A, Bagirova M, Cakir Koc R, Oztel ON, Elcicek S, Ates SC, *et al.* [Approaches and problems in vaccine development against leishmaniasis]. Turkiye Parazitol Derg. 2010; 34(2): 122-30.

[192] Armijos RX, Weigel MM, Calvopina M, Hidalgo A, Cevallos W, Correa J. Safety, immunogenecity, and efficacy of an autoclaved Leishmania amazonensis vaccine plus BCG adjuvant against New World cutaneous leishmaniasis. Vaccine. 2004 Mar 12; 22(9-10): 1320-6.

[193] Nagill R, Kaur S. Vaccine candidates for leishmaniasis: a review. Int Immunopharmacol. 2011 Oct; 11(10): 1464-88.

[194] Palatnik-de-Sousa CB. Vaccines for leishmaniasis in the fore coming 25 years. Vaccine. 2008 Mar 25; 26(14): 1709-24.

[195] Velez ID, Gilchrist K, Arbelaez MP, Rojas CA, Puerta JA, Antunes CM, *et al.* Failure of a killed Leishmania amazonensis vaccine against American cutaneous leishmaniasis in Colombia. Trans R Soc Trop Med Hyg. 2005 Aug; 99(8): 593-8.

[196] Momeni AZ, Jalayer T, Emamjomeh M, Khamesipour A, Zicker F, Ghassemi RL, *et al.* A randomised, double-blind, controlled trial of a killed L. major vaccine plus BCG against zoonotic cutaneous leishmaniasis in Iran. Vaccine. 1999 Feb 5; 17(5): 466-72.

[197] Khalil EA, El Hassan AM, Zijlstra EE, Mukhtar MM, Ghalib HW, Musa B, *et al.* Autoclaved Leishmania major vaccine for prevention of visceral leishmaniasis: a randomised, double-blind, BCG-controlled trial in Sudan. Lancet. 2000 Nov 4; 356(9241): 1565-9.

[198] Sundar S, Jha TK, Thakur CP, Bhattacharya SK, Rai M. Oral miltefosine for the treatment of Indian visceral leishmaniasis. Trans R Soc Trop Med Hyg. 2006 Dec; 100 Suppl 1: S26-33.

[199] Mayrink W, Magalhaes PA, Michalick MS, da Costa CA, Lima Ade O, Melo MN, *et al.* Immunotherapy as a treatment of American cutaneous leishmaniasis: preliminary studies in Brazil. Parassitologia. 1992 Dec; 34(1-3): 159-65.

[200] Genaro O, de Toledo VP, da Costa CA, Hermeto MV, Afonso LC, Mayrink W. Vaccine for prophylaxis and immunotherapy, Brazil. Clin Dermatol. 1996 Sep-Oct; 14(5): 503-12.

[201] Convit J, Castellanos PL, Rondon A, Pinardi ME, Ulrich M, Castes M, *et al.* Immunotherapy *versus* chemotherapy in localised cutaneous leishmaniasis. Lancet. 1987 Feb 21; 1(8530): 401-5.

[202] Convit J, Ulrich M, Polegre MA, Avila A, Rodriguez N, Mazzedo MI, *et al.* Therapy of Venezuelan patients with severe mucocutaneous or early lesions of diffuse cutaneous leishmaniasis with a vaccine containing pasteurized Leishmania promastigotes and bacillus Calmette-Guerin: preliminary report. Mem Inst Oswaldo Cruz. 2004 Feb; 99(1): 57-62.

[203] Ghalib H, Modabber F. Consultation meeting on the development of therapeutic vaccines for post kala azar dermal leishmaniasis. Kinetoplastid Biol Dis. 2007; 6: 7.

[204] Daneshvar H, Coombs GH, Hagan P, Phillips RS. Leishmania mexicana and Leishmania major: attenuation of wild-type parasites and vaccination with the attenuated lines. Journal of Infectious Diseases. 2003; 187(10): 1662-8.

[205] Lemma A, Cole L. Leishmania enriettii: radiation effects and evaluation of radioattenuated organisms for vaccination. Experimental Parasitology. 1974; 35(1): 161-9.

[206] Hogg KG, Kumkate S, Mountford AP. IL-10 regulates early IL-12-mediated immune responses induced by the radiation-attenuated schistosome vaccine. International immunology. 2003; 15(12): 1451-9.

[207] Handman E. Leishmania vaccines: old and new. Parasitology today. 1997; 13(6): 236-8.

[208] Khamesipour A, Dowlati Y, Asilian A, Hashemi-Fesharki R, Javadi A, Noazin S, *et al.* Leishmanization: use of an old method for evaluation of candidate vaccines against leishmaniasis. Vaccine. 2005 May 25; 23(28): 3642-8.

[209] Coler RN, Reed SG. Second-generation vaccines against leishmaniasis. Trends Parasitol. 2005 May; 21(5): 244-9.

[210] Bhowmick S, Ravindran R, Ali N. gp63 in stable cationic liposomes confers sustained vaccine immunity to susceptible BALB/c mice infected with Leishmania donovani. Infect Immun. 2008 Mar; 76(3): 1003-15.

[211] McMahon-Pratt D, Rodriguez D, Rodriguez J, Zhang Y, Manson K, Bergman C, *et al.* Recombinant vaccinia viruses expressing GP46/M-2 protect against Leishmania infection. Infection and immunity. 1993; 61(8): 3351-9.

[212] Borja-Cabrera GP, Cruz Mendes A, Paraguai de Souza E, Hashimoto Okada LY, de A Trivellato FA, Kawasaki JKA, *et al.* Effective immunotherapy against canine visceral leishmaniasis with the FML-vaccine. Vaccine. 2004; 22(17): 2234-43.

[213] Marques-da-Silva EA, Coelho EA, Gomes DC, Vilela MC, Masioli CZ, Tavares CA, *et al.* Intramuscular immunization with p36(LACK) DNA vaccine induces IFN-gamma production but does not protect BALB/c mice against Leishmania chagasi intravenous challenge. Parasitol Res. 2005 Dec; 98(1): 67-74.

[214] Aguilar-Be I, da Silva Zardo R, de Souza EP, Borja-Cabrera GP, Rosado-Vallado M, Mut-Martin M, *et al.* Cross-protective efficacy of a prophylactic Leishmania donovani DNA vaccine against visceral and cutaneous murine leishmaniasis. Infection and immunity. 2005; 73(2): 812-9.

[215] Bedate Alonso C. Chimeric gene encoding the antigenic determinants of four proteins of L. infantum. EP Patent 1,624,063; 2009.

[216] Rafati S, Baba AA, Bakhshayesh M, Vafa M. Vaccination of BALB/c mice with Leishmania major amastigote-specific cysteine proteinase. Clinical & Experimental Immunology. 2000; 120(1): 134-8.

[217] Jensen ATR, Curtis J, Montgomery J, Handman E, Theander TG. Molecular and immunological characterisation of the glucose regulated protein 78 of Leishmania donovani1. Biochimica et Biophysica Acta (BBA)-Protein Structure and Molecular Enzymology. 2001; 1549(1): 73-87.

[218] Breton M, Tremblay MJ, Ouellette M, Papadopoulou B. Live nonpathogenic parasitic vector as a candidate vaccine against visceral leishmaniasis. Infection and immunity. 2005; 73(10): 6372-82.

[219] Stäger S, Smith DF, Kaye PM. Immunization with a recombinant stage-regulated surface protein from Leishmania donovani induces protection against visceral leishmaniasis. The Journal of Immunology. 2000; 165(12): 7064.

[220] Streit JA, Recker TJ, Donelson JE, Wilson ME. BCG expressing LCR1 of Leishmania chagasi induces protective immunity in susceptible mice. Experimental Parasitology. 2000; 94(1): 33-41.

[221] Gomes R, Teixeira C, Teixeira MJ, Oliveira F, Menezes MJ, Silva C, *et al.* Immunity to a salivary protein of a sand fly vector protects against the fatal outcome of visceral leishmaniasis in a hamster model. Proceedings of the National Academy of Sciences. 2008; 105(22): 7845.

[222] Sjölander A, Baldwin TM, Curtis JM, Lövgren Bengtsson K, Handman E. Vaccination with recombinant Parasite Surface Antigen 2 from Leishmania major induces a Th1 type of immune response but does not protect against infection. Vaccine. 1998; 16(20): 2077-84.

[223] Fernandes AP, Costa MMS, Coelho EAF, Michalick MSM, de Freitas E, Melo MN, *et al.* Protective immunity against challenge with Leishmania (Leishmania) chagasi in beagle dogs vaccinated with recombinant A2 protein. Vaccine. 2008; 26(46): 5888-95.

[224] Iborra S, Soto M, Carrión J, Alonso C, Requena JM. Vaccination with a plasmid DNA cocktail encoding the nucleosomal histones of Leishmania confers protection against murine cutaneous leishmaniosis. Vaccine. 2004; 22(29-30): 3865-76.

[225] Darrah PA, Patel DT, De Luca PM, Lindsay RWB, Davey DF, Flynn BJ, *et al.* Multifunctional TH1 cells define a correlate of vaccine-mediated protection against Leishmania major. Nature medicine. 2007; 13(7): 843-50.

[226] Fujiwara RT, Vale AM, da Silva JCF, da Costa RT, da Silva Quetz J, Martins Filho OA, *et al.* Immunogenicity in dogs of three recombinant antigens (TSA, LeIF and LmSTI1) potential vaccine candidates for canine visceral leishmaniasis. Veterinary research. 2005; 36(5-6): 827-38.

[227] Webb JR, Kaufmann D, Campos-Neto A, Reed SG. Molecular cloning of a novel protein antigen of Leishmania major that elicits a potent immune response in experimental murine leishmaniasis. The Journal of Immunology. 1996; 157(11): 5034.

[228] Campos-Neto A, Webb J, Greeson K, Coler R, Skeiky Y, Reed S. Vaccination with plasmid DNA encoding TSA/LmSTI1 leishmanial fusion proteins confers protection against Leishmania major infection in susceptible BALB/c mice. Infection and immunity. 2002; 70(6): 2828-36.

[229] Skeiky YAW, Coler RN, Brannon M, Stromberg E, Greeson K, Thomas Crane R, *et al.* Protective efficacy of a tandemly linked, multi-subunit recombinant leishmanial vaccine (Leish-111f) formulated in MPL® adjuvant. Vaccine. 2002; 20(27-28): 3292-303.

[230] Carrillo E, Crusat M, Nieto J, Chicharro C, Thomas MC, Martínez E, *et al.* Immunogenicity of HSP-70, KMP-11 and PFR-2 leishmanial antigens in the experimental model of canine visceral leishmaniasis. Vaccine. 2008; 26(15): 1902-11.

[231] Gurunathan S, Sacks DL, Brown DR, Reiner SL, Charest H, Glaichenhaus N, *et al.* Vaccination with DNA encoding the immunodominant LACK parasite antigen confers protective immunity to mice infected with Leishmania major. The Journal of experimental medicine. 1997; 186(7): 1137-47.

[232] Russell DG, Alexander J. Effective immunization against cutaneous leishmaniasis with defined membrane antigens reconstituted into liposomes [published erratum appears in J Immunol 1988 Apr 15; 140 (8): 2858]. The Journal of Immunology. 1988; 140(4): 1274.

[233] Gradoni L. An update on antileishmanial vaccine candidates and prospects for a canine Leishmania vaccine. Vet Parasitol. 2001 Sep 12; 100(1-2): 87-103.

[234] Singh B, Sundar S. Leishmaniasis: Vaccine candidates and perspectives. Vaccine. 2012 Jun 6; 30(26): 3834-42.

[235] Paraguai de Souza E, Bernardo RR, Palatnik M, Palatnik de Sousa CB. Vaccination of Balb/c mice against experimental visceral leishmaniasis with the GP36 glycoprotein antigen of Leishmania donovani. Vaccine. 2001 Apr 30; 19(23-24): 3104-15.

[236] Russo DM, Burns JM, Jr., Carvalho EM, Armitage RJ, Grabstein KH, Button LL, *et al.* Human T cell responses to gp63, a surface antigen of Leishmania. J Immunol. 1991 Nov 15; 147(10): 3575-80.

[237] Olobo JO, Anjili CO, Gicheru MM, Mbati PA, Kariuki TM, Githure JI, *et al.* Vaccination of vervet monkeys against cutaneous leishmaniosis using recombinant Leishmania 'major surface glycoprotein' (gp63). Vet Parasitol. 1995 Dec; 60(3-4): 199-212.

[238] Mougneau E, Altare F, Wakil AE, Zheng S, Coppola T, Wang ZE, *et al.* Expression cloning of a protective Leishmania antigen. Science. 1995 Apr 28; 268(5210): 563-6.

[239] Launois P, Maillard I, Pingel S, Swihart KG, Xenarios I, Acha-Orbea H, *et al.* IL-4 rapidly produced by V beta 4 V alpha 8 CD4+ T cells instructs Th2 development and susceptibility to Leishmania major in BALB/c mice. Immunity. 1997 May; 6(5): 541-9.

[240] Evans KJ, Kedzierski L. Development of Vaccines against Visceral Leishmaniasis. J Trop Med. 2012; 2012: 892817.

[241] Ramiro MJ, Zarate JJ, Hanke T, Rodriguez D, Rodriguez JR, Esteban M, *et al.* Protection in dogs against visceral leishmaniasis caused by Leishmania infantum is achieved by immunization with a heterologous prime-boost regime using DNA and vaccinia recombinant vectors expressing LACK. Vaccine. 2003 Jun 2; 21(19-20): 2474-84.

[242] Melby PC, Yang J, Zhao W, Perez LE, Cheng J. Leishmania donovani p36(LACK) DNA vaccine is highly immunogenic but not protective against experimental visceral leishmaniasis. Infect Immun. 2001 Aug; 69(8): 4719-25.

[243] Reis AB, Giunchetti RC, Carrillo E, Martins-Filho OA, Moreno J. Immunity to Leishmania and the rational search for vaccines against canine leishmaniasis. Trends Parasitol. 2010 Jul; 26(7): 341-9.

[244] Parra LE, Borja-Cabrera GP, Santos FN, Souza LO, Palatnik-de-Sousa CB, Menz I. Safety trial using the Leishmune vaccine against canine visceral leishmaniasis in Brazil. Vaccine. 2007 Mar 8; 25(12): 2180-6.

[245]   Borja-Cabrera GP, Santos FN, Santos FB, Trivellato FA, Kawasaki JK, Costa AC, *et al.* Immunotherapy with the saponin enriched-Leishmune vaccine *versus* immunochemotherapy in dogs with natural canine visceral leishmaniasis. Vaccine. 2010 Jan 8; 28(3): 597-603.

[246]   Mukhopadhyay S, Sen P, Bhattacharyya S, Majumdar S, Roy S. Immunoprophylaxis and immunotherapy against experimental visceral leishmaniasis. Vaccine. 1999 Jan 21; 17(3): 291-300.

[247]   Rodriguez-Cortes A, Ojeda A, Lopez-Fuertes L, Timon M, Altet L, Solano-Gallego L, *et al.* Vaccination with plasmid DNA encoding KMPII, TRYP, LACK and GP63 does not protect dogs against Leishmania infantum experimental challenge. Vaccine. 2007 Nov 14; 25(46): 7962-71.

[248]   Rafati S, Nakhaee A, Taheri T, Taslimi Y, Darabi H, Eravani D, *et al.* Protective vaccination against experimental canine visceral leishmaniasis using a combination of DNA and protein immunization with cysteine proteinases type I and II of L. infantum. Vaccine. 2005 May 25; 23(28): 3716-25.

[249]   Rafati S, Kariminia A, Seyde-Eslami S, Narimani M, Taheri T, Lebbatard M. Recombinant cysteine proteinases-based vaccines against Leishmania major in BALB/c mice: the partial protection relies on interferon gamma producing CD8(+) T lymphocyte activation. Vaccine. 2002 Jun 7; 20(19-20): 2439-47.

[250]   Ferreira JH, Gentil LG, Dias SS, Fedeli CE, Katz S, Barbieri CL. Immunization with the cysteine proteinase Ldccys1 gene from Leishmania (Leishmania) chagasi and the recombinant Ldccys1 protein elicits protective immune responses in a murine model of visceral leishmaniasis. Vaccine. 2008 Jan 30; 26(5): 677-85.

[251]   Rafati S, Fasel N, Masina S. Leishmania cysteine proteinases: from gene to subunit vaccine. Current Genomics. 2003; 4(3): 253-61.

[252]   Kavoosi G, Ardestani SK, Kariminia A, Alimohammadian MH. Leishmania major lipophosphoglycan: discrepancy in Toll-like receptor signaling. Exp Parasitol. 2010 Feb; 124(2): 214-8.

[253]   Pinheiro RO, Pinto EF, de Matos Guedes HL, Filho OA, de Mattos KA, Saraiva EM, *et al.* Protection against cutaneous leishmaniasis by intranasal vaccination with lipophosphoglycan. Vaccine. 2007 Mar 30; 25(14): 2716-22.

[254]   Handman E, Goding JW. The Leishmania receptor for macrophages is a lipid-containing glycoconjugate. EMBO J. 1985 Feb; 4(2): 329-36.

[255]   Russell DG, Wright SD. Complement receptor type 3 (CR3) binds to an Arg-Gly-Asp-containing region of the major surface glycoprotein, gp63, of Leishmania promastigotes. J Exp Med. 1988 Jul 1; 168(1): 279-92.

[256]   Smirlis D, Bisti SN, Xingi E, Konidou G, Thiakaki M, Soteriadou KP. Leishmania histone H1 overexpression delays parasite cell-cycle progression, parasite differentiation and reduces Leishmania infectivity in vivo. Mol Microbiol. 2006 Jun; 60(6): 1457-73.

[257]   Masina S, Zangger H, Rivier D, Fasel N. Histone H1 regulates chromatin condensation in Leishmania parasites. Exp Parasitol. 2007 May; 116(1): 83-7.

[258]   Solioz N, Blum-Tirouvanziam U, Jacquet R, Rafati S, Corradin G, Mauel J, *et al.* The protective capacities of histone H1 against experimental murine cutaneous leishmaniasis. Vaccine. 1999 Dec 10; 18(9-10): 850-9.

[259]	Saravia NG, Hazbon MH, Osorio Y, Valderrama L, Walker J, Santrich C, *et al.* Protective immunogenicity of the paraflagellar rod protein 2 of Leishmania mexicana. Vaccine. 2005 Jan 11; 23(8): 984-95.

[260]	Kedzierski L, Zhu Y, Handman E. Leishmania vaccines: progress and problems. Parasitology. 2006; 133 Suppl: S87-112.

[261]	Gradoni L, Foglia Manzillo V, Pagano A, Piantedosi D, De Luna R, Gramiccia M, *et al.* Failure of a multi-subunit recombinant leishmanial vaccine (MML) to protect dogs from Leishmania infantum infection and to prevent disease progression in infected animals. Vaccine. 2005 Nov 1; 23(45): 5245-51.

[262]	Reed SG, Coler RN, Campos-Neto A. Development of a leishmaniasis vaccine: the importance of MPL. Expert Rev Vaccines. 2003 Apr; 2(2): 239-52.

[263]	Rico AI, Angel SO, Alonso C, Requena JM. Immunostimulatory properties of the Leishmania infantum heat shock proteins HSP70 and HSP83. Mol Immunol. 1999 Dec; 36(17): 1131-9.

[264]	Bolhassani A, Rafati S. Heat-shock proteins as powerful weapons in vaccine development. Expert review of vaccines. 2008; 7(8): 1185-99.

[265]	Rafati S, Gholami E, Hassani N, Ghaemimanesh F, Taslimi Y, Taheri T, *et al.* Leishmania major heat shock protein 70 (HSP70) is not protective in murine models of cutaneous leishmaniasis and stimulates strong humoral responses in cutaneous and visceral leishmaniasis patients. Vaccine. 2007 May 22; 25(21): 4159-69.

[266]	Gamboa-Leon R, Paraguai de Souza E, Borja-Cabrera GP, Santos FN, Myashiro LM, Pinheiro RO, *et al.* Immunotherapy against visceral leishmaniasis with the nucleoside hydrolase-DNA vaccine of Leishmania donovani. Vaccine. 2006 May 29; 24(22): 4863-73.

[267]	Rosado-Vallado M, Mut-Martin M, Garcia-Miss Mdel R, Dumonteil E. Aluminium phosphate potentiates the efficacy of DNA vaccines against Leishmania mexicana. Vaccine. 2005 Nov 16; 23(46-47): 5372-9.

[268]	Khamesipour A, Rafati S, Davoudi N, Maboudi F, Modabber F. Leishmaniasis vaccine candidates for development: a global overview. Indian J Med Res. 2006 Mar; 123(3): 423-38.

[269]	Handman E, Symons FM, Baldwin TM, Curtis JM, Scheerlinck JP. Protective vaccination with promastigote surface antigen 2 from Leishmania major is mediated by a TH1 type of immune response. Infect Immun. 1995 Nov; 63(11): 4261-7.

[270]	Kedzierski L, Sakthianandeswaren A, Curtis JM, Andrews PC, Junk PC, Kedzierska K. Leishmaniasis: current treatment and prospects for new drugs and vaccines. Curr Med Chem. 2009; 16(5): 599-614.

[271]	Molano I, Alonso MG, Miron C, Redondo E, Requena JM, Soto M, *et al.* A Leishmania infantum multi-component antigenic protein mixed with live BCG confers protection to dogs experimentally infected with L. infantum. Vet Immunol Immunopathol. 2003 Mar 20; 92(1-2): 1-13.

[272]	Scott P, Pearce E, Natovitz P, Sher A. Vaccination against cutaneous leishmaniasis in a murine model. II. Immunologic properties of protective and nonprotective subfractions of soluble promastigote extract. J Immunol. 1987 Nov 1; 139(9): 3118-25.

[273]	Stager S, Smith DF, Kaye PM. Immunization with a recombinant stage-regulated surface protein from Leishmania donovani induces protection against visceral leishmaniasis. J Immunol. 2000 Dec 15; 165(12): 7064-71.

[274] Jensen AT, Curtis J, Montgomery J, Handman E, Theander TG. Molecular and immunological characterisation of the glucose regulated protein 78 of Leishmania donovani(1). Biochim Biophys Acta. 2001 Sep 10; 1549(1): 73-87.

[275] Jensen AT, Ismail A, Gaafar A, El Hassan AM, Theander TG. Humoral and cellular immune responses to glucose regulated protein 78 -- a novel Leishmania donovani antigen. Trop Med Int Health. 2002 May; 7(5): 471-6.

[276] Elnaiem DE, Meneses C, Slotman M, Lanzaro GC. Genetic variation in the sand fly salivary protein, SP-15, a potential vaccine candidate against Leishmania major. Insect Mol Biol. 2005 Apr; 14(2): 145-50.

[277] Rogers KA, DeKrey GK, Mbow ML, Gillespie RD, Brodskyn CI, Titus RG. Type 1 and type 2 responses to Leishmania major. FEMS Microbiol Lett. 2002 Mar 19; 209(1): 1-7.

[278] Ghosh A, Zhang WW, Matlashewski G. Immunization with A2 protein results in a mixed Th1/Th2 and a humoral response which protects mice against Leishmania donovani infections. Vaccine. 2001 Oct 12; 20(1-2): 59-66.

[279] Coelho EA, Tavares CA, Carvalho FA, Chaves KF, Teixeira KN, Rodrigues RC, *et al.* Immune responses induced by the Leishmania (Leishmania) donovani A2 antigen, but not by the LACK antigen, are protective against experimental Leishmania (Leishmania) amazonensis infection. Infect Immun. 2003 Jul; 71(7): 3988-94.

[280] Fernandes AP, Costa MM, Coelho EA, Michalick MS, de Freitas E, Melo MN, *et al.* Protective immunity against challenge with Leishmania (Leishmania) chagasi in beagle dogs vaccinated with recombinant A2 protein. Vaccine. 2008 Oct 29; 26(46): 5888-95.

[281] Garg R, Dube A. Animal models for vaccine studies for visceral leishmaniasis. Indian J Med Res. 2006 Mar; 123(3): 439-54.

[282] Rachamim N, Jaffe CL. Pure protein from Leishmania donovani protects mice against both cutaneous and visceral leishmaniasis. J Immunol. 1993 Mar 15; 150(6): 2322-31.

[283] Jaffe CL, Rachamim N, Sarfstein R. Characterization of two proteins from Leishmania donovani and their use for vaccination against visceral leishmaniasis. J Immunol. 1990 Jan 15; 144(2): 699-706.

[284] Jakob T, Walker PS, Krieg AM, Udey MC, Vogel JC. Activation of cutaneous dendritic cells by CpG-containing oligodeoxynucleotides: a role for dendritic cells in the augmentation of Th1 responses by immunostimulatory DNA. The Journal of Immunology. 1998; 161(6): 3042.

[285] Moll H, Berberich C. Dendritic cell-based vaccination strategies: induction of protective immunity against leishmaniasis. Immunobiology. 2001 Dec; 204(5): 659-66.

[286] Flohe SB, Bauer C, Flohe S, Moll H. Antigen-pulsed epidermal Langerhans cells protect susceptible mice from infection with the intracellular parasite Leishmania major. Eur J Immunol. 1998 Nov; 28(11): 3800-11.

[287] Berberich C, Ramirez-Pineda JR, Hambrecht C, Alber G, Skeiky YA, Moll H. Dendritic cell (DC)-based protection against an intracellular pathogen is dependent upon DC-derived IL-12 and can be induced by molecularly defined antigens. J Immunol. 2003 Mar 15; 170(6): 3171-9.

[288] Ramirez-Pineda JR, Frohlich A, Berberich C, Moll H. Dendritic cells (DC) activated by CpG DNA *ex vivo* are potent inducers of host resistance to an intracellular pathogen that is independent of IL-12 derived from the immunizing DC. J Immunol. 2004 May 15; 172(10): 6281-9.

[289] Nandan D, Camargo de Oliveira C, Moeenrezakhanlou A, Lopez M, Silverman JM, Subek J, *et al.* Myeloid cell IL-10 production in response to leishmania involves inactivation of glycogen synthase kinase-3beta downstream of phosphatidylinositol-3 kinase. J Immunol. 2012 Jan 1; 188(1): 367-78.

[290] Baldwin T, Henri S, Curtis J, O'Keeffe M, Vremec D, Shortman K, *et al.* Dendritic cell populations in Leishmania major-infected skin and draining lymph nodes. Infect Immun. 2004 Apr; 72(4): 1991-2001.

[291] Croft SL, Barrett MP, Urbina JA. Chemotherapy of trypanosomiases and leishmaniasis. Trends Parasitol. 2005 Nov; 21(11): 508-12.

[292] Natera S, Machuca C, Padron-Nieves M, Romero A, Diaz E, Ponte-Sucre A. Leishmania spp.: proficiency of drug-resistant parasites. Int J Antimicrob Agents. 2007 Jun; 29(6): 637-42.

[293] Davis AJ, Kedzierski L. Recent advances in antileishmanial drug development. Curr Opin Investig Drugs. 2005 Feb; 6(2): 163-9.

[294] Perez-Victoria FJ, Sanchez-Canete MP, Seifert K, Croft SL, Sundar S, Castanys S, *et al.* Mechanisms of experimental resistance of Leishmania to miltefosine: Implications for clinical use. Drug Resist Updat. 2006 Feb-Apr; 9(1-2): 26-39.

[295] Rakotomanga M, Saint-Pierre-Chazalet M, Loiseau PM. Alteration of fatty acid and sterol metabolism in miltefosine-resistant Leishmania donovani promastigotes and consequences for drug-membrane interactions. Antimicrob Agents Chemother. 2005 Jul; 49(7): 2677-86.

[296] Salem MM, Werbovetz KA. Natural products from plants as drug candidates and lead compounds against leishmaniasis and trypanosomiasis. Current medicinal chemistry. 2006; 13(21): 2571-98.

[297] Croft SL, Seifert K, Yardley V. Current scenario of drug development for leishmaniasis. Indian J Med Res. 2006 Mar; 123(3): 399-410.

[298] Sundar S, Chatterjee M. Visceral leishmaniasis - current therapeutic modalities. Indian J Med Res. 2006 Mar; 123(3): 345-52.

[299] Werbovetz K. Diamidines as antitrypanosomal, antileishmanial and antimalarial agents. Curr Opin Investig Drugs. 2006 Feb; 7(2): 147-57.

[300] Linares GE, Ravaschino EL, Rodriguez JB. Progresses in the field of drug design to combat tropical protozoan parasitic diseases. Curr Med Chem. 2006; 13(3): 335-60.

[301] Cortes-Selva F, Jimenez IA, Munoz-Martinez F, Campillo M, Bazzocchi IL, Pardo L, *et al.* Dihydro-beta-agarofuran sesquiterpenes: a new class of reversal agents of the multidrug resistance phenotype mediated by P-glycoprotein in the protozoan parasite Leishmania. Curr Pharm Des. 2005; 11(24): 3125-39.

[302] Pink R, Hudson A, Mouries MA, Bendig M. Opportunities and challenges in antiparasitic drug discovery. Nat Rev Drug Discov. 2005 Sep; 4(9): 727-40.

[303] Rocha LG, Almeida JR, Macedo RO, Barbosa-Filho JM. A review of natural products with antileishmanial activity. Phytomedicine. 2005 Jun; 12(6-7): 514-35.

[304] Singh RK, Pandey HP, Sundar S. Visceral leishmaniasis (kala-azar): challenges ahead. Indian J Med Res. 2006 Mar; 123(3): 331-44.

[305] Wyllie S, Cunningham ML, Fairlamb AH. Dual action of antimonial drugs on thiol redox metabolism in the human pathogen Leishmania donovani. J Biol Chem. 2004 Sep 17; 279(38): 39925-32.

[306] Rosen BP. Biochemistry of arsenic detoxification. FEBS Lett. 2002 Oct 2; 529(1): 86-92.

[307] Denton H, McGregor JC, Coombs GH. Reduction of antileishmanial pentavalent antimonial drugs by a parasite-specific thiol-dependent reductase, TDR1. Biochem J. 2004 Jul 15; 381(Pt 2): 405-12.

[308] Zhou Y, Messier N, Ouellette M, Rosen BP, Mukhopadhyay R. Leishmania major LmACR2 is a pentavalent antimony reductase that confers sensitivity to the drug pentostam. J Biol Chem. 2004 Sep 3; 279(36): 37445-51.

[309] Ferreira Cdos S, Martins PS, Demicheli C, Brochu C, Ouellette M, Frezard F. Thiol-induced reduction of antimony(V) into antimony(III): a comparative study with trypanothione, cysteinyl-glycine, cysteine and glutathione. Biometals. 2003 Sep; 16(3): 441-6.

[310] Gourbal B, Sonuc N, Bhattacharjee H, Legare D, Sundar S, Ouellette M, et al. Drug uptake and modulation of drug resistance in Leishmania by an aquaglyceroporin. J Biol Chem. 2004 Jul 23; 279(30): 31010-7.

[311] El Fadili K, Messier N, Leprohon P, Roy G, Guimond C, Trudel N, et al. Role of the ABC transporter MRPA (PGPA) in antimony resistance in Leishmania infantum axenic and intracellular amastigotes. Antimicrob Agents Chemother. 2005 May; 49(5): 1988-93.

[312] Croft SL, Sundar S, Fairlamb AH. Drug resistance in leishmaniasis. Clin Microbiol Rev. 2006 Jan; 19(1): 111-26.

[313] Mehta A, Shaha C. Apoptotic death in Leishmania donovani promastigotes in response to respiratory chain inhibition: complex II inhibition results in increased pentamidine cytotoxicity. J Biol Chem. 2004 Mar 19; 279(12): 11798-813.

[314] Croft SL, Olliaro P. Leishmaniasis chemotherapy--challenges and opportunities. Clin Microbiol Infect. 2011 Oct; 17(10): 1478-83.

[315] Jhingran A, Chawla B, Saxena S, Barrett MP, Madhubala R. Paromomycin: uptake and resistance in Leishmania donovani. Mol Biochem Parasitol. 2009 Apr; 164(2): 111-7.

[316] Yeates C. Sitamaquine (GlaxoSmithKline/Walter Reed Army Institute). Curr Opin Investig Drugs. 2002 Oct; 3(10): 1446-52.

[317] Singh N, Kumar M, Singh RK. Leishmaniasis: Current status of available drugs and new potential drug targets. Asian Pac J Trop Med. 2012 Jun; 5(6): 485-97.

[318] Papadopoulou B, Kündig C, Singh A, Ouellette M. Drug resistance in Leishmania: similarities and differences to other organisms. Drug Resistance Updates. 1998; 1(4): 266-78.

[319] Croft SL, Neal RA, Pendergast W, Chan JH. The activity of alkyl phosphorylcholines and related derivatives against Leishmania donovani. Biochem Pharmacol. 1987 Aug 15; 36(16): 2633-6.

[320] Kuhlencord A, Maniera T, Eibl H, Unger C. Hexadecylphosphocholine: oral treatment of visceral leishmaniasis in mice. Antimicrob Agents Chemother. 1992 Aug; 36(8): 1630-4.

[321] Wheelan P, Clay KL. Albumin and fatty acid effects on the stimulated production of 1-O-hexadecyl-2-acetyl-sn-glycero-3-phosphocholine (PAF) by human polymorphonuclear leukocytes. Biochim Biophys Acta. 1992 Aug 19; 1127(3): 284-92.

[322] Loiseau PM, Bories C. Mechanisms of drug action and drug resistance in Leishmania as basis for therapeutic target identification and design of antileishmanial modulators. Curr Top Med Chem. 2006; 6(5): 539-50.

[323] Poli A, Sozzi S, Guidi G, Bandinelli P, Mancianti F. Comparison of aminosidine (paromomycin) and sodium stibogluconate for treatment of canine leishmaniasis. Vet Parasitol. 1997 Aug; 71(4): 263-71.

[324] Maarouf M, Lawrence F, Croft SL, Robert-Gero M. Ribosomes of Leishmania are a target for the aminoglycosides. Parasitol Res. 1995; 81(5): 421-5.

[325] Hirokawa G, Kaji H, Kaji A. Inhibition of antiassociation activity of translation initiation factor 3 by paromomycin. Antimicrob Agents Chemother. 2007 Jan; 51(1): 175-80.

[326] Coimbra ES, Goncalves-da-Costa SC, Costa BL, Giarola NL, Rezende-Soares FA, Fessel MR, et al. A Leishmania (L.) amazonensis ATP diphosphohydrolase isoform and potato apyrase share epitopes: antigenicity and correlation with disease progression. Parasitology. 2008 Mar; 135(3): 327-35.

[327] Pfaller MA, Marr JJ. Antileishmanial effect of allopurinol. Antimicrob Agents Chemother. 1974 May; 5(5): 469-72.

[328] Shapiro TA, Were JB, Danso K, Nelson DJ, Desjardins RE, Pamplin CL, 3rd. Pharmacokinetics and metabolism of allopurinol riboside. Clin Pharmacol Ther. 1991 May; 49(5): 506-14.

[329] Najarian D, English J. Imiquimod cream: a new multipurpose topical therapy for dermatology. P AND T. 2003; 28(2): 122-6.

[330] Freitas-Junior LH, Chatelain E, Kim HA, Siqueira-Neto JL. Visceral leishmaniasis treatment: What do we have, what do we need and how to deliver it? Int J Parasitol Drugs Drug Resist. 2012 Jan 28; 2: 11-19. eCollection 2012 Dec. Review.

[331] van Griensven J, Balasegaram M, Meheus F, Alvar J, Lynen L, Boelaert M. Combination therapy for visceral leishmaniasis. Lancet Infect Dis. 2010Mar; 10(3): 184-94.

[332] Melaku Y, Collin S.M., Keus K, Gatluak F, Ritmeijer K, et al. (2007) Treatment of kala-azar in Southern Sudan using a 17 dasy regimen of Sodium Stibogluconate combined with Paromomycin: A retrospective comparison with 30-day Sodium Stibogluconate monotherapy. Am J Trop Med Hyg 77(1), 2007, 89–94.

[333] Pal C, Raha M, Basu A, Roy KC, Gupta A, Ghosh M, Sahu NP, Banerjee S, Mandal NB, Bandyopadhyay S. Combination therapy with indolylquinoline derivative and sodium antimony gluconate cures established visceral leishmaniasis in hamsters. Antimicrob Agents Chemother. 2002 Jan; 46(1): 259-61.

[334] Thakur CP, Olliaro P, Gothoskar S, Bhowmick S, Choudhury BK, Prasad S, Kumar M, Verma BB. Treatment of visceral leishmaniasis (kala-azar) with aminosidine (=paromomycin)-antimonial combinations, a pilot study in Bihar, India. Trans R Soc Trop Med Hyg. 1992 Nov-Dec; 86(6): 615-6.

[335] Sundar S, Rai M, Chakravarty J, Agarwal D, Agrawal N, Vaillant M, Olliaro P, Murray HW. New treatment approach in Indian visceral leishmaniasis: single-dose liposomal amphotericin B followed by short-course oral miltefosine. Clin Infect Dis. 2008 Oct 15; 47(8): 1000-6.

[336] Alkhawajah A. Recent trends in the treatment of cutaneous leishmaniasis. Ann Saudi Med. 1998; 18(5): 412-6.

[337] Anjili C, Langat B, Ngumbi P, Mbati PA, Githure J, Tonui WK. Effects of anti-Leishmania monoclonal antibodies on the development of Leishmania major in Phlebotomus duboscqi (Diptera: Psychodidae). East Afr Med J. 2006 Feb; 83(2): 72-8.

[338] Carmody M, Murphy B, Byrne B, Power P, Rai D, Rawlings B, et al. Biosynthesis of amphotericin derivatives lacking exocyclic carboxyl groups. J Biol Chem. 2005 Oct 14; 280(41): 34420-6.

[339] Besteiro S, Williams RAM, Coombs GH, Mottram JC. Protein turnover and differentiation in Leishmania. International journal for parasitology. 2007; 37(10): 1063-75.

[340] Ivens AC, Peacock CS, Worthey EA, Murphy L, Aggarwal G, Berriman M, *et al*. The genome of the kinetoplastid parasite, Leishmania major. Science. 2005 Jul 15; 309(5733): 436-42.

[341] Robertson CD. The *Leishmania mexicana* proteasome. Molecular and biochemical parasitology. 1999; 103(1): 49-60.

[342] Mottram JC, Coombs GH, Alexander J. Cysteine peptidases as virulence factors of *Leishmania*. Current opinion in microbiology. 2004; 7(4): 375-81.

[343] Withers-Martinez C, Jean L, Blackman MJ. Subtilisin like proteases of the malaria parasite. Molecular microbiology. 2004; 53(1): 55-63.

[344] Silva-Lopez RE, Morgado-Diaz JA, Chavez MA, Giovanni-De-Simone S. Effects of serine protease inhibitors on viability and morphology of Leishmania (Leishmania) amazonensis promastigotes. Parasitol Res. 2007 Nov; 101(6): 1627-35.

[345] Tavares J, Ouaissi A, Lin PK, Tomas A, Cordeiro-da-Silva A. Differential effects of polyamine derivative compounds against Leishmania infantum promastigotes and axenic amastigotes. Int J Parasitol. 2005 May; 35(6): 637-46.

[346] Vannier-Santos MA, Menezes D, Oliveira MF, de Mello FG. The putrescine analogue 1,4-diamino-2-butanone affects polyamine synthesis, transport, ultrastructure and intracellular survival in Leishmania amazonensis. Microbiology. 2008 Oct; 154(Pt 10): 3104-11.

[347] Kandpal M, Tekwani BL, Chauhan P, Bhaduri A. Correlation between inhibition of growth and arginine transport of *Leishmania donovani* promastigotes *in vitro* by diamidines. Life sciences. 1996; 59(7): PL175-PL80.

[348] Roberts SC, Jiang Y, Gasteier J, Frydman B, Marton LJ, Heby O, *et al*. Leishmania donovani polyamine biosynthetic enzyme overproducers as tools to investigate the mode of action of cytotoxic polyamine analogs. Antimicrobial agents and chemotherapy. 2007; 51(2): 438-45.

[349] Baiocco P, Colotti G, Franceschini S, Ilari A. Molecular basis of antimony treatment in leishmaniasis. J Med Chem. 2009 Apr 23; 52(8): 2603-12.

[350] Heby O, Persson L, Rentala M. Targeting the polyamine biosynthetic enzymes: a promising approach to therapy of African sleeping sickness, Chagas' disease, and leishmaniasis. Amino Acids. 2007 Aug; 33(2): 359-66.

[351] Reguera RM, Tekwani BL, Balana-Fouce R. Polyamine transport in parasites: a potential target for new antiparasitic drug development. Comp Biochem Physiol C Toxicol Pharmacol. 2005 Feb; 140(2): 151-64.

[352] Plewes KA, Barr SD, Gedamu L. Iron superoxide dismutases targeted to the glycosomes of Leishmania chagasi are important for survival. Infection and immunity. 2003; 71(10): 5910-20.

[353] Bringaud F, Riviere L, Coustou V. Energy metabolism of trypanosomatids: adaptation to available carbon sources. Mol Biochem Parasitol. 2006 Sep; 149(1): 1-9.

[354] Krauth-Siegel RL, Inhoff O. Parasite-specific trypanothione reductase as a drug target molecule. Parasitology research. 2003; 90: 77-85.

[355] Krauth-Siegel RL, Meiering SK, Schmidt H. The parasite-specific trypanothione metabolism of trypanosoma and leishmania. Biological chemistry. 2003; 384(4): 539.

[356] Cunningham ML, Titus RG, Turco SJ, Beverley SM. Regulation of differentiation to the infective stage of the protozoan parasite Leishmania major by tetrahydrobiopterin. Science. 2001 Apr 13; 292(5515): 285-7.

[357]   Ascenzi P, Bocedi A, Visca P, Antonini G, Gradoni L. Catalytic properties of cysteine proteinases from Trypanosoma cruzi and Leishmania infantum: a pre-steady-state and steady-state study. Biochem Biophys Res Commun. 2003 Sep 26; 309(3): 659-65.

[358]   Grant KM, Dunion MH, Yardley V, Skaltsounis AL, Marko D, Eisenbrand G, *et al.* Inhibitors of Leishmania mexicana CRK3 cyclin-dependent kinase: chemical library screen and antileishmanial activity. Antimicrob Agents Chemother. 2004 Aug; 48(8): 3033-42.

[359]   Affranchino JL, Gonzalez SA, Pays E. Isolation of a mitotic-like cyclin homologue from the protozoan Trypanosoma brucei. Gene. 1993 Sep 30; 132(1): 75-82.

[360]   Hassan P, Fergusson D, Grant KM, Mottram JC. The CRK3 protein kinase is essential for cell cycle progression of Leishmania mexicana. Molecular and biochemical parasitology. 2001; 113(2): 189-98.

[361]   Xingi E, Smirlis D, Myrianthopoulos V, Magiatis P, Grant KM, Meijer L, *et al.* 6-Br-5methylindirubin-3'oxime (5-Me-6-BIO) targeting the leishmanial glycogen synthase kinase-3 (GSK-3) short form affects cell-cycle progression and induces apoptosis-like death: exploitation of GSK-3 for treating leishmaniasis. Int J Parasitol. 2009 Oct; 39(12): 1289-303.

[362]   Wiese M, Wang Q, Gorcke I. Identification of mitogen-activated protein kinase homologues from Leishmania mexicana. Int J Parasitol. 2003 Dec; 33(14): 1577-87.

[363]   Wiese M. Leishmania MAP kinases-Familiar proteins in an unusual context. International journal for parasitology. 2007; 37(10): 1053-62.

[364]   Wiese M, Görcke I. Homologues of LMPK, a mitogen-activated protein kinase from Leishmania mexicana, in different Leishmania species. Medical Microbiology and Immunology. 2001; 190(1): 19-22.

[365]   Lorente SO, Jimenez CJ, Gros L, Yardley V, de Luca-Fradley K, Croft SL, *et al.* Preparation of transition-state analogues of sterol 24-methyl transferase as potential anti-parasitics. Bioorg Med Chem. 2005 Sep 15; 13(18): 5435-53.

[366]   Liang PH, Anderson KS. Substrate channeling and domain-domain interactions in bifunctional thymidylate synthase-dihydrofolate reductase. Biochemistry. 1998; 37(35): 12195-205.

[367]   Senkovich O, Schormann N, Chattopadhyay D. Structures of dihydrofolate reductase-thymidylate synthase of Trypanosoma cruzi in the folate-free state and in complex with two antifolate drugs, trimetrexate and methotrexate. Acta Crystallogr D Biol Crystallogr. 2009 Jul; 65(Pt 7): 704-16.

[368]   Zuccotto F, Martin AC, Laskowski RA, Thornton JM, Gilbert IH. Dihydrofolate reductase: a potential drug target in trypanosomes and leishmania. J Comput Aided Mol Des. 1998 May; 12(3): 241-57.

[369]   Kuntz ID. Structure-based strategies for drug design and discovery. Science. 1992 Aug 21; 257(5073): 1078-82.

[370]   Veras P, Brodskyn C, Balestieri F, Freitas LAR, Ramos A, Queiroz A, *et al.* A dhfr-ts-Leishmania major knockout mutant cross-protects against Leishmania amazonensis. Memórias do Instituto Oswaldo Cruz. 1999; 94(4): 491-6.

[371]   Bello AR, Nare B, Freedman D, Hardy L, Beverley SM. PTR1: a reductase mediating salvage of oxidized pteridines and methotrexate resistance in the protozoan parasite Leishmania major. Proc Natl Acad Sci U S A. 1994 Nov 22; 91(24): 11442-6.

[372] Wang J, Leblanc E, Chang CF, Papadopoulou B, Bray T, Whiteley JM, *et al*. Pterin and folate reduction by the Leishmania tarentolae H locus short-chain dehydrogenase/reductase PTR1. Arch Biochem Biophys. 1997 Jun 15; 342(2): 197-202.

[373] Schneider E, Hsiang YH, Liu LF. DNA topoisomerases as anticancer drug targets. Adv Pharmacol. 1990; 21(7): 149-83.

[374] Heisig P. Inhibitors of bacterial topoisomerases: mechanisms of action and resistance and clinical aspects. Planta medica. 2001; 67(1): 3-12.

[375] Singh G, Jayanarayan KG, Dey CS. Novobiocin induces apoptosis-like cell death in topoisomerase II over-expressing arsenite resistant Leishmania donovani. Mol Biochem Parasitol. 2005 May; 141(1): 57-69.

[376] Rosypal AC, Tripp S, Lewis S, Francis J, Stoskopf MK, Larsen RS, *et al*. Survey of antibodies to Trypanosoma cruzi and Leishmania spp. in gray and red fox populations from North Carolina and Virginia. J Parasitol. 2010 Dec; 96(6): 1230-1.

[377] Kosec G, Alvarez VE, Aguero F, Sanchez D, Dolinar M, Turk B, *et al*. Metacaspases of Trypanosoma cruzi: possible candidates for programmed cell death mediators. Mol Biochem Parasitol. 2006 Jan; 145(1): 18-28.

[378] Lee N, Gannavaram S, Selvapandiyan A, Debrabant A. Characterization of metacaspases with trypsin-like activity and their putative role in programmed cell death in the protozoan parasite Leishmania. Eukaryotic cell. 2007; 6(10): 1745-57.

[379] Denise H, Poot J, Jimenez M, Ambit A, Herrmann DC, Vermeulen AN, *et al*. Studies on the CPA cysteine peptidase in the Leishmania infantum genome strain JPCM5. BMC Mol Biol. 2006; 7: 42.

[380] González IJ, Desponds C, Schaff C, Mottram JC, Fasel N. *Leishmania major* metacaspase can replace yeast metacaspase in programmed cell death and has arginine-specific cysteine peptidase activity. International journal for parasitology. 2007; 37(2): 161-72.

[381] Meslin B, Zalila H, Fasel N, Picot S, Bienvenu AL. Are protozoan metacaspases potential parasite killers? Parasit Vectors. 2011; 4: 26.

[382] Alvar J, Aparicio P, Aseffa A, Den Boer M, Canavate C, Dedet JP, *et al*. The relationship between leishmaniasis and AIDS: the second 10 years. Clinical microbiology reviews. 2008 Apr; 21(2): 334-59, table of contents.

[383] Desjeux P, Alvar J. Leishmania/HIV co-infections: epidemiology in Europe. Annals of tropical medicine and parasitology. 2003 Oct; 97 Suppl 1: 3-15.

[384] Lyons S, Veeken H, Long J. Visceral leishmaniasis and HIV in Tigray, Ethiopia. Tropical medicine & international health: TM & IH. 2003 Aug; 8(8): 733-9.

[385] Laguna F. Treatment of leishmaniasis in HIV-positive patients. Annals of tropical medicine and parasitology. 2003 Oct; 97 Suppl 1: 135-42.

[386] Hurissa Z, Gebre-Silassie S, Hailu W, Tefera T, Lalloo DG, Cuevas LE, *et al*. Clinical characteristics and treatment outcome of patients with visceral leishmaniasis and HIV co-infection in northwest Ethiopia. Tropical medicine & international health: TM & IH. 2010 Jul; 15(7): 848-55.

[387] Waheed AA, Ablan SD, Soheilian F, Nagashima K, Ono A, Schaffner CP, *et al*. Inhibition of human immunodeficiency virus type 1 assembly and release by the cholesterol-binding compound amphotericin B methyl ester: evidence for Vpu dependence. Journal of virology. 2008 Oct; 82(19): 9776-81.

[388] Jimenez-Exposito MJ, Alonso-Villaverde C, Sarda P, Masana L. Visceral leishmaniasis in HIV-infected patients with non-detectable HIV-1 viral load after highly active antiretroviral therapy. AIDS. 1999 Jan 14; 13(1): 152-3.

[389] Sinha PK, van Griensven J, Pandey K, Kumar N, Verma N, Mahajan R, *et al*. Liposomal amphotericin B for visceral leishmaniasis in human immunodeficiency virus-coinfected patients: 2-year treatment outcomes in Bihar, India. Clin Infect Dis. 2011 Oct; 53(7): e91-8.

[390] Balana-Fouce R, Reguera RM, Cubria JC, Ordonez D. The pharmacology of leishmaniasis. Gen Pharmacol. 1998 Apr; 30(4): 435-43.

[391] Knighton DR, Kan CC, Howland E, Janson CA, Hostomska Z, Welsh KM, *et al*. Structure of and kinetic channelling in bifunctional dihydrofolate reductase-thymidylate synthase. Nat Struct Biol. 1994 Mar; 1(3): 186-94.

[392] Krieger S, Schwarz W, Ariyanayagam MR, Fairlamb AH, Krauth-Siegel RL, Clayton C. Trypanosomes lacking trypanothione reductase are avirulent and show increased sensitivity to oxidative stress. Mol Microbiol. 2000 Feb; 35(3): 542-52.

[393] Dumas C, Ouellette M, Tovar J, Cunningham ML, Fairlamb AH, Tamar S, *et al*. Disruption of the trypanothione reductase gene of Leishmania decreases its ability to survive oxidative stress in macrophages. EMBO J. 1997 May 15; 16(10): 2590-8.

[394] Fairlamb AH, Henderson GB, Cerami A. Trypanothione is the primary target for arsenical drugs against African trypanosomes. Proc Natl Acad Sci U S A. 1989 Apr; 86(8): 2607-11.

[395] McKerrow JH, Sun E, Rosenthal PJ, Bouvier J. The proteases and pathogenicity of parasitic protozoa. Annu Rev Microbiol. 1993; 47: 821-53.

[396] McKerrow JH, McGrath ME, Engel JC. The cysteine protease of Trypanosoma cruzi as a model for antiparasite drug design. Parasitol Today. 1995 Aug; 11(8): 279-82.

[397] Coombs GH, Mottram JC. Parasite proteinases and amino acid metabolism: possibilities for chemotherapeutic exploitation. Parasitology. 1997; 114 Suppl: S61-80.

[398] Brochu C, Haimeur A, Ouellette M. The heat shock protein HSP70 and heat shock cognate protein HSC70 contribute to antimony tolerance in the protozoan parasite leishmania. Cell Stress Chaperones. 2004 Autumn; 9(3): 294-303.

[399] Maltezou HC. Drug resistance in visceral leishmaniasis. J Biomed Biotechnol. 2010; 2010: 617521.

[400] Ouellette M, Drummelsmith J, Papadopoulou B. Leishmaniasis: drugs in the clinic, resistance and new developments. Drug Resist Update. 2004 Aug-Oct; 7(4-5): 257-66.

[401] Hay RJ. Antifungal therapy and the new azole compounds. J Antimicrob Chemother. 1991 Jul; 28 Suppl A: 35-46.

[402] Ouellette M, Légaré D, Haimeur A, Grondin K, Roy G, Brochu C, *et al*. ABC transporters in Leishmania and their role in drug resistance. Drug Resistance Updates. 1998; 1(1): 43-8.

[403] Singh AK, Papadopoulou B, Ouellette M. Gene amplification in amphotericin B-resistant Leishmania tarentolae. Exp Parasitol. 2001 Nov; 99(3): 141-7.

[404] Mbongo N, Loiseau PM, Billion MA, Robert-Gero M. Mechanism of amphotericin B resistance in Leishmania donovani promastigotes. Antimicrob Agents Chemother. 1998 Feb; 42(2): 352-7.

[405] Perez-Victoria FJ, Gamarro F, Ouellette M, Castanys S. Functional cloning of the miltefosine transporter. A novel P-type phospholipid translocase from Leishmania involved in drug resistance. J Biol Chem. 2003 Dec 12; 278(50): 49965-71.

[406] Perez-Victoria JM, Parodi-Talice A, Torres C, Gamarro F, Castanys S. ABC transporters in the protozoan parasite Leishmania. Int Microbiol. 2001 Sep; 4(3): 159-66.

[407]   Basselin M, Denise H, Coombs GH, Barrett MP. Resistance to pentamidine in Leishmania mexicana involves exclusion of the drug from the mitochondrion. Antimicrob Agents Chemother. 2002 Dec; 46(12): 3731-8.

[408]   Coelho AC, Beverley SM, Cotrim PC. Functional genetic identification of PRP1, an ABC transporter superfamily member conferring pentamidine resistance in Leishmania major. Mol Biochem Parasitol. 2003 Aug 31; 130(2): 83-90.

[409]   Roberts CW, McLeod R, Rice DW, Ginger M, Chance ML, Goad LJ. Fatty acid and sterol metabolism: potential antimicrobial targets in apicomplexan and trypanosomatid parasitic protozoa. Mol Biochem Parasitol. 2003 Feb; 126(2): 129-42.

[410]   Ouellette M, Drummelsmith J, Papadopoulou B. Leishmaniasis: drugs in the clinic, resistance and new developments. Drug Resist Updat. 2004 Aug-Oct; 7(4-5): 257-66.

[411]   Rakotomanga M, Loiseau PM, Saint-Pierre-Chazalet M. Hexadecylphosphocholine interaction with lipid monolayers. Biochim Biophys Acta. 2004 Mar 9; 1661(2): 212-8.

[412]   Dodge MA, Waller RF, Chow LM, Zaman MM, Cotton LM, McConville MJ, *et al.* Localization and activity of multidrug resistance protein 1 in the secretory pathway of Leishmania parasites. Mol Microbiol. 2004 Mar; 51(6): 1563-75.

[413]   Maarouf M, de Kouchkovsky Y, Brown S, Petit PX, Robert-Gero M. In vivo interference of paromomycin with mitochondrial activity of Leishmania. Exp Cell Res. 1997 May 1; 232(2): 339-48.

[414]   Gueiros-Filho FJ, Beverley SM. On the introduction of genetically modified Leishmania outside the laboratory. Exp Parasitol. 1994 Jun; 78(4): 425-8.

[415]   Bories C, Cojean S, Huteau F, Loiseau PM. Selection and phenotype characterisation of sitamaquine-resistant promastigotes of Leishmania donovani. Biomed Pharmacother. 2008 Mar; 62(3): 164-7.

[416]   Garnier T, Brown MB, Lawrence MJ, Croft SL. In-vitro and in-vivo studies on a topical formulation of sitamaquine dihydrochloride for cutaneous leishmaniasis. J Pharm Pharmacol. 2006 Aug; 58(8): 1043-54.

[417]   Sanglard D, Kuchler K, Ischer F, Pagani JL, Monod M, Bille J. Mechanisms of resistance to azole antifungal agents in Candida albicans isolates from AIDS patients involve specific multidrug transporters. Antimicrob Agents Chemother. 1995 Nov; 39(11): 2378-86.

[418]   Sanglard D, Ischer F, Koymans L, Bille J. Amino acid substitutions in the cytochrome P-450 lanosterol 14alpha-demethylase (CYP51A1) from azole-resistant Candida albicans clinical isolates contribute to resistance to azole antifungal agents. Antimicrob Agents Chemother. 1998 Feb; 42(2): 241-53.

[419]   Ramos H, Saint-Pierre-Chazalet M, Bolard J, Cohen BE. Effect of ketoconazole on lethal action of amphotericin B on Leishmania mexicana promastigotes. Antimicrob Agents Chemother. 1994 May; 38(5): 1079-84.

[420]   Basselin M, Coombs GH, Barrett MP. Putrescine and spermidine transport in Leishmania. Mol Biochem Parasitol. 2000 Jun; 109(1): 37-46.

[421]   Aronow B, Kaur K, McCartan K, Ullman B. Two high affinity nucleoside transporters in Leishmania donovani. Mol Biochem Parasitol. 1987 Jan 2; 22(1): 29-37.

[422]   Kerby BR, Detke S. Reduced purine accumulation is encoded on an amplified DNA in Leishmania mexicana amazonensis resistant to toxic nucleosides. Mol Biochem Parasitol. 1993 Aug; 60(2): 171-85.

[423] Wilson K, Berens RL, Sifri CD, Ullman B. Amplification of the inosinate dehydrogenase gene in Trypanosoma brucei gambiense due to an increase in chromosome copy number. J Biol Chem. 1994 Nov 18; 269(46): 28979-87.

[424] Ouellette M, Leblanc E, Kundig C, Papadopoulou B. Antifolate resistance mechanisms from bacteria to cancer cells with emphasis on parasites. Adv Exp Med Biol. 1998; 456: 99-113.

[425] Minodier P, Parola P. Cutaneous leishmaniasis treatment. Travel medicine and infectious disease. 2007; 5(3): 150-8.

[426] Uzun S, Durdu M, Culha G, Allahverdiyev AM, Memisoglu HR. Clinical features, epidemiology, and efficacy and safety of intralesional antimony treatment of cutaneous leishmaniasis: recent experience in Turkey. J Parasitol. 2004 Aug; 90(4): 853-9.

[427] Panagiotopoulos A, Stavropoulos PG, Hasapi V, Papakonstantinou AM, Petridis A, Katsambas A. Treatment of cutaneous leishmaniasis with cryosurgery. Int J Dermatol. 2005 Sep; 44(9): 749-52.

[428] al-Majali O, Routh HB, Abuloham O, Bhowmik KR, Muhsen M, Hebeheba H. A 2-year study of liquid nitrogen therapy in cutaneous leishmaniasis. Int J Dermatol. 1997 Jun; 36(6): 460-2.

[429] Asilian A, Sadeghinia A, Faghihi G, Momeni A. Comparative study of the efficacy of combined cryotherapy and intralesional meglumine antimoniate (Glucantime) *vs* cryotherapy and intralesional meglumine antimoniate (Glucantime) alone for the treatment of cutaneous leishmaniasis. Int J Dermatol. 2004 Apr; 43(4): 281-3.

[430] Navin TR, Arana BA, Arana FE, de Merida AM, Castillo AL, Pozuelos JL. Placebo-controlled clinical trial of meglumine antimonate (glucantime) *vs* localized controlled heat in the treatment of cutaneous leishmaniasis in Guatemala. Am J Trop Med Hyg. 1990 Jan; 42(1): 43-50.

[431] Babajev KB, Babajev OG, Korepanov VI. Treatment of cutaneous leishmaniasis using a carbon dioxide laser. Bull World Health Organ. 1991; 69(1): 103-6.

[432] Asilian A, Sharif A, Faghihi G, Enshaeieh S, Shariati F, Siadat AH. Evaluation of CO laser efficacy in the treatment of cutaneous leishmaniasis. Int J Dermatol. 2004 Oct; 43(10): 736-8.

[433] Iwu MM, Jackson JE, Schuster BG. Medicinal plants in the fight against leishmaniasis. Parasitol Today. 1994 Feb; 10(2): 65-8.

[434] Rates S. Plants as source of drugs. Toxicon. 2001; 39(5): 603-13.

[435] Ganguly S, Bandyopadhyay S, Sarkar A, Chatterjee M. Development of a semi-automated colorimetric assay for screening antileishmanial agents. J Microbiol Methods. 2006 Jul; 66(1): 79-86.

[436] Mandal S, Maharjan M, Ganguly S, Chatterjee M, Singh S, Buckner FS, *et al.* High-throughput screening of amastigotes of Leishmania donovani clinical isolates against drugs using a colorimetric beta-lactamase assay. Indian J Exp Biol. 2009 Jun; 47(6): 475-9.

[437] Kigondu EV, Rukunga GM, Keriko JM, Tonui WK, Gathirwa JW, Kirira PG, *et al.* Anti-parasitic activity and cytotoxicity of selected medicinal plants from Kenya. J Ethnopharmacol. 2009 Jun 25; 123(3): 504-9.

[438] Santos AO, Santin AC, Yamaguchi MU, Cortez LE, Ueda-Nakamura T, Dias-Filho BP, *et al.* Antileishmanial activity of an essential oil from the leaves and flowers of Achillea millefolium. Ann Trop Med Parasitol. 2010 Sep; 104(6): 475-83.

[439] Karioti A, Skaltsa H, Kaiser M, Tasdemir D. Trypanocidal, leishmanicidal and cytotoxic effects of anthecotulide-type linear sesquiterpene lactones from Anthemis auriculata. Phytomedicine. 2009 Aug; 16(8): 783-7.

[440] da Silva Filho AA, Resende DO, Fukui MJ, Santos FF, Pauletti PM, Cunha WR, *et al.* In vitro antileishmanial , antiplasmodial and cytotoxic activities of phenolics and triterpenoids from Baccharis dracunculifolia D. C. (Asteraceae). Fitoterapia. 2009 Dec; 80(8): 478-82.

[441] Valadeau C, Pabon A, Deharo E, Alban-Castillo J, Estevez Y, Lores FA, *et al.* Medicinal plants from the Yanesha (Peru): evaluation of the leishmanicidal and antimalarial activity of selected extracts. J Ethnopharmacol. 2009 Jun 25; 123(3): 413-22.

[442] Gachet MS, Lecaro JS, Kaiser M, Brun R, Navarrete H, Muñoz RA, *et al.* Assessment of anti-protozoal activity of plants traditionally used in Ecuador in the treatment of leishmaniasis. Journal of ethnopharmacology. 2010; 128(1): 184-97.

[443] Tiuman TS, Ueda-Nakamura T, Filho B, Cortez DAG, Nakamura CV. Studies on the effectiveness of Tanacetum parthenium against Leishmania amazonensis. Acta protozoologica. 2005; 44(3): 245.

[444] Tiuman TS, Ueda-Nakamura T, Garcia Cortez DA, Dias Filho BP, Morgado-Diaz JA, de Souza W, *et al.* Antileishmanial activity of parthenolide, a sesquiterpene lactone isolated from Tanacetum parthenium. Antimicrob Agents Chemother. 2005 Jan; 49(1): 176-82.

[445] da Silva BP, Cortez DA, Violin TY, Dias Filho BP, Nakamura CV, Ueda-Nakamura T, *et al.* Antileishmanial activity of a guaianolide from Tanacetum parthenium (L.) Schultz Bip. Parasitol Int. 2010 Dec; 59(4): 643-6.

[446] Braga FG, Bouzada MLM, Fabri RL, de O Matos M, Moreira FO, Scio E, *et al.* Antileishmanial and antifungal activity of plants used in traditional medicine in Brazil. Journal of ethnopharmacology. 2007; 111(2): 396-402.

[447] Tempone AG, Borborema SE, de Andrade HF, Jr., de Amorim Gualda NC, Yogi A, Carvalho CS, *et al.* Antiprotozoal activity of Brazilian plant extracts from isoquinoline alkaloid-producing families. Phytomedicine. 2005 May; 12(5): 382-90.

[448] Osorio E, Arango GJ, Jimenez N, Alzate F, Ruiz G, Gutierrez D, *et al.* Antiprotozoal and cytotoxic activities in vitro of Colombian Annonaceae. J Ethnopharmacol. 2007 May 22; 111(3): 630-5.

[449] Lamidi M, DiGiorgio C, Delmas F, Favel A, Eyele Mve-Mba C, Rondi ML, *et al.* In vitro cytotoxic, antileishmanial and antifungal activities of ethnopharmacologically selected Gabonese plants. J Ethnopharmacol. 2005 Nov 14; 102(2): 185-90.

[450] Castillo D, Arevalo J, Herrera F, Ruiz C, Rojas R, Rengifo E, *et al.* Spirolactone iridoids might be responsible for the antileishmanial activity of a Peruvian traditional remedy made with Himatanthus sucuuba (Apocynaceae). Journal of ethnopharmacology. 2007; 112(2): 410-4.

[451] Billo M, Fournet A, Cabalion P, Waikedre J, Bories C, Loiseau P, *et al.* Screening of New Caledonian and Vanuatu medicinal plants for antiprotozoal activity. J Ethnopharmacol. 2005 Jan 15; 96(3): 569-75.

[452] Brenzan MA, Nakamura CV, Prado Dias Filho B, Ueda-Nakamura T, Young MC, Aparicio Garcia Cortez D. Antileishmanial activity of crude extract and coumarin from Calophyllum brasiliense leaves against Leishmania amazonensis. Parasitol Res. 2007 Aug; 101(3): 715-22.

[453]   Muzitano MF, Tinoco LW, Guette C, Kaiser CR, Rossi-Bergmann B, Costa SS. The antileishmanial activity assessment of unusual flavonoids from Kalanchoe pinnata. Phytochemistry. 2006 Sep; 67(18): 2071-7.

[454]   Jullian V, Bonduelle C, Valentin A, Acebey L, Duigou AG, Prevost MF, *et al.* New clerodane diterpenoids from Laetia procera (Poepp.) Eichler (Flacourtiaceae), with antiplasmodial and antileishmanial activities. Bioorg Med Chem Lett. 2005 Nov 15; 15(22): 5065-70.

[455]   Santos AO, Ueda-Nakamura T, Dias Filho BP, Veiga Junior VF, Pinto AC, Nakamura CV. Effect of Brazilian copaiba oils on Leishmania amazonensis. J Ethnopharmacol. 2008 Nov 20; 120(2): 204-8.

[456]   Desrivot J, Waikedre J, Cabalion P, Herrenknecht C, Bories C, Hocquemiller R, *et al.* Antiparasitic activity of some New Caledonian medicinal plants. Journal of ethnopharmacology. 2007; 112(1): 7-12.

[457]   Weniger B, Vonthron-Sénécheau C, Kaiser M, Brun R, Anton R. Comparative antiplasmodial, leishmanicidal and antitrypanosomal activities of several biflavonoids. Phytomedicine. 2006; 13(3): 176-80.

[458]   Danelli MG, Soares DC, Abreu HS, Pecanha LM, Saraiva EM. Leishmanicidal effect of LLD-3 (1), a nor-triterpene isolated from Lophanthera lactescens. Phytochemistry. 2009 Mar; 70(5): 608-14.

[459]   Lakshmi V, Pandey K, Kapil A, Singh N, Samant M, Dube A. In vitro and in vivo leishmanicidal activity of Dysoxylum binectariferum and its fractions against Leishmania donovani. Phytomedicine. 2007 Jan; 14(1): 36-42.

[460]   Arango V, Robledo S, Seìon-Meìniel B, Figadeìre B, Cardona W, Saìez J, *et al.* Coumarins from Galipea panamensis and Their Activity against Leishmania panamensis. Journal of Natural Products. 2010; 73(5): 1012-4.

[461]   Tasdemir D, Brun R, Franzblau SG, Sezgin Y, Calis I. Evaluation of antiprotozoal and antimycobacterial activities of the resin glycosides and the other metabolites of Scrophularia cryptophila. Phytomedicine. 2008 Mar; 15(3): 209-15.

[462]   Iranshahi M, Arfa P, Ramezani M, Jaafari MR, Sadeghian H, Bassarello C, *et al.* Sesquiterpene coumarins from Ferula szowitsiana and in vitro antileishmanial activity of 7-prenyloxycoumarins against promastigotes. Phytochemistry. 2007 Feb; 68(4): 554-61.

[463]   Capranico G, Zagotto G, Palumbo M. Development of DNA topoisomerase-related therapeutics: a short perspective of new challenges. Curr Med Chem Anticancer Agents. 2004 Jul; 4(4): 335-45.

[464]   Sen N, Majumder HK. Mitochondrion of protozoan parasite emerges as potent therapeutic target: exciting drugs are on the horizon. Curr Pharm Des. 2008; 14(9): 839-46.

[465]   Balana-Fouce R, Redondo CM, Perez-Pertejo Y, Diaz-Gonzalez R, Reguera RM. Targeting atypical trypanosomatid DNA topoisomerase I. Drug Discov Today. 2006 Aug; 11(15-16): 733-40.

[466]   Fairlamb AH, Cerami A. Metabolism and functions of trypanothione in the Kinetoplastida. Annu Rev Microbiol. 1992; 46: 695-729.

[467]   Schmidt A, Krauth-Siegel RL. Enzymes of the trypanothione metabolism as targets for antitrypanosomal drug development. Curr Top Med Chem. 2002 Nov; 2(11): 1239-59.

[468]   Sen R, Saha P, Sarkar A, Ganguly S, Chatterjee M. Iron enhances generation of free radicals by Artemisinin causing a caspase-independent, apoptotic death in Leishmania donovani promastigotes. Free Radic Res. 2010 Nov; 44(11): 1289-95.

[469] Murray HW. Clinical and experimental advances in treatment of visceral leishmaniasis. Antimicrob Agents Chemother. 2001 Aug; 45(8): 2185-97.

[470] Zhai L, Blom J, Chen M, Christensen SB, Kharazmi A. The antileishmanial agent licochalcone A interferes with the function of parasite mitochondria. Antimicrob Agents Chemother. 1995 Dec; 39(12): 2742-8.

[471] Chen M, Zhai L, Christensen SB, Theander TG, Kharazmi A. Inhibition of fumarate reductase in Leishmania major and L. donovani by chalcones. Antimicrob Agents Chemother. 2001 Jul; 45(7): 2023-9.

[472] Mittra B, Saha A, Chowdhury AR, Pal C, Mandal S, Mukhopadhyay S, *et al.* Luteolin, an abundant dietary component is a potent antileishmanial agent that acts by inducing topoisomerase II-mediated kinetoplast DNA cleavage leading to apoptosis. MOLECULAR MEDICINE-CAMBRIDGE MA THEN NEW YORK-. 2000; 6(6): 527-41.

[473] Gomes DC, Muzitano MF, Costa SS, Rossi-Bergmann B. Effectiveness of the immunomodulatory extract of Kalanchoe pinnata against murine visceral leishmaniasis. Parasitology. 2010 Apr; 137(4): 613-8.

[474] Sarkar A, Sen R, Saha P, Ganguly S, Mandal G, Chatterjee M. An ethanolic extract of leaves of Piper betle (Paan) Linn mediates its antileishmanial activity *via* apoptosis. Parasitol Res. 2008 May; 102(6): 1249-55.

[475] Misra P, Kumar A, Khare P, Gupta S, Kumar N, Dube A. Pro-apoptotic effect of the landrace Bangla Mahoba of Piper betle on Leishmania donovani may be due to the high content of eugenol. J Med Microbiol. 2009 Aug; 58(Pt 8): 1058-66.

[476] Ridoux O, Di Giorgio C, Delmas F, Elias R, Mshvildadze V, Dekanosidze G, *et al.* In vitro antileishmanial activity of three saponins isolated from ivy, alpha-hederin, beta-hederin and hederacolchiside A(1), in association with pentamidine and amphotericin B. Phytother Res. 2001 Jun; 15(4): 298-301.

[477] Tandon JS, Srivastava V, Guru PY. Iridoids: a new class of leishmanicidal agents from Nyctanthes arbortristis. J Nat Prod. 1991 Jul-Aug; 54(4): 1102-4.

[478] del Rayo Camacho M, Kirby GC, Warhurst DC, Croft SL, Phillipson JD. Oxoaporphine alkaloids and quinones from Stephania dinklagei and evaluation of their antiprotozoal activities. Planta medica. 2000; 66(5): 478-80.

[479] Fournet A, Barrios AA, Munoz V, Hocquemiller R, Cave A. Effect of natural naphthoquinones in BALB/c mice infected with Leishmania amazonensis and L. venezuelensis. Trop Med Parasitol. 1992 Dec; 43(4): 219-22.

[480] Hazra B, Sarkar R, Bhattacharyya S, Ghosh PK, Chel G, Dinda B. Synthesis of plumbagin derivatives and their inhibitory activities against Ehrlich ascites carcinoma in vivo and Leishmania donovani promastigotes in vitro. Phytotherapy Research. 2002; 16(2): 133-7.

[481] Ghosh AK, Bhattacharyya FK, Ghosh DK. Leishmania donovani: amastigote inhibition and mode of action of berberine. Exp Parasitol. 1985 Dec; 60(3): 404-13.

[482] Saha P, Sen R, Hariharan C, Kumar D, Das P, Chatterjee M. Berberine chloride causes a caspase-independent, apoptotic-like death in Leishmania donovani promastigotes. Free Radic Res. 2009; 43(11): 1101-10.

[483] Soares DC, Pereira CG, Meireles MÂA, Saraiva EM. Leishmanicidal activity of a supercritical fluid fraction obtained from< i> Tabernaemontana catharinensis</i>. Parasitology International. 2007; 56(2): 135-9.

[484] Ozer L, El-On J, Golan-Goldhirsh A, Gopas J. Leishmania major: antileishmanial activity of Nuphar lutea extract mediated by the activation of transcription factor NF-kappaB. Exp Parasitol. 2010 Dec; 126(4): 510-6.

[485] Guimaraes LR, Rodrigues AP, Marinho PS, Muller AH, Guilhon GM, Santos LS, *et al*. Activity of the julocrotine, a glutarimide alkaloid from Croton pullei var. glabrior, on Leishmania (L.) amazonensis. Parasitol Res. 2010 Oct; 107(5): 1075-81.

[486] Ponte-Sucre A, Faber JH, Gulder T, Kajahn I, Pedersen SE, Schultheis M, *et al*. Activities of naphthylisoquinoline alkaloids and synthetic analogs against Leishmania major. Antimicrob Agents Chemother. 2007 Jan; 51(1): 188-94.

[487] Mishra BB, Kale RR, Singh RK, Tiwari VK. Alkaloids: future prospective to combat leishmaniasis. Fitoterapia. 2009 Mar; 80(2): 81-90.

[488] Srivastava A, Singh N, Mishra M, Kumar V, Gour JK, Bajpai S, *et al*. Identification of TLR inducing Th1-responsive Leishmania donovani amastigote-specific antigens. Mol Cell Biochem. 2012 Jan; 359(1-2): 359-68.

[489] Salem MM, Werbovetz KA. Natural products from plants as drug candidates and lead compounds against leishmaniasis and trypanosomiasis. Curr Med Chem. 2006; 13(21): 2571-98.

[490] Dube A, Singh N, Saxena A, Lakshmi V. Antileishmanial potential of a marine sponge, Haliclona exigua (Kirkpatrick) against experimental visceral leishmaniasis. Parasitol Res. 2007 Jul; 101(2): 317-24.

[491] Simmons TL, Engene N, Urena LD, Romero LI, Ortega-Barria E, Gerwick L, *et al*. Viridamides A and B, lipodepsipeptides with antiprotozoal activity from the marine cyanobacterium Oscillatoria nigro-viridis. J Nat Prod. 2008 Sep; 71(9): 1544-50.

[492] Di Giorgio C, Delmas F, Akhmedjanova V, Ollivier E, Bessonova I, Riad E, *et al*. In vitro antileishmanial activity of diphyllin isolated from Haplophyllum bucharicum. Planta Med. 2005 Apr; 71(4): 366-9.

[493] Sauvain M, Dedet JP, Kunesch N, Poisson J. Isolation of flavins from the Amazonian shrub Faramea guianesis. J Nat Prod. 1994 Mar; 57(3): 403-6.

[494] Kolodziej H, Kayser O, Kiderlen AF, Ito H, Hatano T, Yoshida T, *et al*. Proanthocyanidins and related compounds: antileishmanial activity and modulatory effects on nitric oxide and tumor necrosis factor-alpha-release in the murine macrophage-like cell line RAW 264.7. Biol Pharm Bull. 2001 Sep; 24(9): 1016-21.

[495] Kolodziej H, Kayser O, Kiderlen A, Ito H, Hatano T, Yoshida T, *et al*. Antileishmanial Activity of Hydrolyzable Tannins and their Modulatory Effects on Nitric Oxide and Tumour Necrosis Factor-alpha-Release in Macrophages in Vitro. Planta medica. 2001; 67(9): 825-32.

[496] do Socorro SRMS, Mendonca-Filho RR, Bizzo HR, de Almeida Rodrigues I, Soares RM, Souto-Padron T, *et al*. Antileishmanial activity of a linalool-rich essential oil from Croton cajucara. Antimicrob Agents Chemother. 2003 Jun; 47(6): 1895-901.

[497] Krishna S, Uhlemann AC, Haynes RK. Artemisinins: mechanisms of action and potential for resistance. Drug Resist Updat. 2004 Aug-Oct; 7(4-5): 233-44.

[498] Yang Z, Ding J, Yang C, Gao Y, Li X, Chen X, Peng Y, Fang J, Xiao S. Immunomodulatory and anti-inflammatory properties of artesunate in experimental colitis. Curr Med Chem. 2012; 19(26): 4541-51.

[499] Sen R, Ganguly S, Saha P, Chatterjee M. Efficacy of artemisinin in experimental visceral leishmaniasis. International Journal of Antimicrobial Agents. 2010; 36(1): 43-9.

[500] Ukil A, Biswas A, Das T, Das PK. 18 Beta-glycyrrhetinic acid triggers curative Th1 response and nitric oxide up-regulation in experimental visceral leishmaniasis associated with the activation of NF-kappa B. J Immunol. 2005 Jul 15; 175(2): 1161-9.

[501] Misra P, Sashidhara KV, Singh SP, Kumar A, Gupta R, Chaudhaery SS, *et al*. 16alpha-Hydroxycleroda-3,13 (14)Z-dien-15,16-olide from Polyalthia longifolia: a safe and orally active antileishmanial agent. Br J Pharmacol. 2010 Mar; 159(5): 1143-50.

[502] Martin-Quintal Z, del Rosario Garcia-Miss M, Mut-Martin M, Matus-Moo A, Torres-Tapia LW, Peraza-Sanchez SR. The leishmanicidal effect of (3S)-16,17-didehydrofalcarinol, an oxylipin isolated from Tridax procumbens, is independent of NO production. Phytother Res. 2010 Jul; 24(7): 1004-8.

[503] Gupta S, Raychaudhuri B, Banerjee S, Das B, Mukhopadhaya S, Datta SC. Momordicatin purified from fruits of Momordica charantia is effective to act as a potent antileishmania agent. Parasitol Int. 2010 Jun; 59(2): 192-7.

[504] Jaeger T, Flohe L. The thiol-based redox networks of pathogens: unexploited targets in the search for new drugs. Biofactors. 2006; 27(1-4): 109-20.

[505] Singh N, Kumar A, Gupta P, Chand K, Samant M, Maurya R, *et al*. Evaluation of antileishmanial potential of Tinospora sinensis against experimental visceral leishmaniasis. Parasitol Res. 2008 Feb; 102(3): 561-5.

[506] Soares DC, Andrade AL, Delorenzi JC, Silva JR, Freire-de-Lima L, Falcao CA, *et al*. Leishmanicidal activity of Himatanthus sucuuba latex against Leishmania amazonensis. Parasitol Int. 2010 Jun; 59(2): 173-7.

[507] Sharma U, Velpandian T, Sharma P, Singh S. Evaluation of antileishmanial activity of selected Indian plants known to have antimicrobial properties. Parasitol Res. 2009 Oct; 105(5): 1287-93.

[508] Ghazanfari T, Hassan ZM, Ebtekar M, Ahmadiani A, Naderi G, Azar A. Garlic induces a shift in cytokine pattern in Leishmania major-infected BALB/c mice. Scand J Immunol. 2000 Nov; 52(5): 491-5.

[509] Dutta A, Mandal G, Mandal C, Chatterjee M. In vitro antileishmanial activity of Aloe vera leaf exudate: a potential herbal therapy in leishmaniasis. Glycoconj J. 2007 Jan; 24(1): 81-6.

[510] Dutta A, Bandyopadhyay S, Mandal C, Chatterjee M. Aloe vera leaf exudate induces a caspase-independent cell death in Leishmania donovani promastigotes. J Med Microbiol. 2007 May; 56(Pt 5): 629-36.

[511] Patricio FJ, Costa GC, Pereira PV, Aragao-Filho WC, Sousa SM, Frazao JB, *et al*. Efficacy of the intralesional treatment with Chenopodium ambrosioides in the murine infection by Leishmania amazonensis. J Ethnopharmacol. 2008 Jan 17; 115(2): 313-9.

[512] Monzote L, Garcia M, Montalvo AM, Linares R, Scull R. Effect of oral treatment with the essential oil from Chenopodium ambrosioides against cutaneous leishmaniasis in BALB/c mice, caused by Leishmania amazonensis. Forsch Komplementmed. 2009 Oct; 16(5): 334-8.

[513] Guimaraes ET, Lima MS, Santos LA, Ribeiro IM, Tomassini TB, Ribeiro dos Santos R, *et al*. Activity of physalins purified from Physalis angulata in in vitro and in vivo models of cutaneous leishmaniasis. J Antimicrob Chemother. 2009 Jul; 64(1): 84-7.

[514] Khaliq T, Misra P, Gupta S, Reddy KP, Kant R, Maulik PR, *et al*. Peganine hydrochloride dihydrate an orally active antileishmanial agent. Bioorg Med Chem Lett. 2009 May 1; 19(9): 2585-6.

[515]   Poddar A, Banerjee A, Ghanta S, Chattopadhyay S. In vivo efficacy of calceolarioside A against experimental visceral leishmaniasis. Planta Med. 2008 Apr; 74(5): 503-8.

[516]   Medda S, Mukhopadhyay S, Basu MK. Evaluation of the in-vivo activity and toxicity of amarogentin, an antileishmanial agent, in both liposomal and niosomal forms. J Antimicrob Chemother. 1999 Dec; 44(6): 791-4.

[517]   Bhattacharjee S, Gupta G, Bhattacharya P, Mukherjee A, Mujumdar SB, Pal A, *et al.* Quassin alters the immunological patterns of murine macrophages through generation of nitric oxide to exert antileishmanial activity. Journal of antimicrobial chemotherapy. 2009; 63(2): 317-24.

[518]   Gupta S, Ramesh SC, Srivastava VM. Efficacy of picroliv in combination with miltefosine, an orally effective antileishmanial drug against experimental visceral leishmaniasis. Acta Trop. 2005 Apr; 94(1): 41-7.

[519]   Wagner H, Ulrich-Merzenich G. Synergy research: approaching a new generation of phytopharmaceuticals. Phytomedicine. 2009 Mar; 16(2-3): 97-110.

[520]   Kayser O, Kiderlen AF, Bertels S, Siems K. Antileishmanial activities of aphidicolin and its semisynthetic derivatives. Antimicrob Agents Chemother. 2001 Jan; 45(1): 288-92.

[521]   Ma G, Khan SI, Jacob MR, Tekwani BL, Li Z, Pasco DS, *et al.* Antimicrobial and antileishmanial activities of hypocrellins A and B. Antimicrobial agents and chemotherapy. 2004; 48(11): 4450-2.

[522]   Delorenzi JC, Attias M, Gattass CR, Andrade M, Rezende C, da Cunha Pinto Â, *et al.* Antileishmanial Activity of an Indole Alkaloid fromPeschiera australis. Antimicrobial agents and chemotherapy. 2001; 45(5): 1349-54.

[523]   Evangelou G, Krasagakis K, Giannikaki E, Kruger-Krasagakis S, Tosca A. Successful treatment of cutaneous leishmaniasis with intralesional aminolevulinic acid photodynamic therapy. Photodermatol Photoimmunol Photomed. 2011 Oct; 27(5): 254-6.

[524]   Henderson BW, Dougherty TJ. How does photodynamic therapy work? Photochemistry and photobiology. 1992; 55(1): 145-57.

[525]   Ericson MB, Wennberg AM, Larkö O. Review of photodynamic therapy in actinic keratosis and basal cell carcinoma. Therapeutics and clinical risk management. 2008; 4(1): 1-9.

[526]   van Bowen Z. Ruimere toepassing van fotodynamische therapie in de dermatologie. Ned Tijdschr Geneeskd. 2005; 149: 232-7.

[527]   van der Snoek EM, Robinson DJ, van Hellemond JJ, Neumann HA. A review of photodynamic therapy in cutaneous leishmaniasis. J Eur Acad Dermatol Venereol. 2008 Aug; 22(8): 918-22.

[528]   Fritsch C, Goerz G, Ruzicka T. Photodynamic therapy in dermatology. Arch Dermatol. 1998 Feb; 134(2): 207-14.

[529]   Taylor EL, Brown SB. The advantages of aminolevulinic acid photodynamic therapy in dermatology. J Dermatolog Treat. 2002; 13 Suppl 1: S3-11.

[530]   Angell-Petersen E, Sorensen R, Warloe T, Soler AM, Moan J, Peng Q, *et al.* Porphyrin formation in actinic keratosis and basal cell carcinoma after topical application of methyl 5-aminolevulinate. J Invest Dermatol. 2006 Feb; 126(2): 265-71.

[531]   LAR T. Terapia fotodinâmica em dermatologia. Laser em Dermatologia São Paulo: Editora Roca. 2002: 121-36.

[532]   Leman JA, Morton CA. Photodynamic therapy: applications in dermatology. Expert Opin Biol Ther. 2002 Jan; 2(1): 45-53.

[533] Braathen LR, Szeimies RM, Basset-Seguin N, Bissonnette R, Foley P, Pariser D, *et al*. Guidelines on the use of photodynamic therapy for nonmelanoma skin cancer: an international consensus. Journal of the American Academy of Dermatology. 2007; 56(1): 125-43.

[534] Peng Q, Berg K, Moan J, Kongshaug M, Nesland JM. 5-Aminolevulinic acid-based photodynamic therapy: principles and experimental research. Photochem Photobiol. 1997 Feb; 65(2): 235-51.

[535] Salva KA. Photodynamic therapy: unapproved uses, dosages, or indications. Clin Dermatol. 2002 Sep-Oct; 20(5): 571-81.

[536] Riddle RD, Yamamoto M, Engel JD. Expression of delta-aminolevulinate synthase in avian cells: separate genes encode erythroid-specific and nonspecific isozymes. Proc Natl Acad Sci U S A. 1989 Feb; 86(3): 792-6.

[537] Anderson PM, Desnick RJ. Purification and properties of delta-aminolevulinate dehydrase from human erythrocytes. J Biol Chem. 1979 Aug 10; 254(15): 6924-30.

[538] Jarret C, Stauffer F, Henz ME, Marty M, Luond RM, Bobalova J, *et al*. Inhibition of Escherichia coli porphobilinogen synthase using analogs of postulated intermediates. Chem Biol. 2000 Mar; 7(3): 185-96.

[539] Shoolingin-Jordan PM, Al-Dbass A, McNeill LA, Sarwar M, Butler D. Human porphobilinogen deaminase mutations in the investigation of the mechanism of dipyrromethane cofactor assembly and tetrapyrrole formation. Biochem Soc Trans. 2003 Jun; 31(Pt 3): 731-5.

[540] Jordan PM, Seehra JS. The biosynthesis of uroporphyrinogen III: order of assembly of the four porphobilinogen molecules in the formation of the tetrapyrrole ring. FEBS Lett. 1979 Aug 15; 104(2): 364-6.

[541] Munakata H, Sun JY, Yoshida K, Nakatani T, Honda E, Hayakawa S, *et al*. Role of the heme regulatory motif in the heme-mediated inhibition of mitochondrial import of 5-aminolevulinate synthase. J Biochem. 2004 Aug; 136(2): 233-8.

[542] Srivastava G, Borthwick IA, Maguire DJ, Elferink CJ, Bawden MJ, Mercer JF, *et al*. Regulation of 5-aminolevulinate synthase mRNA in different rat tissues. J Biol Chem. 1988 Apr 15; 263(11): 5202-9.

[543] Surinya KH, Cox TC, May BK. Transcriptional regulation of the human erythroid 5-aminolevulinate synthase gene. Identification of promoter elements and role of regulatory proteins. J Biol Chem. 1997 Oct 17; 272(42): 26585-94.

[544] Collaud S, Juzeniene A, Moan J, Lange N. On the selectivity of 5-aminolevulinic acid-induced protoporphyrin IX formation. Curr Med Chem Anticancer Agents. 2004 May; 4(3): 301-16.

[545] Kurwa H, Barlow R. The role of photodynamic therapy in dermatology. Clinical and experimental dermatology. 1999; 24(3): 143-8.

[546] Farah J, Ralston J, Zeitouni N, Oseroff A. ALA-PDT treatment of pre-skin cancer. Photodynamic Therapy Philadelphia: Elsevier Saunders. 2005: 1-12.

[547] Morton CA, Brown SB, Collins S, Ibbotson S, Jenkinson H, Kurwa H, *et al*. Guidelines for topical photodynamic therapy: report of a workshop of the British Photodermatology Group. Br J Dermatol. 2002 Apr; 146(4): 552-67.

[548] Kalka K, Merk H, Mukhtar H. Photodynamic therapy in dermatology. J Am Acad Dermatol. 2000 Mar; 42(3): 389-413; quiz 4-6.

[549] Gardlo K, Horska Z, Enk CD, Rauch L, Megahed M, Ruzicka T, *et al.* Treatment of cutaneous leishmaniasis by photodynamic therapy. J Am Acad Dermatol. 2003 Jun; 48(6): 893-6.

[550] Enk CD, Fritsch C, Jonas F, Nasereddin A, Ingber A, Jaffe CL, *et al.* Treatment of cutaneous leishmaniasis with photodynamic therapy. Arch Dermatol. 2003 Apr; 139(4): 432-4.

[551] Gardlo K, Hanneken S, Ruzicka T, Neumann NJ. [Photodynamic therapy of cutaneous leishmaniasis. A promising new therapeutic modality]. Hautarzt. 2004 Apr; 55(4): 381-3.

[552] Asilian A, Davami M. Comparison between the efficacy of photodynamic therapy and topical paromomycin in the treatment of Old World cutaneous leishmaniasis: a placebo-controlled, randomized clinical trial. Clinical and experimental dermatology. 2006; 31(5): 634-7.

[553] Ghaffarifar F, Jorjani O, Mirshams M, Miranbaygi M, Hosseini Z. Photodynamic therapy as a new treatment of cutaneous leishmaniasis. Eastern Mediterranean Health Journal. 2006; 12(6): 902.

[554] Sohl S, Kauer F, Paasch U, Simon JC. Photodynamic treatment of cutaneous leishmaniasis. J Dtsch Dermatol Ges. 2007 Feb; 5(2): 128-30.

[555] Akilov OE, Kosaka S, O'Riordan K, Hasan T. Parasiticidal effect of delta-aminolevulinic acid-based photodynamic therapy for cutaneous leishmaniasis is indirect and mediated through the killing of the host cells. Exp Dermatol. 2007 Aug; 16(8): 651-60.

[556] Akilov OE, Kosaka S, O'Riordan K, Hasan T. Photodynamic therapy for cutaneous leishmaniasis: the effectiveness of topical phenothiaziniums in parasite eradication and Th1 immune response stimulation. Photochem Photobiol Sci. 2007 Oct; 6(10): 1067-75.

[557] Akilov OE, Yousaf W, Lukjan SX, Verma S, Hasan T. Optimization of topical photodynamic therapy with 3,7-bis(di-n-butylamino)phenothiazin-5-ium bromide for cutaneous leishmaniasis. Lasers Surg Med. 2009 Jul; 41(5): 358-65.

[558] Gardner DM, Taylor VM, Cedeno DL, Padhee S, Robledo SM, Jones MA, *et al.* Association of acenaphthoporphyrins with liposomes for the photodynamic treatment of leishmaniasis. Photochem Photobiol. 2010 May-Jun; 86(3): 645-52.

[559] Latorre-Esteves E, Akilov OE, Rai P, Beverley SM, Hasan T. Monitoring the efficacy of antimicrobial photodynamic therapy in a murine model of cutaneous leishmaniasis using L. major expressing GFP. J Biophotonics. 2010 Jun; 3(5-6): 328-35.

[560] Peloi LS, Biondo CE, Kimura E, Politi MJ, Lonardoni MV, Aristides SM, *et al.* Photodynamic therapy for American cutaneous leishmaniasis: the efficacy of methylene blue in hamsters experimentally infected with Leishmania (Leishmania) amazonensis. Exp Parasitol. 2011 Aug; 128(4): 353-6.

[561] Song D, Lindoso JAL, Oyafuso LK, Kanashiro EHY, Cardoso JL, Uchoa AF, *et al.* Photodynamic Therapy Using Methylene Blue to Treat Cutaneous Leishmaniasis. Photomedicine and Laser Surgery. 2011; 29(10): 711-5.

[562] Allahverdiyev AM, Koc RC, Ates SC, Bagirova M, Elcicek S, Oztel ON. Leishmania tropica: the effect of darkness and light on biological activities in vitro. Exp Parasitol. 2011 Aug; 128(4): 318-23.

[563] Jin S, Ye K. Nanoparticle-mediated drug delivery and gene therapy. Biotechnol Prog. 2007 Jan-Feb; 23(1): 32-41.

[564] Riboh JC, Haes AJ, McFarland AD, Yonzon CR, Van Duyne RP. A nanoscale optical biosensor: real-time immunoassay in physiological buffer enabled by improved nanoparticle adhesion. The Journal of Physical Chemistry B. 2003; 107(8): 1772-80.

[565] Sondi I, Salopek-Sondi B. Silver nanoparticles as antimicrobial agent: a case study on< i> E. coli</i> as a model for Gram-negative bacteria. Journal of colloid and interface science. 2004; 275(1): 177-82.

[566] Zhang AP, Sun YP. Photocatalytic killing effect of TiO2 nanoparticles on Ls-174-t human colon carcinoma cells. World J Gastroenterol. 2004 Nov 1; 10(21): 3191-3.

[567] Blake DM, Maness PC, Huang Z, Wolfrum EJ, Huang J, Jacoby WA. Application of the photocatalytic chemistry of titanium dioxide to disinfection and the killing of cancer cells. Separation and Purification Methods. 1999; 28(1): 1-50.

[568] Raffi M, Hussain F, Bhatti T, Akhter J, Hameed A, Hasan M. Antibacterial characterization of silver nanoparticles against E. coli ATCC-15224. Journal of Materials Science and Technology. 2008; 24(2): 192-6.

[569] Lara HH, Ayala-Núnez NV, Ixtepan Turrent LC, Rodríguez Padilla C. Bactericidal effect of silver nanoparticles against multidrug-resistant bacteria. World Journal of Microbiology and Biotechnology. 2010; 26(4): 615-21.

[570] Nanda A, Saravanan M. Biosynthesis of silver nanoparticles from Staphylococcus aureus and its antimicrobial activity against MRSA and MRSE. Nanomedicine. 2009 Dec; 5(4): 452-6.

[571] Allahverdiyev AM, Abamor ES, Bagirova M, Rafailovich M. Antimicrobial effects of TiO(2) and Ag(2)O nanoparticles against drug-resistant bacteria and leishmania parasites. Future Microbiol. 2011 Aug; 6(8): 933-40.

[572] Allahverdiyev AM, Abamor ES, Bagirova M, Ustundag CB, Kaya C, Kaya F, *et al.* Antileishmanial effect of silver nanoparticles and their enhanced antiparasitic activity under ultraviolet light. International Journal of Nanomedicine. 2011; 6: 2705.

[573] Arruebo M, Fernández-Pacheco R, Ibarra MR, Santamaría J. Magnetic nanoparticles for drug delivery. Nano Today. 2007; 2(3): 22-32.

[574] Kumari A, Yadav SK, Yadav SC. Biodegradable polymeric nanoparticles based drug delivery systems. Colloids Surf B Biointerfaces. 2010 Jan 1; 75(1): 1-18.

[575] Chellat F, Merhi Y, Moreau A, Yahia L. Therapeutic potential of nanoparticulate systems for macrophage targeting. Biomaterials. 2005 Dec; 26(35): 7260-75.

[576] Date AA, Joshi MD, Patravale VB. Parasitic diseases: Liposomes and polymeric nanoparticles *versus* lipid nanoparticles. Adv Drug Deliv Rev. 2007 Jul 10; 59(6): 505-21.

[577] Muller RH, Jacobs C, Kayser O. Nanosuspensions as particulate drug formulations in therapy. Rationale for development and what we can expect for the future. Adv Drug Deliv Rev. 2001 Mar 23; 47(1): 3-19.

[578] Kayser O, Olbrich C, Yardley V, Kiderlen A, Croft S. Formulation of amphotericin B as nanosuspension for oral administration. International journal of pharmaceutics. 2003; 254(1): 73-5.

[579] Santangelo R, Paderu P, Delmas G, Chen ZW, Mannino R, Zarif L, *et al.* Efficacy of oral cochleate-amphotericin B in a mouse model of systemic candidiasis. Antimicrob Agents Chemother. 2000 Sep; 44(9): 2356-60.

[580] MendozamEstella-Hermoso de A, Rayo M, Mollinedo F, Blanco-Prieto MJ. Lipid nanoparticles for alkyl lysophospholipid edelfosine encapsulation: development and in vitro characterization. Eur J Pharm Biopharm. 2008 Feb; 68(2): 207-13.

[581]　Carvalho Ade O, Gomes VM. Role of plant lipid transfer proteins in plant cell physiology-a concise review. Peptides. 2007 May; 28(5): 1144-53.

[582]　Zaman U, Abbasi A. Isolation, purification and characterization of a nonspecific lipid transfer protein from Cuminum cyminum. Phytochemistry. 2009 May; 70(8): 979-87.

[583]　Pato C, Le Borgne M, Le Baut G, Le Pape P, Marion D, Douliez JP. Potential application of plant lipid transfer proteins for drug delivery. Biochem Pharmacol. 2001 Sep 1; 62(5): 555-60.

[584]　Ben Salah A, Buffet PA, Morizot G, Ben Massoud N, Zaatour A, Ben Alaya N, *et al.* WR279,396, a third generation aminoglycoside ointment for the treatment of Leishmania major cutaneous leishmaniasis: a phase 2, randomized, double blind, placebo controlled study. PLoS Negl Trop Dis. 2009; 3(5): e432.

[585]　Tallarida RJ. The interaction index: a measure of drug synergism. Pain. 2002 Jul; 98(1-2): 163-8.

[586]　Monzote L, Montalvo AM, Scull R, Miranda M, Abreu J. Combined effect of the essential oil from Chenopodium ambrosioides and antileishmanial drugs on promastigotes of Leishmania amazonensis. Rev Inst Med Trop Sao Paulo. 2007 Jul-Aug; 49(4): 257-60.

CHAPTER 6

In Silico Study Verifying Antiviral Activity of Proanthocyanidins with Special Reference to Dengue Virus

Lakshmi Chandrasekaran[1], Koji Ichiyama[1], Vivian Feng Chen[1], Akiko Saito[2], Yoshiyuki Yoshinaka[3] and Naoki Yamamoto[*,1]

[1]*Translational ID Lab, Department of Microbiology, Yong Loo Lin School of Medicine, National University of Singapore, 14 Medical Drive, #15-02 Centre for Translational Medicine (MD6), 117599 Singapore;* [2]*Graduate School of Engineering, Osaka Electro-Communication University (OECU), Osaka 572-8530, Japan; and* [3]*Department of Molecular Virology, Graduate 15 School, Tokyo Medical and Dental University, Tokyo 113-5819, Japan*

Abstract: Proanthocyanidins exist as a part of a particular group of polyphenolic compounds known as flavanols. They are commonly occurring plant metabolites generally available in many sources such as fruits, bark, leaves and seeds of plants. They possess monomers, oligomers and polymers of varying molecular sizes composed of flavan-3-ols that serve as the building blocks. These compounds have been reported to have anti-carcinogenic, anti-inflammatory, anti-allergic, antioxidant, antibacterial and antiviral properties in human beings. This review will primarily focus on the *in silico* and *in vitro* analyses that verify antiviral activity of proanthocyanidins against several viruses, primarily the dengue virus.

Keywords: Antiviral activity, catechin, dengue virus, epicatechin, flavonoids, *in silico, in vitro,* proanthocyanidins.

INTRODUCTION

Proanthocyanidins

Flavonoids also known as bioflavonoids exist as a class of plant secondary metabolites that are classified into flavonoids, isoflavonoids and neoflavonoids. They remain broadly dispersed in plants and are the utmost prevalent class of polyphenolic compounds in the human diet [1]. Tannins also called as tannic acid

*Corresponding Author Naoki Yamamoto: Translational ID Lab, Department of Microbiology, Yong Loo Lin School of Medicine, National University of Singapore, 14 Medical Drive, #15-02 Centre for Translational Medicine (MD6), 117599 Singapore; Tel: (+65) 6516-3332; Fax: (+65) 6776-6872; E-mails: micny@nus.edu.sg/ naoki_yamamoto@nuhs.edu.sg

are polyphenols which are obtained from various plants [2]. These polyphenols are able to form interconnection with proteins and other macromolecules because of the presence of huge quantity of hydroxyl or other functional groups. Tannins are classified into two major classes: hydrolyzable tannins and condensed tannins. Condensed tannins are also known as proanthocyanidins (PCs). PCs belong to a class of polyphenols called flavanols, which are a type of flavonoid. The structures of PCs are a combination of monomers, dimers, and trimers of catechins, which is a 4x-hydroxylated flavan-3-ol. PCs are commonly distributed in many plants, fruits, vegetables, seeds, flowers, bark, wine, cranberries, and tea [3]. Pycnogenol (PG), a patented extract of maritime pine bark contains nearly 70% PCs [4]. PCs are high molecular weight polymers whose structures depend upon the stereochemistry and hydroxylation pattern of flavan-3-ol units. They are classified into subtypes based on the flavan-3-ol units and they are procyanidins, prodelphinidins, propelargonidins, profisetinidins and prorobinetidins. Procyanidins is a type of condensed tannin found in grapes [5]. These features make them potential sources for drug production, as natural plant extracts generally they have low side effects when ingested. In recent years, researchers have shown interest towards catechin compounds due to their broad spectrum of antiviral activity and additional merits such as antibacterial, anti-cancer, and antioxidant effects. Current treatments for viral diseases have proven to be limited due to the many types and subtypes of pathogenic viruses, which mutate easily to form drug-resistant strains. Thus, development of safe antiviral drugs with broad-spectrum activity and high selectivity for viruses over mammalian cells is strongly desired in the modern world and PCs may prove to be worth candidates. This review focuses on the antiviral activity of catechins, in particular their interactions with the dengue virus (DENV) [6]. The figure shows the structures of catechin and the four main PCs present in green tea: (−)-epigallocatechin (EGC), (−)-epicatechin gallate (ECG), (−)-epigallocatechin gallate (EGCG), and (−)-epicatechin (EC) (Fig. 1). The galloyl moiety present in EGC, ECG, and EGCG was found to be important for the antiviral activity and the aforementioned additional merits of catechin compounds.

Dengue

Dengue has been ranked as one of the important infectious diseases by the World Health Organization (WHO) [7]. The WHO has estimated that about 40% of the world's population is at the threat of dengue, infecting millions of people annually [8]. This number has been estimated to increase by three times annually by Bhatt *et al.* [9]. The infection, risk factors and the severity vary based on factors such as age, ethnicity and complications with other diseases [10]. The DENV is a member of the Flaviviridae family and Flavivirus genus. It is an arthropod-borne virus transmitted by mosquitoes of the Aedes genus. There are four serotypes in DENV (DENV-1 to DENV-4), and these four serotypes result in diseases such as dengue fever (DF), dengue hemorrhagic fever (DHF), and dengue shock syndrome. In humans, infections with one of the four serotypes result in self-limited DF; however, a secondary infection with a different serotype increases the risk of the disease escalating to the lethal DHF [11]. This presents itself as a challenge for anti-DENV drug and vaccine research. The structure of the DENV is that of an enveloped virus. The mature virion consists of a capsid which contains a single stranded, positive sense RNA [12].

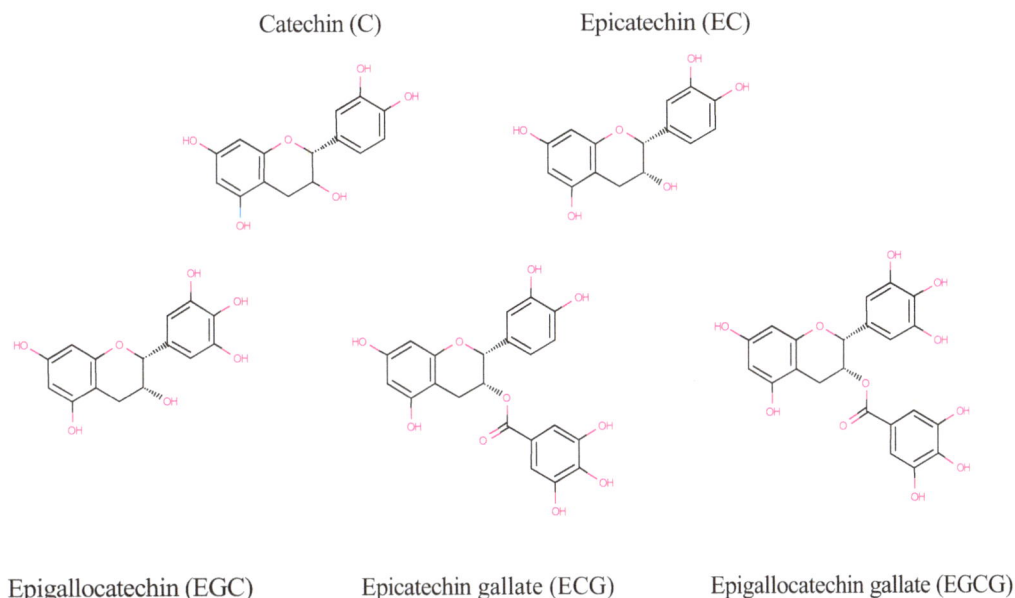

Fig. (1). Structure of catechin (C), epicatechin (EC), epigallocatechin (EGC), epicatechin gallate (ECG) and epigallocatechin gallate (EGCG).

The RNA genome encodes for 10 proteins, of which three are structural proteins (capsid, pre-membrane, and envelope (C, prM, E)), and seven are non-structural proteins (NS1, NS2A, NS2B, NS3, NS4A, NS4B, and NS5) (Fig. **2**) [13]. In the virus replication cycle, the structural proteins are responsible for virion formation and non-structural proteins are responsible for replication, functioning at different steps of the cycle [14]. The DENV replication cycle has several steps involved. The life cycle of DENV starts *via* the attachment of the structural proteins (E and prM) from the viral envelope to the cell receptor(s) which is unknown at the moment [15]. Through membrane fusion, the virus internalizes into the cell cytoplasm *via* endocytosis. The acidification of the endocytic vesicles is followed by the exposure of the fusion loop, enabling the trimerization of the E protein which initiates the fusion of virus and cell membrane [16]. The nucleocapsid then enters the cytoplasm, releasing the viral genome (Fig. **3**). A single long polyprotein is produced by the translation of the RNA strand. The viral and host proteases further process the polyprotein, yielding all components necessary for the budding of new DENV units. This process synthesizes a negative RNA strand from a positive RNA genome [17]. Currently, research is focused on the structural and non-structural proteins of DENV for finding new viral inhibitors.

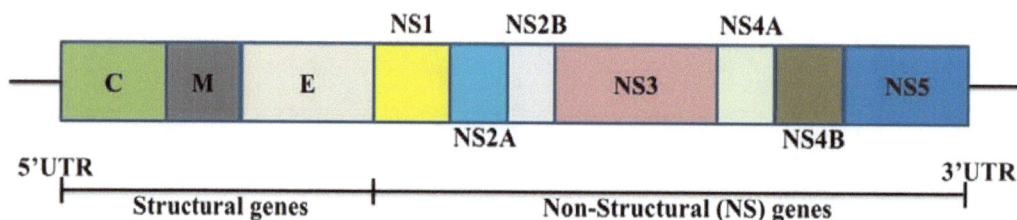

Fig. (2). The structure of DENV genome. DENV encodes three structural and seven nonstructural proteins.

Antiviral Activities of PCs – *In Silico* and *In Vitro* Studies of Catechin

Antiviral activities of catechins on various viruses have been demonstrated in many papers, whether *in silico* or *in vitro*. The mechanisms of the inhibitory effect on various RNA and DNA viruses are also being studied, especially for tea catechins. Current antiviral therapies in use do increase the success rate of the treatments but they often have undesirable side effects, and there are no universal therapies for all viral genotypes. Therefore, scientists are in search of new compounds, which could provide more effective antiviral treatment with little side effect, and could be further used as potent vaccines against viral infection. The *in silico* methods used in this study are 3D structure prediction, molecular docking, molecular dynamics (MD) simulation and binding free energy calculation.

Dengue Virus

In silico study involving flexible receptor docking was performed for the various catechins against DENV E protein. We analyzed the differences in binding energy and interaction between the four catechins present in green tea and the E protein. The 3D structure of the DENV E protein was obtained from protein data bank (PDB) (PDB ID: 1OKE). The 2D ligand structures were obtained from PubChem database and were converted to 3D using open babel. The molegro virtual docker (MVD) software was used for the detection of cavities and blind docking. The results of the blind docking are summarized below in Table **1**. The order of the Moldock score is: EGCG < ECG < EGC < EC and the order of the interaction is: EGCG > ECG > EGC > EC (Figs. **4** & **5**). Among the four catechins, the EGCG showed the least binding energy for one of the five cavities detected by the MVD software. The binding site of EGCG on E protein is predicted to lie at the crossing point of domain II and domain III of the dimer and adjacent to the fusion loop of the monomer [18]. The amino acids involved in hydrogen bond interaction on EGCG are Leu 277, Ile 46, Leu 45, His 27, His 244 and Lys 247.

We hypothesize that the highly effective binding interactions between EGCG and the E protein may be due to the presence of the galloyl moiety and high molecular weight. To test this hypothesis, we performed blind docking study for other catechins varying in molecular weight (monomer, dimer, trimer, tetramer, pentamer and hexamer) on DENV E protein. The results show that the binding energy decreases as the molecular weight increases. Thus, we hypothesize that as the molecular weight of the catechin compound increases, the efficacy and strength of its binding interactions with the DENV E protein also increases. In addition to the observations above, we also found that oligomeric PCs have better antiviral activity when compared to the monomeric units (unpublished data). To further study this phenomenon, PC-rich factions were isolated from various sources of plants, including Vigna angularis beans, Persea Americana, Cinnamomum verum J. Presl, Lindera umbellta Ramus, Cinnamomum camphora, and Pycnogenol. These extracts were tested for their anti-DENV activity *via* the conventional MTT assay using LLC-MK2 cells infected with DENV-2 virus. They all exhibited favorable anti-DENV activity in a dose-dependent manner, with the selectivity index (SI, ratio of CC50/EC50) values ranging between 10-50.

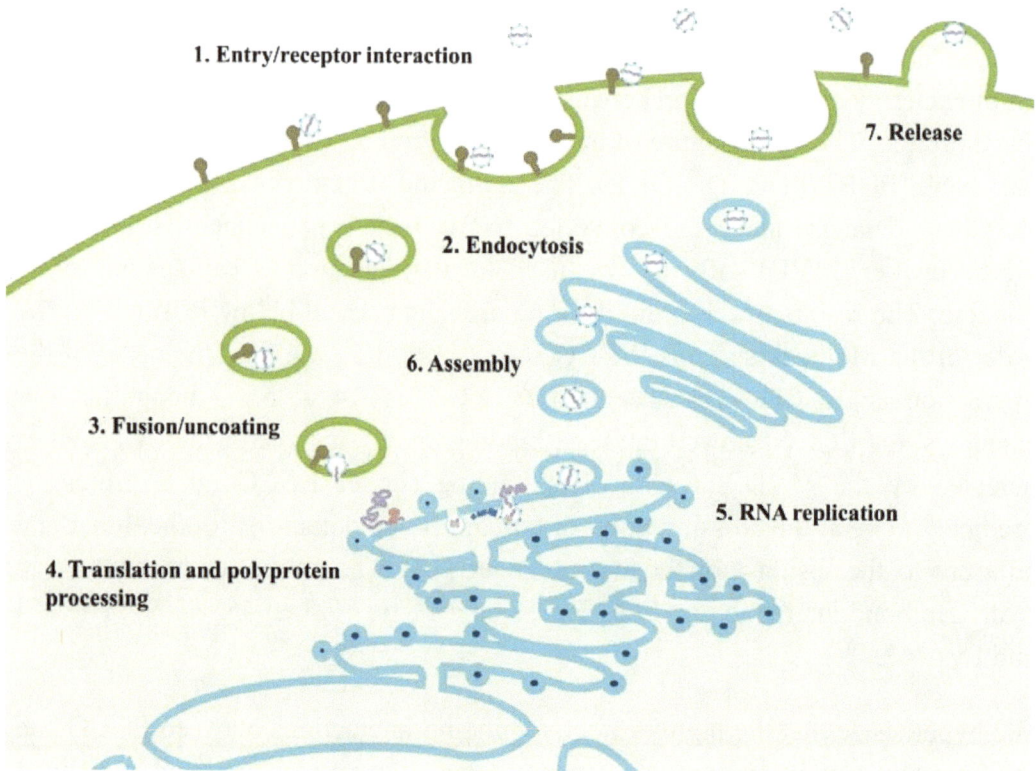

Fig. (3). The Dengue virus replication cycle.

To determine the relationship between molecular size and the antiviral activity of PCs, the extract obtained from Cinnamomum camphora was further separated by silica gel-thin layer chromatography into LMW (low molecular weight) oligomer and HMW (high molecular weight) fractions. Results indicated that all fractions showed anti-DENV activity. However, cellular cytotoxicity (CC50) increases with increase of molecular size of PCs. They were then subjected to 'Time of addition' experiment to get a rough estimate for mechanism of action of the compounds. Antiviral activity was observed when cells were pretreated with compounds from all fractions, suggesting that these compounds act at the entry stage of the virus. We also observed that these fractions, especially LMW, showed antiviral activity even when they were added a few hours later than viral infection. Thus, we believe that these fractions remain potent even after viral entry. This was further proven using a dengue virus replicon system, in which the Cinnamomum camphora extract exhibited anti-DENV activity against BHK cells constantly expressing DENV NS proteins (Replicon cell system). Data obtained using DENV enzymes are also consistent with our observations thus far. Activities of NS5 RNA-dependent RNA polymerase (RdRp) and NS3-NS2b protease were significantly inhibited by the Cinnamomum camphora oligomer (unpublished data). Identification and dissection of active components are underway using chemical fractionation and purification.

Table 1.   The Docking Result for Various Catechins

Ligand	Molecular Formula	Molecular Weight	MolDock Score	No of h Bond
EGCG	$C_{22}H_{18}O_{11}$	458.37172	-169.94	6
ECG	$C_{22}H_{18}O_{10}$	442.37232	-143.58	3
EGC	$C_{15}H_{14}O_7$	306.26746	-118.30	3
EC	$C_{15}H_{14}O_6$	290.26806	-114.19	2

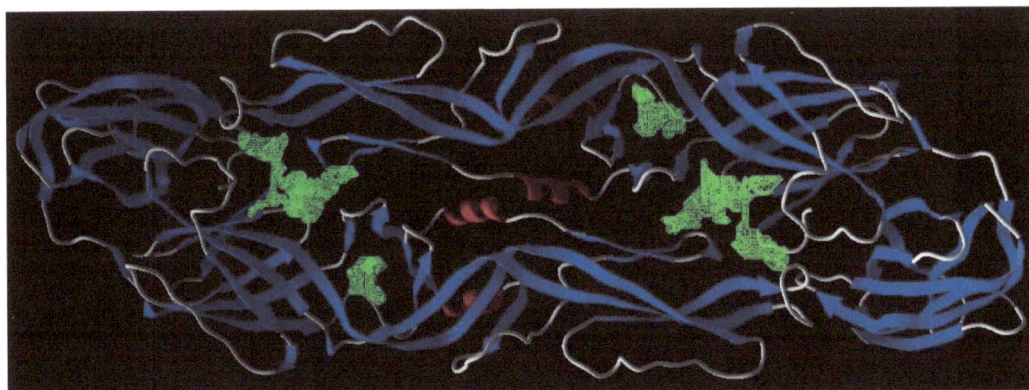

Fig. (4). Cavities (five) detected in DENV E protein by MVD software. (Green: cavities).

We also explored the possibility for combination treatment using 2 or 3 drugs with different mechanisms of anti-DENV actions. Ribavirin (RV) is widely known to inhibit multiple viruses *in vitro* as well as *in vivo*, and anti-DENV activity has been documented. Indeed, our MTT assay using LLC-MK2 cells shows *in vitro* anti-DENV activity with a SI value at approximately 80. However, its significant *in vivo* toxicity hinders the implementation of this broad-spectrum antiviral drug in clinical settings. To overcome this, synergism between crude PCs extracted from Cinnamomum camphora (S1) and RV was tested. As compared to a single-drug treatment with RV, addition of low concentrations of S1 (5 μg/ml) significantly enhanced anti-viral activity of RV at all concentrations tested. EC50 of RV was enhanced by nearly 100 times in the presence of low doses of S1, indicating that concentration of RV could be reduced in such dual-drug treatment. Similar study has been conducted with PCs and chloroquine (CQ), which also has a mild anti-DENV activity, and similar results were obtained (unpublished data). Thus, these data suggest that PCs can be used as a secondary compound to stimulate anti-viral activity of either RV or CQ or even in triple combination with these drugs. Another advantage of S1 is its availability in various methods of administration, oral, intravenous, intramuscular, topical, and inhalation. We have initiated *in vitro* experiments using synthetic PCs with distinct molecular structures, with or without galloyl moieties, ranging from monomer to hexamer. They will be followed by enzyme inhibition assays and *in silico* study. These studies will aid in clarifying which types of PCs inhibit DENV efficiently and can be further used as therapeutics.

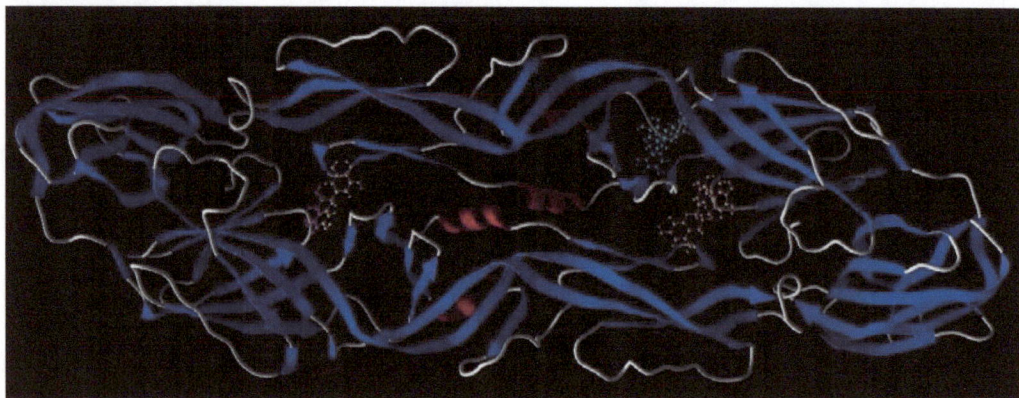

Fig. (5). The binding site of Ligands in DENV E protein (Orange: EGCG, Green: ECG, Yellow: EGC, Pink: EC).

Kimmel *et al*. reports that the oligomeric procyanidins (OPCs) show antiviral activity in DENV infected human peripheral blood mononuclear cells. The OPCs were extracted from non-ripe apple peel, and they reduced dengue virus titers and exhibited direct antiviral activity *in vitro*. Innate immune responses to viral infection were observed for the OPCs and this study was reported as the first to characterize the antiviral innate responses by OPCs which is relevant to infection *in vivo* [19]. The monomeric forms did not show reduction in DENV titers when compared to the OPCs, hence the authors suggest that due to the direct interaction of OPCs with the virus, the trimers and tetramers have more effect that the monomeric forms. Several papers report the direct antiviral effect of OPCs in many viruses, effectively blocking the early entry steps in viral life cycle [20, 21]. Other than targeting the early entry steps of the DENV infection cycle, Senthilvil *et al.* have also listed NS2B-NS3 protein as a potential anti-DENV target because of its importance in the virus replication cycle. Leaf extract from the Carica papaya was tested for antiviral activity using docking study. Quercetin was found to have good binding energy with 6 hydrogen bonds. They hypothesized that the flavonoids from the Carica papaya might have anti-DENV activity [22]. Zandi *et al.* have also reported anti-DENV activity of flavonoids in Vero cells [23].

HIV

Human immunodeficiency virus (HIV) causes AIDS (acquired immunodeficiency syndrome) by preferential destruction of the T cells in humans [24]. HIV is a member of the retroviridae family and it is a single strand enveloped RNA virus. The genome encodes three enzymes: reverse transcriptase, protease and integrase. The reverse transcriptase is an important prerequisite for the virus replication; hence the first antiretroviral drug approved by FDA for HIV-1 is a reverse transcriptase inhibitor, AZT. Since then, several classes of antiretroviral agents that perform on various steps of the HIV life cycle have been recognized. A combination of drugs acting on different viral targets is identified as highly active antiretroviral therapy (HAART) [25]. Since there is no available vaccine or cure for HIV, antiretroviral treatment and its prophylactic use for prevention are the only ways to treat HIV, with the risk of side effects as well as the development of drug-resistant viruses. In the article by Fassina *et al.* EGCG is reported to have antiviral effects against HIV-1 infection [26]. The molecular docking and MD simulations performed on HIV-1 by Hamza *et al.* suggest that EGCG binds favorably to CD4 on cells and gp120 on HIV-1 [27]. The ligand-binding pocket of CD4 contains amino acid residues necessary in the gp120-CD4 interaction. The galloyl moiety of EGCG was found to be similar to the residues and the calculated results obtained are similar to *in vitro* data, suggesting that EGCG binds effectively to the gp120-CD4 complex, preventing HIV-1 infection [28].

The *in silico* study performed by Jiang *et al.* provides a novel and effective method for the planning and development of potent inhibitors of HIV-1. Blind docking study predicted the binding sites of raltegravir (integrase inhibitor) and catechins for the HIV-1 integrase and the viral RNA. The catechins with galloyl moiety interfere with the interaction between raltegravir and viral RNA. Since the Mg ion function is important in this interaction, specific binding was performed around the Mg ion sites in both the models. According to the results published, EGCG has the best docking results in HIV-1 integrase and GCG has the best docking results in viral RNA. The binding sites for the antiretroviral drug and the catechins were similar. The authors concluded that the catechins with the galloyl moiety have better docking energy compared to the catechins without the galloyl moiety. This correlated with the inhibitory potency measured by ELISA test [29]. The 50% inhibitory concentration values of EGCG and ECG were slightly higher than raltegravir and EC showed weak effect. Hence the *in silico* data is supported by the experimental data and they concluded that the binding and inhibitory efficacies reveal that the catechins with galloyl moiety show better inhibition of HIV-1 integrase. It was mentioned that raltegravir and catechins share an analogous inhibitory mechanism and they have effect on the loop domain which may affect the mode of inhibition. Also we reported that a procyanidin extracted from French maritime pine (Pycnogenol), which also binds to the host cells, can block the HIV-1 replication [21].

Influenza Virus

Influenza is one of the most common infectious diseases caused by the RNA viruses belonging to the family Orthomyxoviridae. Based on the antigenic features of the core proteins, Influenza viruses are separated into three categories A, B, and C, each infecting a large variety of species including humans, pigs, horses, sea mammals and birds. There are several subtypes like H1N1 and H5N1, causing pandemics, which often have high mortality rates [30]. The search for anti-influenza virus drugs often focuses on the surface glycoprotein of influenza virus, hemagglutinin (HA), as it plays a major role in the virus infection. Current vaccines are becoming inactive or less effective due to the antigenic shift in the virus, which leads to new strains. Thus, current researches focus on the discovery of broad-spectrum antiviral drugs that can simultaneously treat several influenza virus strains.

The antiviral activity of EGCG in influenza virus was first reported in 1993 by Song *et al.* The catechin molecule affects the infectivity of the virus and showed an inhibitory effect. The same group also performed the structure activity relationship study for the green tea catechins, EGCG, EGC, and ECG. They tested the tea catechins for inhibition of the influenza A and B viruses *in vitro*. The results demonstrated that among catechins, EGCG and ECG inhibit many influenza virus subtypes effectively in MDCK cell culture. The EC50 value confirms the strong inhibitory activity of EGCG. These compounds inhibited Neuraminidase (NA) and HA, in which the 3-galloyl group plays a major role and trihydroxybenzoic acid plays a minor role. They also mentioned that the inhibitory effect is observed throughout the cycle; hence these compounds may have antiviral effect not only in the initial stages of the virus life cycle but also at other stages [31]. To better understand the mechanism of inhibition, Liu *et al.* studied the interactions between the H5N1 of influenza A virus and the various catechins using the flexible docking and MD simulations. They reported the order of the binding specificity and interaction with HA as EGCG > ECG > EGC > EC. The results suggest that the four catechin compounds have similar binding pockets on HA protein. Compared to the other two catechins, EGCG and ECG have strong inhibitory effect for HA with differences in strength of interactions. These results are confirmed by the experimental data that EGCG and ECG have better inhibition than EGC and EC. Residues LysA269, ArgB68, IleA267 and GluB78 show robust interactions and hence they might be responsible for the catechin inhibition against HA [32]. In contrast to the previous paper, this paper reports that due to the presence of the trihydroxybenzoic acid groups, which leads to more H bond interactions, EGCG and ECG are more effective in binding specificity and strength of interaction.

Nakayama *et al.* proposed that the tea polyphenols, EGCG and theaflavin digallate (TF3) bind to the HA of influenza virus and block infection of influenza virus in MDCK cells at the entry stage [33]. A previous report by the same group suggested that the tea extract used the same mechanism for the inhibition of influenza A and B viruses [34]. They also demonstrated that the EGCG inactivates influenza virus directly, but Imanishi *et al.* hypothesized that there is unforeseen effect on host cell which may affect the virus cell membrane fusion. In this study, the authors focused on green tea catechins inhibition on the viral endonuclease activity of influenza A virus RdRp. They reported that the inhibition is due to the presence of the galloyl group. The inhibitory activity of EGCG was stronger than other catechins with the galloyl group and catechins with no galloyl group showed weak or no inhibition. The structure function study revealed that the presence of the galloyl group plays an important role in the inhibition activity. These results were further validated using the *in silico* docking simulations, which confirmed that catechins fit exactly into the active pocket of the domain of influenza A virus with stable binding [35]. Among the tea catechins, EGCG fits better than EGC due to the presence of the galloyl group. Hence this reveals that galloyl moiety is important for the binding of catechins to the pocket. These results may contribute significantly to the further advancement of potent anti-influenza drugs based on modification of catechins. Lu *et al.* studied the inhibition of NA of 2009 H1N1 influenza virus by 20 flavonoid derivatives. The possible binding modes and docked poses for the inhibitors were predicted using the molecular docking and simulation studies. The predicted binding energy is confirmed by the experimental data suggesting that flavonoids are good inhibitors for the NA of H1N1 influenza virus [36].

HCV

Hepatitis C virus (HCV) which causes chronic hepatitis is a universal health complication affecting millions of people worldwide [37]. It is also a common co-infection in HIV infected patients, resulting in cirrhosis and liver cancer [38]. It is a member of the flaviviridae family and has a single stranded RNA genome. They encode six non-structural proteins (NS2, NS3, NS4A, NS4B, NS5A & NS5B) and three structural proteins (core, E1 & E2). The non-structural proteins, mainly NS3/4A are considered to be important targets for anti-HCV drugs, since they play a main role in replication cycle [39]. Though combination of Sovaldi, ribavirin and pegylated interferon is recommended by American Association for the Study of Liver Diseases (AASLD), new inhibitors have to be identified due to the side effects, cost, and low efficacy of the current available treatment. Few groups have found out that EGCG could be used as an inhibitor for the HCV entry pathway [40]. Ciesek *et al.* identified EGCG as an entry inhibitor for HCV. This molecule acts on virus particles and inhibits the virus entry by preventing the virus binding to the cell surface [41]. The EC isomer exerts inhibitory effects on HCV replication without causing host cellular toxicity as reported by Takeshita *et al.* [20]. However, Calland *et al.* reported different observations in which the compound showed no anti-HCV activity [42]. Li *et al.* also reported that the procyanidin B1 suppressed HCV replication but the epicatechin and catechin did not inhibit the HCV replication [43].

Various studies reveal that EGCG shows different mechanisms of action for the inhibition of HCV infection as compared to other catechins [40]. According to the authors, EGCG is effective in inhibiting HCV entry but not effective on the other stages of the life cycle. Anti-HCV molecule screening assay has been used which confirms the effect of EGCG on HCV entry blockage. Hence, EGCG could be used as an anti-HCV drug for preventing the virus entry into the host cells independent of the genotypes. Quercetin is reported to have anti-HCV activity and it is also nontoxic [41, 44-46]. This study focuses on screening the phytochemicals from Acacia nilotica for possible drug candidate which can inhibit the HCV infection. Docking studies were carried out for the phytochemicals and NS3/4A protease of HCV in order to predict the binding interactions. From the interaction it was hypothesized that the phytochemical can act as a potential inhibitor for HCV [47].

Other Viruses

The effect of EGCG was tested against hepatitis B virus (HBV)-infected cell lines and the results show that the green tea catechins inhibit the HBV markers HBsAg and HBeAg in a dose dependent manner [48]. The inhibition of HBV by EGCG suggests that the green tea extract could be a candidate for anti-HBV drug target. It has also been shown that EGCG also suppresses the HCV [49]. Studies reveal that herpes simplex virus (HSV) is also inactivated by green tea catechins. The antiviral activity of EGCG with the clinical isolates of HSV-1 and HSV-2 was effective and in the presence of EGCG, the envelopes of HSV particles were damaged [50]. Antiviral effects are also reported for several other viruses like enterovirus, rotavirus, SARS Co-V, HTLV-1, Sindbis virus, EBV and human papillomavirus (HPV) [51-54]. However, the mechanism of action is unknown and it is believed to differ between viruses.

The number of human studies directly examining the effect of catechins or PCs on prevention of cancer progression is limited. This is mainly due to almost no approved compounds with defined chemical entity. Thus, clinical studies have been mainly performed with crude extracts, such as green tea extracts. Green tea extract is currently used in mouth wash as a preventative for tooth decay and periodontal disease because of its strong antibacterial properties [55, 56]. For viral infections, it should be noted that EGCG topical ointment has been approved by the FDA as protection against HPV infection and eventually cervical cancer [54]. The 15% ointment of sinecatechins, containing a mixture of EGCG and other catechin compounds has been examined for the topical treatment of condylomata acuminata, caused by HPV, mainly HPV types 6 and 11. Although the clearance rate of wart lesions after treatment with sinecatechins was similar to other topical drugs like imiquimod and podophyllotoxin, recurrences are less frequent after treatment with sinecatechins. This suggests that it is a safe and effective treatment option for condylomata acuminata. Therefore, this product has a potential for application to other viral and tumor lesions in the future. According to some clinical studies on the progress of cancers, green tea may reduce risk of breast cancer. This effect has been ascribed mostly to the modification of the estrogen metabolism by phytochemicals including polyphenols such as EGCG, EGC, and EC [57]. More recent meta-analysis shows that the consumption of green tea and coffee seems to reduce esophageal cancer [58]. In summary, these data indicate that potency of tea and tea extracts may not be sufficient to serve as first-line chemotherapeutic compounds but do have a role to play in both primary prevention and prevention of cancer recurrence.

Interference of Catechin Oligomer with Host Cell Factors and Pleiotropic Antiviral Effects of PCs

As mentioned above, PCs apparently show inhibitory effect on entry of various species of viruses such as HCV, HIV, HSV, adenovirus and influenza virus. PCs have been shown to bind directly to viral anti-receptors (envelope or coat proteins) or to target cells possessing viral receptors and other molecules necessary for viral binding. During this process, PCs may directly result in the damage and inactivation of virions. Other than its effect on viral entry, PCs have been reported to act as antiviral agents inside the cells *via* mechanisms including inhibition of viral enzymes (*e.g.* integrase and reverse transcriptase (RT) of HIV-1, NS3/4A serine protease of adenovirus) [29, 59, 60] and viral transcription and replication (*e.g.* immediate early genes of EBV and picorna viral replication) [53]. Suppression of viral replication *via* modulation of cellular redox milieu has also been reported [61]. Regarding the functional importance of PCs for cellular defense against virus infections, oxidative stress induced by viral infection appears to play an important role. Production of reactive oxygen species (ROS) results in activation of several key molecules for host cell activation and signal transduction such as NF-kB, p38MAPK, JNK, *etc.* which lead to inhibition of macromolecular synthesis of the cells and enhancement of virus replication [62]. If the cells are highly susceptible allowing active viral replication, infected cells undergo apoptotic cell death, which represents the typical pattern of acute symptomatic infection. However, if anti-oxidating enzyme Mn-SOD is induced in virus infected cells, these cells may survive the infection [63]. It has been found that Mn-SOD can suppress viral replication, which prompted us to speculate that this protein might be an antiviral host factor and may potentially be a broad-spectrum antiviral drug.

Further study into the mechanism of Mn-SOD shows that virus replication is not affected by growth suppression of cells, because SARS-CoV or influenza virus replication is not suppressed even in the confluent cultures where cellular growth were retarded with contact inhibition. Therefore it seems that Mn-SOD induction could be responsible for the inhibition of virus replication. Macromolecular synthesis and growth of the cells would be suppressed by PCs treatments followed by accumulation of Mn-SOD leading to induction of static state of cells and inhibition of virus replication (Fig. **6**). In order to look for active components of polyphenol ingredients useful for the functions of human and to determine which kind of catechin units are important for antiviral activity of PCs, we initially attempted to isolate single entities of catechin. But using SARS-CoV and DENV, we found most antiviral activity in the fraction of 3-6mer PCs but not as a single molecule. However, there exist hundreds of natural polyphenols and PCs are composed of multiple types of molecules even in a single plant species. It is very difficult to obtain each substance in sufficient quantity and purity, thus making it difficult to study each individual compound. Because of their chemical complexity due to isomeric states, modifications by sugars, and different oxidation states, we found it impossible to isolate pure compounds as single entities, suggesting difficulty in developing drugs by this approach. Hence, we changed our strategy to examine their effects using single species of polyphenols through chemical synthesis [64]. For our purposes, we chose the natural polyphenols, B type PCs (polymer of flavan 3 ol (catechin)), which is distributed widely and involved in regulatory functions of the living body. Preliminary experimental results show that protein astringency and the inhibitory action of cell growth become stronger with the increase of degree of polymerization. This is consistent with our original hypothesis that oligomer PCs s affect cellular functions to a greater extent than monomers and dimers.

Trimers and tetramers regulate cellular functions and inhibit replication of SARS-CoV, and induce intracellular anti-oxidants such as Mn-SOD without influencing cell growth. However, inhibitory effect on cellular functions increases with the increase of polymerization beyond these polymers. It seems that the abilities of PCs to bind proteins such as collagen and to inhibit cell-growth are closely related. If growth inhibition of the cells is slight or limited by time even when it is strong, this growth inhibition recovers upon its removal. This is significantly different from the cell damages caused by common drugs and important from a medical point of view. Thus, it may not be an overstatement that the 'preferable polyphenol effects' exists in a trimer/tetramer (a product of nature C1). It is possible that with better understanding of low molecular weight PCs, favorable polyphenol effects may be achieved under a less cytotoxic condition. These effects including improvements in antioxidative actions, antibacterial activities, as well as better efficacies as modulators for the intestinal cells, anticaries, deodorant, active oxygen eliminator, anti-cholesterol agent, inhibitor for blood sugar rise and hypertension, antitumor agent, anti-hay fever agent, anti-allergic agent, platelet aggregation inhibitor, ultraviolet absorber, and as an antiviral drug.

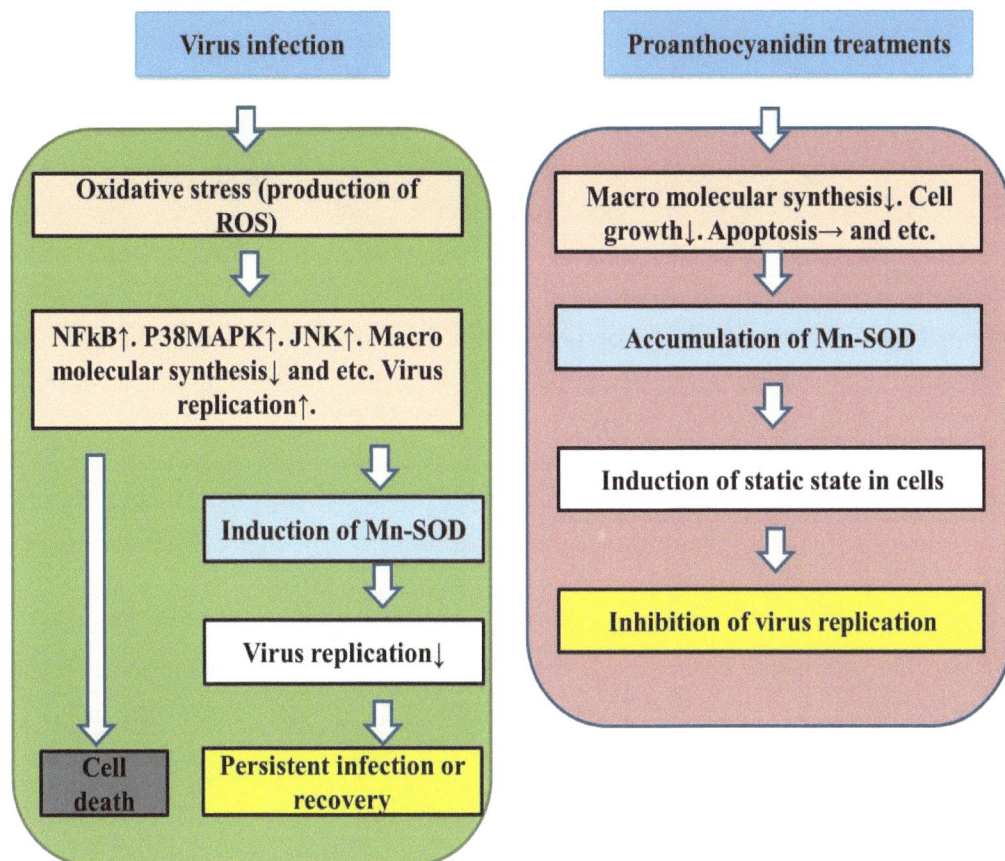

Fig. (6). Induction of Mn-SOD in the cells by PC treatment and viral infection.

CURRENT AND FUTURE DEVELOPMENTS

PCs are being studied for their anti-inflammatory, anticancer, antimicrobial, antioxidant and antiviral properties. Numerous antiviral activity studies are being carried out using catechins against different RNA and DNA viruses. The mechanisms by which the catechins inhibit the viruses are not sufficiently understood due to the fact that most of the studies have been performed with either purified monomers or mixtures of crude PCs as described above. Nevertheless, in most studies these compounds are shown to inhibit the virus by preventing viral entry into cells. Besides, additional effects of PCs are reported in several different viral systems; prevention of the manifestation of specific antigens in EBV, hindrance of the binding of the envelope protein to its receptors in influenza virus and HIV, obstruction of viral enzyme activity in influenza virus and DENV and manipulation of certain host regulative factors [48]. Of the four monomeric tea catechins, EGCG demonstrates the strongest viral inhibitory effects. The molecular basis of this difference can partly be explained by *in silico* docking studies. In this review, the antiviral effects of catechins against viruses like DENV, HCV, HIV, influenza virus, HSV, and others were discussed. However, the bioavailability, side effects, cytotoxicity, dosage and other properties of catechins are yet to be studied in detail. Catechins used in combination with other antiviral compounds should also be explored. Although *in vitro* and *in silico* studies are being carried out generally, *in vivo* studies should also be considered in the near future.

The *in silico* technique described in this review along with *in vitro* studies may present as a better drug design methodology. One of the apparent advantages of this method is enabling us to estimate and design ideal PC molecules matching to pockets residing on surface protein of each virus critical for infection. Molecular docking has been developed as a valuable method to study protein-ligand interactions, which may contribute significantly to the design of effective drugs in the future. However in the immediate future, catechin derivatives can be used as novel antiviral drugs due to their low toxicity and fewer side effects [32]. Phase I clinical trial was conducted for the evaluation of safety, toxicity, dosage and antiviral effect for crude catechins in HIV-1 patients. Also, monomer EGCG has been approved as a safe compound by the FDA for the treatment of HPV and cervical cancer. Possible inhibitors which prevent the viruses to enter into the cells will be considered as useful next-generation anti-viral drugs. A potent inhibitor which blocks the viruses in the initial stages of entry into the cells will have to be developed and also the mechanism of inhibition should be well known. We hypothesize that the good binding interactions and antiviral effects of these PCs are brought about by the presence of the galloyl moiety and high molecular weights. With technical improvement of chemical synthesis of PCs, the mechanisms of action of these compounds will be clarified in more detail. Thus, further research needs to be carried out based on previously reported works, in order to modify catechin compounds into highly efficient broad-spectrum antiviral drugs with little to no side effect.

ACKNOWLEDGEMENTS

The authors are grateful to members of laboratory for helpful comments and discussions. This work was supported by NUS SoM Start-up Grant (R-182-000-160-733, R-182-000-160-133) and NMRC Grant (R-182-000-182-213) to NY.

CONFLICT OF INTEREST

The authors confirm that this chapter contents have no conflict of interest.

REFERENCES

[1]　Middleton Jr E, Kandaswami C. Effects of flavonoids on immune and inflammatory cell functions. Biochemical Pharmacology 1992; 43(6): 1167-79.

[2]　Bagchi D, Garg A, Krohn R, *et al.* Oxygen free radical scavenging abilities of vitamins C and E, and a grape seed proanthocyanidin extract *in vitro*. Research Communications in Molecular Pathology and Pharmacology 1997; 95(2): 179.

[3]　Ricardo da Silva JM, Rigaud J, Cheynier V, Cheminat A, Moutounet M. Procyanidin dimers and trimers from grape seeds. Phytochemistry 1991; 30(4): 1259-64.

[4]　Rohdewald P. A review of the French maritime pine bark extract (Pycnogenol), a herbal medication with a diverse clinical pharmacology. International journal of clinical pharmacology and therapeutics 2002; 40(4): 158-68.

[5]　Rice-Evans CA, Miller NJ, Paganga G. Structure-antioxidant activity relationships of flavonoids and phenolic acids. Free radical biology and medicine 1996; 20(7): 933-56.

[6]　Balentine DA, Wiseman SA, Bouwens LC. The chemistry of tea flavonoids. Critical Reviews in Food Science & Nutrition 1997; 37(8): 693-704.

[7]　Guzmán MG, Kouri G. Dengue: an update. The Lancet Infectious Diseases 2002; 2(1): 33-42.

[8]　Mackenzie JS, Gubler DJ, Petersen LR. Emerging flaviviruses: the spread and resurgence of Japanese encephalitis, West Nile and dengue viruses. Nature medicine 2004; 10: S98-S109.

[9]　Bhatt S, Gething PW, Brady OJ, *et al.* The global distribution and burden of dengue. Nature 2013.

[10]　Bravo J, Guzman M, Kouri G. Why dengue haemorrhagic fever in Cuba? I. Individual risk factors for dengue haemorrhagic fever/dengue shock syndrome (DHF/DSS). Transactions of the Royal Society of Tropical Medicine and Hygiene 1987; 81(5): 816-20.

[11]　Takahashi H, Takahashi C, Moreland NJ, *et al.* Establishment of a robust dengue virus NS3–NS5 binding assay for identification of protein–protein interaction inhibitors. Antiviral research 2012; 96(3): 305-14.

[12]　Kuhn RJ, Zhang W, Rossmann MG, *et al.* Structure of dengue virus: implications for flavivirus organization, maturation, and fusion. Cell 2002; 108(5): 717-25.

[13]　Kümmerer BM, Rice CM. Mutations in the yellow fever virus nonstructural protein NS2A selectively block production of infectious particles. Journal of virology 2002; 76(10): 4773-84.

[14] Guzman MG, Halstead SB, Artsob H, *et al.* Dengue: a continuing global threat. Nature Reviews Microbiology 2010; 8: S7-S16.

[15] Chen Y-C, Wang S-Y, King C-C. Bacterial lipopolysaccharide inhibits dengue virus infection of primary human monocytes/macrophages by blockade of virus entry *via* a CD14-dependent mechanism. Journal of virology 1999; 73(4): 2650-7.

[16] Allison SL, Schalich J, Stiasny K, *et al.* Oligomeric rearrangement of tick-borne encephalitis virus envelope proteins induced by an acidic pH. Journal of virology 1995; 69(2): 695-700.

[17] Tomlinson S, Malmstrom R, Watowich S. New approaches to structure-based discovery of dengue protease inhibitors. Infectious Disorders-Drug Targets (Formerly Current Drug Targets-Infectious Disorders) 2009; 9(3): 327-43.

[18] Ichiyama K, Reddy SBG, Zhang LF, *et al.* Sulfated Polysaccharide, Curdlan Sulfate, Efficiently Prevents Entry/Fusion and Restricts Antibody-Dependent Enhancement of Dengue Virus Infection *In Vitro*: A Possible Candidate for Clinical Application. PLoS neglected tropical diseases 2013; 7(4): e2188.

[19] Kimmel EM, Jerome M, Holderness J, *et al.* Oligomeric procyanidins stimulate innate antiviral immunity in dengue virus infected human PBMCs. Antiviral research 2011; 90(1): 80-6.

[20] Takeshita M, Ishida Y-i, Akamatsu E, *et al.* Proanthocyanidin from blueberry leaves suppresses expression of subgenomic hepatitis C virus RNA. Journal of biological chemistry 2009; 284(32): 21165-76.

[21] Feng WY, Tanaka R, Inagaki Y, *et al.* Pycnogenol, a procyanidin-rich extract from French maritime pine, inhibits intracellular replication of HIV-1 as well as its binding to host cells. Jpn J Infect Dis 2008; 61(4): 279-85.

[22] Senthilvel P, Lavanya P, Kumar KM, *et al.* Flavonoid from Carica papaya inhibits NS2B-NS3 protease and prevents Dengue 2 viral assembly. Bioinformation 2013; 9(18): 889.

[23] Zandi K, Teoh B-T, Sam S-S, *et al.* Antiviral activity of four types of bioflavonoid against dengue virus type-2. Virol J 2011; 8: 560.

[24] Sleasman JW, Goodenow MM. 13. HIV-1 infection. The Journal of allergy and clinical immunology 2003; 111(2): S582-S92.

[25] Vlietinck A, De Bruyne T, Apers S, Pieters L. Plant-derived leading compounds for chemotherapy of human immunodeficiency virus (HIV) infection. Planta Medica 1998; 64(02): 97-109.

[26] Fassina G, Buffa A, Benelli R, *et al.* Polyphenolic antioxidant (-)-epigallocatechin-3-gallate from green tea as a candidate anti-HIV agent. Aids 2002; 16(6): 939-41.

[27] Hamza A, Zhan C-G. How can (-)-epigallocatechin gallate from green tea prevent HIV-1 infection? Mechanistic insights from computational modeling and the implication for rational design of anti-HIV-1 entry inhibitors. The Journal of Physical Chemistry B 2006; 110(6): 2910-7.

[28] Kawai K, Tsuno NH, Kitayama J, *et al.* Epigallocatechin gallate, the main component of tea polyphenol, binds to CD4 and interferes with gp120 binding. Journal of allergy and clinical immunology 2003; 112(5): 951-7.

[29] Jiang F, Chen W, Yi K, *et al.* The evaluation of catechins that contain a galloyl moiety as potential HIV-1 integrase inhibitors. Clinical Immunology 2010; 137(3): 347-56.

[30] Miller M, Viboud C, Simonsen L, Olson DR, Russell C. Mortality and morbidity burden associated with A/H1N1pdm influenza virus: Who is likely to be infected, experience clinical symptoms, or die from the H1N1pdm 2009 pandemic virus? PLoS currents 2009; 1.

[31]   Song J-M, Lee K-H, Seong B-L. Antiviral effect of catechins in green tea on influenza virus. Antiviral research 2005; 68(2): 66-74.

[32]   Liu J, Yang Z, Wang S, *et al.* Exploring the molecular basis of H5N1 hemagglutinin binding with catechins in green tea: A flexible docking and molecular dynamics study. Journal of Theoretical and Computational Chemistry 2012; 11(01): 111-25.

[33]   Nakayama M, Suzuki K, Toda M, *et al.* Inhibition of the infectivity of influenza virus by tea polyphenols. Antiviral research 1993; 21(4): 289-99.

[34]   Nakayama M, Toda M, Okubo S, Shimamura T. Inhibition of influenza virus infection by tea. Letters in Applied Microbiology 1990; 11(1): 38-40.

[35]   Kuzuhara T, Iwai Y, Takahashi H, Hatakeyama D, Echigo N. Green tea catechins inhibit the endonuclease activity of influenza A virus RNA polymerase. PLoS currents 2009; 1.

[36]   Lu S-J, Chong F-C. Combining Molecular docking and molecular dynamics to predict the binding modes of flavonoid derivatives with the neuraminidase of the 2009 H1N1 influenza a virus. International journal of molecular sciences 2012; 13(4): 4496-507.

[37]   Alter MJ. Epidemiology of hepatitis C virus infection. World Journal of Gastroenterology 2007; 13(17): 2436.

[38]   Levrero M. Viral hepatitis and liver cancer: the case of hepatitis C. Oncogene 2006; 25(27): 3834-47.

[39]   Penin F, Dubuisson J, Rey FA, Moradpour D, Pawlotsky JM. Structural biology of hepatitis C virus. Hepatology 2004; 39(1): 5-19.

[40]   Lin Y-T, Wu Y-H, Tseng C-K, *et al.* Green tea phenolic epicatechins inhibit hepatitis C virus replication *via* cycloxygenase-2 and attenuate virus-induced inflammation. PloS one 2013; 8(1): e54466.

[41]   Ciesek S, von Hahn T, Colpitts CC, *et al.* The green tea polyphenol, epigallocatechin-3-gallate, inhibits hepatitis C virus entry. Hepatology 2011; 54(6): 1947-55.

[42]   Calland N, Albecka A, Belouzard S, *et al.* (−)-Epigallocatechin-3-gallate is a new inhibitor of hepatitis C virus entry. Hepatology 2012; 55(3): 720-9.

[43]   Li S, Kodama EN, Inoue Y, *et al.* Procyanidin B1 purified from Cinnamomi cortex suppresses hepatitis C virus replication. Antivir Chem Chemother 2010; 20(6): 239-48.

[44]   Fukazawa H, Suzuki T, Wakita T, Murakami Y. A cell-based, microplate colorimetric screen identifies 7, 8-benzoflavone and green tea gallate catechins as inhibitors of the hepatitis C virus. Biological & pharmaceutical bulletin 2011; 35(8): 1320-7.

[45]   Gonzalez O, Fontanes V, Raychaudhuri S, *et al.* The heat shock protein inhibitor Quercetin attenuates hepatitis C virus production. Hepatology 2009; 50(6): 1756-64.

[46]   Bachmetov L, Gal-Tanamy M, Shapira A, *et al.* Suppression of hepatitis C virus by the flavonoid quercetin is mediated by inhibition of NS3 protease activity. Journal of viral hepatitis 2012; 19(2): e81-e8.

[47]   Khan M, Qasim M, Ashfaq UA, Idrees S, Shah M. Computer aided screening of Accacia nilotica phytochemicals against HCV NS3/4a. Bioinformation 2013; 9(14): 710.

[48]   Xu J, Wang J, Deng F, Hu Z, Wang H. Green tea extract and its major component epigallocatechin gallate inhibits hepatitis B virus *in vitro*. Antiviral research 2008; 78(3): 242-9.

[49]   Chen C, Qiu H, Gong J, *et al.* (−)-Epigallocatechin-3-gallate inhibits the replication cycle of hepatitis C virus. Archives of virology 2012; 157(7): 1301-12.

[50]   Isaacs CE, Wen GY, Xu W, *et al.* Epigallocatechin gallate inactivates clinical isolates of herpes simplex virus. Antimicrobial agents and chemotherapy 2008; 52(3): 962-70.

[51]   Mukoyama A, Ushijima H, Nishimura S, *et al*. Inhibition of rotavirus and enterovirus infections by tea extracts. Japanese journal of medical science & biology 1991; 44(4): 181-6.

[52]   Sonoda J, Koriyama C, Yamamoto S, *et al*. HTLV-1 provirus load in peripheral blood lymphocytes of HTLV-1 carriers is diminished by green tea drinking. Cancer science 2004; 95(7): 596-601.

[53]   Chang L-K, Wei T-T, Chiu Y-F, *et al*. Inhibition of Epstein–Barr virus lytic cycle by (−)-epigallocatechin gallate. Biochemical and biophysical research communications 2003; 301(4): 1062-8.

[54]   Blumenthal M. FDA approves special green tea extract as a new topical drug for genital warts. HerbalGram 2007; 2007.

[55]   Araghizadeh A, Kohanteb J, Fani MM. Inhibitory activity of green tea (Camellia sinensis) extract on some clinically isolated cariogenic and periodontopathic bacteria. Medical Principles and Practice 2013; 22(4): 368-72.

[56]   Steinmann J, Buer J, Pietschmann T, Steinmann E. Anti-infective properties of epigallocatechin-3-gallate (EGCG), a component of green tea. British journal of pharmacology 2013; 168(5): 1059-73.

[57]   Fuhrman BJ, Pfeiffer RM, Wu AH, *et al*. Green tea intake is associated with urinary estrogen profiles in Japanese-American women. Nutrition journal 2013; 12(1): 25.

[58]   Zheng J-S, Yang J, Fu Y-Q, *et al*. Effects of green tea, black tea, and coffee consumption on the risk of esophageal cancer: a systematic review and meta-analysis of observational studies. Nutrition and cancer 2013; 65(1): 1-16.

[59]   Nakane H, Ono K, editors. Differential inhibition of HIV-reverse transcriptase and various DNA and RNA polymerases by some catechin derivatives. Nucleic acids symposium series 1988.

[60]   Weber JM, Ruzindana-Umunyana A, Imbeault L, Sircar S. Inhibition of adenovirus infection and adenain by green tea catechins. Antiviral research 2003; 58(2): 167-73.

[61]   Ho H-Y, Cheng M-L, Weng S-F, Leu Y-L, Chiu DT-Y. Antiviral effect of epigallocatechin gallate on enterovirus 71. Journal of agricultural and food chemistry 2009; 57(14): 6140-7.

[62]   Nakatsue T, Katoh I, Nakamura S, *et al*. Acute infection of Sindbis virus induces phosphorylation and intracellular translocation of small heat shock protein HSP27 and activation of p38 MAP kinase signaling pathway. Biochemical and biophysical research communications 1998; 253(1): 59-64.

[63]   Yoshinaka Y, Takahashi Y, Nakamura S, *et al*. Induction of Manganese-Superoxide Dismutase in MRC-5 Cells Persistently Infected with an Alphavirus, Sindbis. Biochemical and biophysical research communications 1999; 261(1): 139-43.

[64]   Saito A, Mizushina Y, Tanaka A, Nakajima N. Versatile synthesis of epicatechin series procyanidin oligomers, and their antioxidant and DNA polymerase inhibitory activity. Tetrahedron 2009; 65(36): 7422-8.

INDEX

E

L

LACK proteins 215
Lactams 42, 43, 78, 94, 95
Langerhans cells (LC) 222
Latent state 4, 11
L. chagasi 198, 219, 249, 250, 262
L. donovani 198, 211, 216, 218, 220, 224, 238, 249-51, 255-59, 275, 278
L. donovani cells 241, 243
L. donovani infection 207, 214, 215, 218, 221
L. donovani promastigotes 229, 254, 255
Leishmania 194-96, 202, 204, 207-10, 216, 217, 220, 221, 226, 229, 236-38, 241, 243-46, 248, 259, 276, 278
    amastigotes 228, 240, 268
    antigens 205, 208, 275
    cells 226, 239
    histone H1 218
    infections 206, 208, 209, 222, 223, 243
    parasites 194, 195, 197, 199-201, 204, 207, 212, 213, 216, 218, 219, 221, 222, 233, 237-39, 242, 247, 252, 253, 259, 261, 266, 273, 276, 277
    promastigotes 201, 204, 248, 254, 258
Leishmaniasis 194-97, 199, 200, 205, 206, 210-15, 217-19, 222, 224, 228, 235, 236, 238, 239, 248, 262, 265, 266, 273-75, 277, 278, 280
    clinical variants of 197
    diagnosis of 200, 201, 203, 280
    diffuse cutaneous 197-99
    treatment of 210, 211, 219, 224, 225, 247, 248, 255, 273-75, 278
Leishmania species 197, 202, 209, 212, 232, 244, 246, 248, 267
Leishmania spp 227, 237, 238, 245, 280
Leishmania vaccines 211, 212
Leishmanization 213
Lentivirus 142, 161
Lentiviruses 154, 156, 157, 161
Lentivirus vectors (LVs) 143, 154-56

Q

S

T

www.ingramcontent.com/pod-product-compliance
Lightning Source LLC
Chambersburg PA
CBHW050803220326
41598CB00006B/105